DRUG USE

in

AMERICAN SOCIETY

AN EDITED ANTHOLOGY

Preliminary Edition

Edited by Robert Slisz and JoAnne C. Bunnage

Indiana University Bloomington

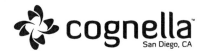

cognella
San Diego, CA

Bassim Hamadeh, Publisher
Michael Simpson, Vice President of Acquisitions
Christopher Foster, Vice President of Marketing
Jessica Knott, Managing Editor
Stephen Milano, Creative Director
Kevin Fahey, Cognella Marketing Program Manager
Al Grisante, Acquisitions Editor
Jamie Giganti, Project Editor
Luiz Fererria, Licensing Associate

16 15 14 13 12   1 2 3 4 5

Printed in the United States of America

ISBN: 978-1-60927-123-7

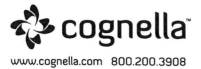

www.cognella.com   800.200.3908

Contents

An Introduction to Drug Abuse

By Howard Abadinsky

There is probably one thing, and one thing only, on which the leaders of all modern states agree; on which Catholics, Protestants, Jews, Mohammedans, and atheists agree; on which Democrats, Republicans, Socialists, Communists, Liberals, and Conservatives agree; on which medical and scientific authorities throughout the world agree. That thing is the "scientific fact" that certain substances which people like to ingest or inject are "dangerous" both to those who use them and to others; and that the use of such substances constitutes "drug abuse" or "drug addiction—a disease whose control and eradication are the duty of the combined forces of the medical profession and the state. However, there is little agreement on which substances are acceptable and which substances are unacceptable.

—ADAPTED FROM THOMAS SZASZ
(1974, p. xi)

Public Morals and Private Vices

Drug abuse rains individual lives and families and drains billions of dollars each year from the U.S. economy. The violence and corruption associated with drug trafficking erodes the nation's quality of life—a not surprising observation by the President's Commission on Organized Crime (1986). Drug abuse implies the misuse of certain substances—it is a moral, not a scientific, term, an "unstandardized, value-laden, and highly relative term used with a great deal of imprecision and confusion, generally implying drug use that is excessive, dangerous, or undesirable to the individual or community and that ought to be modified" (Nelson et al, 1982, p. 33). Norman Zinberg (1984) points out that there are numerous definitions of drug abuse that reflect social values and not scientific insight: "One reason for the prevalence of definitions of drug abuse that are neither logical nor scientific is the strength of Puritan moralism in American culture which frowns on the pleasure and recreation provided by intoxicants" (p. 27). Such definitions typically refer to (1) the nonmedical use of a substance (2) to alter the mental state (3) in a manner that is detrimental to the individual or the community, or (4) that is illegal. For example, the American Social Health Association (1972) defines drug abuse as "the use of mood modifying chemicals outside of medical supervision, and in a manner which is harmful to the person and the community" (p. 1). Other definitions, such as those offered by the World Health Organization and the American Medical Association, include references to physical and/or psychological dependency (Zinberg, 1984).

Drug abuse may be defined from a number of perspectives:

> The legal definition equates drug use with the mere act of using a proscribed drug or using a drug under proscribed conditions. The moral definition is similar, but greater emphasis is placed on the motivation or purpose for which the drug is used. The medical model opposes unsupervised usage but emphasizes the physical and mental consequences for the user, and the social definition stresses social responsibility and adverse effects on others. (Baiter, 1974, p. 5)

The National Commission on Marijuana and Drug Abuse (1973) states that drug abuse "must be deleted from official pronouncements and public policy dialogue" because the "term has no functional utility and has become no more than an arbitrary codeword for that drug use which is presently considered wrong" (p. 13).

In this text, moderate use of a drug will be defined as "abuse" and illegal, if society so determines, or it will be socially acceptable and lawful if society so determines regardless of the relative danger inherent in the substance (see chapter 2). Alcohol is clearly a potentially harmful drug used by mainstream religions such as Judaism and Catholicism (although prohibited by Islam and several Protestant denominations), but recreational use of alcohol in moderation is an accepted part of U.S. culture. The cost of alcohol abuse is twice the social cost of all illegal drug abuse (McNulty, 1986). Alcohol is reputed to be the direct cause of 80,000 to 100,000 deaths annually, and alcohol-related auto accidents are the leading cause of death for teenagers (Wicker, 1987). In 1986 there were 23,990 alcohol-related traffic deaths (Stevens, 1987). Alcohol is a factor in nearly half of America's murders, suicides, and accidental deaths ("Coming to Grips with Alcoholism," 1987)} In fact, notes G. Douglas Talbott, a physician specializing in the treatment of alcohol- and drug-abusing physicians, "under every scientific and pharmacological constraint existing today for the protection of society, alcohol most certainly would be a class 2 narcotic and would be available only with a Government Narcotic Registry Number[1] (quoted in Gonzales 1988: 27). Thus, while the use of alcohol is a major social problem in the United States, where reputedly there are more than 13 million alcoholics (D. Smith, 1986), alcohol for recreational use may be legally manufactured, imported, sold, and possessed. Because of this reality, trafficking in alcohol has not been associated with violence and corruption since the repeal of Prohibition in 1933.

There is another drug that meets the rigorous criteria for abuse liability and dependence potential, a drug that strongly stimulates the central nervous system. Heavy doses produce disturbed vision, confusion, convulsions, and eventually death. Small doses of the drug cause irritation of the mouth, throat, and bronchi, high blood

---

1   For an examination of the relationship between alcohol and crime, see Collins (1981).

pressure, and increased risk of heart disease and cancer, and are a health threat to the fetuses of pregnant women. Treatment for the drug is quite difficult, and relapses are frequent. Tolerance develops, producing withdrawal symptoms when the substance is discontinued. This drug is nicotine, a substance found in tobacco.

Cigarette smoking, notes Jack Henningfield (1986, p. 28), shares certain critical features with classic forms of drug dependence. Nicotine is a psychoactive substance that can function as a euphoriant, and it serves as a reinforcer for humans and laboratory test animals. On May 16, 1988, C. Everett Koop, the U.S. surgeon general, declared that nicotine was as addicting as heroin and cocaine (Tolchin, 1988). According to the Centers for Disease Control, at least 320,000 people die each year from causes directly linked to cigarette smoking. And, the financial cost of smoking-induced illness is staggering, accounting for nearly 18 percent of health-care costs in the United States for an annual total of $365 billion (Sachs, 1986).

There are also a variety of lawful substances that are addicting and have been abused by any number of "respectable persons," including government officials (Shabecoff, 1987); these substances—sedatives and tranquilizers (benzodiazapenes)—have led to the deaths of major public figures. Erich Goode (1972) points out that social expectations and definitions determine what kind of drug-taking is appropriate, as well as the social situations that are approved or disapproved for drug use. The use of drugs is neither inherently bad nor inherently good—these are socially determined values. Thus, Mormons and Christian Scientists consider the use of tea and coffee abusive.

This text will be concerned only with those substances that are prohibited by law in the United States, outside of accepted medical procedures. While recognizing the incongruities discussed in this chapter, we will accept the societal definition of drug abuse—a definition that excludes the widely used, but licit, psychoactive substances caffeine, nicotine, and alcohol: Drug abuse is the use of psychoactive substances in a manner that is illegal or outside of accepted medical practice.

Drugs of Abuse

Erich Goode (1972) points out that there is no completely satisfying way of delineating what is and what is not a drug. Some feel that the term "drug abuse" is inappropriate; a better term would be chemical or substance abuse. "Imprecision of the term 'drug,'" note Gerald Uelmen and Victor Haddox (1983) has had serious social consequences.

> Because alcohol is excluded, the public is conditioned to regard a martini as something fundamentally different from a marijuana cigarette, and barbiturate capsule, or a bag of heroin. Similarly, because the referents of the word "drug" differ so widely in the therapeutic and social contexts, the public is conditioned to believe that "street" drugs act according to entirely different principles than "medical" drugs. The result is that the risks of the former are exaggerated and the risks of the latter are overlooked. (pp.1–3)

"In contemporary society," write Kenneth Jones, Louis Shainberg, and Curtis Byer (1979), "the word drug has two connotations—one positive, explaining its crucial role in medicine, and one negative, reflecting not the natural and synthetic makeup of these chemicals, but the self-destruction and socially deleterious patterns of misuse" (p. 1). In this text, the word drug will refer to substances having mood-altering or psychoactive effects. This definition includes caffeine as well as cocaine. The word addiction, from the Latin verb addicere, meaning to bind a person to one thing or another, is often used to mean chronic drug use. In this text, addiction will be used to label psychological and physiological dependence, the latter referring to an objective and measurable withdrawal syndrome. Once physiological dependence is established, "maintenance doses of the drug must be taken or the drug-accommodated equilibrium will be upset and symptoms of withdrawal will appear" (Biernacki, 1986, p. 9). These symptoms continue until a maintenance dose is administered, or until the physiological processes readjust and bring about a drug-free state of equilibrium.

Some nonaddicting drugs are referred to as "habituating," producing psychological but not physiological dependence (although, as we shall see in chapter 3, the difference between addicting and habituating may be difficult to determine). Drugs that have a legitimate medical use may be marketed under a variety of trade names. In this text, trade names begin with a capital letter, while chemical or generic names do not.

Drug abuse can be viewed as occurring on a continuum. At one end is the nonuser who has never used prohibited drugs; at the other end is the compulsive user whose life revolves around obtaining, maintaining, and using a supply of drugs. For the compulsive user, failure to secure an adequate supply of the desired drug results in psychological stress and discomfort, and if the substance craved is addicting, the user experiences withdrawal symptoms. "While compulsive users constitute only a very small proportion of the overall population, they consume a disproportionate share of the drugs in this society—and contribute disproportionately to the society's 'drug problem'" (Drug Abuse and Drug Abuse Research, 1987, p. 14; hereafter, "Drug Abuse").

The major drugs may be arranged in four categories according to their effects on the central nervous system: depressants, stimulants, hallucinogens, and cannabis. The Institute for the Study of Drug Dependence (1987, hereafter, ISDD) offers some cautions, however: "Drug effects are strongly influenced by the amount taken, how much has been taken before, what the user wants and expects to happen, the surroundings in which it is taken, and the reactions of other people. All of these influences are themselves tied up with social and cultural attitudes and beliefs about drugs as well as more general social conditions. Even the same person will react differently at different times" (p. 1). A brief look at the most important substances in each category is necessary in order to examine some larger questions about drug abuse.

1. **Depressants.** These drugs depress the central nervous system (CNS) and reduce pain. The most frequently used drug in this category is alcohol; the most frequently used illegal drug is the opiate derivative heroin. Other depressants, all of which have some medical use, include morphine, codeine, methadone, barbiturates, methaqualone, and tranquilizers. These substances can cause physical and psychological dependence, a craving, and withdrawal symptoms resulting in physical and psychological stress. Opiate derivatives (heroin, morphine. codeine) and opiumlike drugs such as methadone are addicting and are often referred to as narcotics. (Drug laws frequently label cocaine a narcotic, although it is clearly a stimulant.)

2. **Stimulants.** These drugs elevate a persons mood (produce feelings of well-being) by stimulating the central nervous system. The most frequently used drugs in this

category are caffeine and nicotine. The most frequently used illegal stimulant is cocaine, while amphetamines have limited medical use. These drugs are habituating, that is, they can produce Dsychological dependence.

3. **Hallucinogens**. These drugs alter perceptual functions, and the term "hallucinogen" as opposed to, for example, "psychoactive" or "psychedelic" is value laden. The most frequently used are LSD (lysergic acid diethylamide) and PGP (phencyclidme), both produced artificially. Neither has legitimate medical use. 'Ihere are also organic hallucinogens such as mescaline, which is found in the peyote cactus. The lawful use of peyote is limited to the religious ceremonies of Native Americans.

4. **Cannabis.** Frequently used in the form of marijuana, cannabis exhibits some of the characteristics of hallucinogens, depressants, and even stimulants. Its lawful use (in the liquid form of its psychoactive ingredient, THC) is limited to treating glaucoma and to reducing some side-effects of cancer chemotherapy.

Polydrug Use

Drug abuse is made more complicated by the phenomenon of polydrug use, consuming more than one type of psychoactive chemical. George Vaiilant (1970, p. 492) notes that "in contradiction to the public's view of narcotics addiction as existing discretely apart from other addictions, the heroin addict is a multiple drug user" who is often an alcohol abuser. The New York State Division of Substance Abuse Services (1986) reports that the "use of more than one substance continues to be the predominant pattern of abuse. Both heroin and cocaine are commonly used with one drug ameliorating the undesired effects of the other; PGP is used by some heroin abusers to heighten the effect of heroin. Alcohol use is almost always involved" (pp. 14-15). In San Antonio, Texas, the medical examiner found that in 70 percent of the cases in which heroin was the primary cause of death, cocaine was also present in the body. Drug treatment programs in that city report that many clients test positive for both heroin and cocaine (Texas Commission on Alcohol and Drug Abuse, 1987). In Minnesota, polydrug use, which includes alcohol, is widespread among that states chemical abusing population (Minnesota Department of Human Services. 1987). Almost 19 percent of the persons admitted to hospitals for heroin abuse treatment in Colorado reported the use of cocaine (Colorado Alcohol and Drug Abuse Division, 1987).

Bruce Johnson and his colleagues (1985) round that 90 percent of the heroin addicts they studied also abused alcohol and cocaine. Heroin and cocaine abusers do not limit their drug consumption to heroin or cocaine. Much evidence shows that heroin addicts and cocaine abusers are also heavy polydrug abusers: they frequently use marijuana, pills, and alcohol. Many such abusers consume large amounts of alcohol daily" (Johnson. Lipton. and Wish, 1986b, p. 2). Mark Gold and his colleagues (1986) found that most cocaine abusers are concurrently abusing alcohol or other sedative-hypnotics to alleviate the unpleasant side effects of cocaine (p. 55). For example, an autopsy on ballet star Patrick Bissell. thirty years old. who died December 29. 1987 indicated that he overdosed on cocaine, codeine, methadone, and several other substances. (Michael Stone [1988] states that drug use, particularly cocaine, is endemic in the ballet world.) Drug abusers who are unable to get their preferred substance due to lack of funds or connections often seek substitutes.

Responding to the Problem of Drug Abuse

David Musto (1973) provides a summary of the history of U.S. policy toward drug abuse:

> American concern with narcotics is more than a medical or legal problem—it is in the fullest sense a political problem. The energy that has given impetus to drug control and prohibition came from profound tensions among socioeconomic groups, ethnic minorities, and generations—as well as the psychological attraction of certain drugs. The form of this control has been shaped by the gradual evolution of federal police powers. The bad results of drug use and the number of drug users have often been exaggerated for partisan advantage. Public demand for action against drug abuse has led to regulative decisions that lack a true regard for the reality of drug use. Regulations with foreign nations, often the sources of the drugs, have been a theme in the domestic scene from the beginning of the American antinarcotic movement. Narcotics addiction has proven to be one of the most intractable medical inquiries ever faced by American clinicians and scientists (p. 244).

Out of this developed two basic models for responding to dangerous substances. The first is the disease or public health model, which defines substance abuse as a disease to be prevented or treated, just as any other public health problem. The second is the moral-legal model, which defines alcohol and other psychoactive drugs as either legal or illegal and attempts to control availability through penalties. The moral–legal model utilizes three methods to control potentially dangerous drugs in the United States:

1. **Regulation.** Certain substances that may be harmful to their users can be sold but with restrictions. These substances are heavily taxed, providing the government with an important source of revenue. Alcoholic beverages and tobacco products are subjected to disproportionate taxation, and their sale is restricted to those above a certain chronological age. Special licenses are usually required for the manufacture, distribution, and sale of regulated substances.

2. **Medical auspices.** Certain potentially harmful substances may be used under medical supervision. John Kaplan (1985) notes that "this model seems to be the preferred one for drugs having medical uses, in that taken under the direction of a physician, their value outweighs their danger" (p. 644). Under this model the medical profession is given control over legal access to specific substances. In this category are barbiturates, amphetamines, certain opiates (morphine and codeine), and heroin substitutes such as methadone.

3. **Law enforcement.** Statutes make the manufacture or possession of certain dangerous substances a crime and empower specific public officials to enforce the statutes. Certain substances are permitted for medical use, but punishment is specified for persons possessing these substances outside of accepted medical practice. Thus, heroin has no permissible use in the United States—it is absolutely prohibited. Other psychoactive substances, for example, morphine and Seconal (secobarbital sodium), are permissible

for medical use, but are illegal under any other circumstances.

From Civil War times until the 1920s, the U.S. response to dangerous drugs moved from permissiveness to one of rigid legal control, from the public health model to the moral-legal model. Edwin Schur (1965. p. 130) says that the practical effect of this change was "to define the addict as a criminal offender": it has led to the creation of a vast black market. Drug entrepreneurs quickly filled the void left by the withdrawal of lawful sources:

> In the 1920s this country had a large number of addicts, but they were not regarded as criminals by the law: in general, they did not commit crimes and conducted their lives much the same way as the nonaddict population did. Clinics and private physicians were free to prescribe maintenance doses. It was the outlawing of the addictive drug that gave rise to an illegal market controlled by organized crime: and it is the exorbitant cost of the outlawed drug that has driven addicts into criminal activity to support their habit. (National Council on Crime and Delinquency, 1974, p. 4)

"The social importance of drugs," state Norman ZInberg and John Robertson (1972) "does not lie In their capacity to injure and reduce the capabilities of drug users, though when misused drugs can inflict psychological and physical harm. These casualties are a small minority, and in most cases they could be treated if less punitive legal policy were operating" (p. 11). A "clearer case of misapplication of the criminal sanction," writes Herbert Packer (1968), "would be difficult to imagine" (p. 333).

This approach may be contrasted with that of England, where in 1926 the Ministry of Health recommended providing those dependent on drugs with prescriptions for heroin and other chemicals. While the long- range goal was to withdraw abusers from their dependency, the system for decades simply provided maintenance doses of morphine and heroin to addicts. The British system was popularized in the United States with the publication, in 1962, of Edwin Schur's Narcotic Addiction in Britain and America. James Inciardi (1986) states that the well-researched arguments provided by Schur created a climate that led to the promotion of methadone maintenance programs in the United States. (Methadone maintenance is discussed in chapter 5.)

For many decades the British approach to drug abuse appeared to be quite successful—the drug-dependent population was older and relatively stable, and drug abuse was not associated with crime. During the 1960s, however, the drug scene changed; more and younger drug abusers were becoming part of a drug subculture closely resembling that of the United States during the 1950s. In response, the British system was overhauled in 1967. Drug abusers could no longer receive maintenance prescriptions from private physicians. Regulations restricted the authority to prescribe narcotics for the treatment of drug dependency to a few specially licensed doctors (ISDD, 1987). During the 1970s the system moved away from opiates (morphine and heroin) and toward methadone maintenance. An extensive black market developed not only in opiates but also in cocaine, barbiturates, and amphetamines. British physicians are currently prohibited from prescribing cocaine as a way of dealing with abuse of that drug (ISDD, 1987). (The implications of the "British system" for the United States are discussed in chapter 8.) England has also strengthened its law enforcement response to illegal drug trafficking. British police officers have special powers to stop, detain, and search persons on the "reasonable suspicion" that they are in possession of a controlled drug, and statutes provide for the seizure of assets and penalties for the "laundering" of drug revenues. (Laundering will be discussed in chapter 6.)

Success in the struggle against drug abuse is difficult if not impossible to measure. In England, for example, doctors must report the names of patients receiving controlled substances for their addiction; how many drug abusers there are who are not part of any medical program, of course, is not known. In the United States no one knows with any degree of accuracy how many persons are abusing drugs or are addicted to any substance (including alcohol). This is a significant handicap in attempting to determine the effectiveness of any approach to drug abuse, whether it is an approach that stresses law enforcement or one that seeks to reduce demand by treating abusers.

This deficiency, however, provides the basis for important political posturing. For example, in his 1980 State of the Union message. President Jimmy Carter told Congress: "At the beginning of my administration there were over a half million heroin addicts in the United States. Our continued emphasis on reducing the supply of heroin, as well as providing for the treatment and rehabilitation of its victims, has reduced the heroin population to 380,000" (Trebach, 1982). Three years earlier, President Richard Nixon had proclaimed: "We have turned the comer on drug addiction in the United States" (Trebach, 1982). The Nixon administration referred to its achievements in decreasing the rate of increase, a measure that, David Bellis (1981) notes, "allows bureaucrats and line programs (addiction treatment and drug law enforcement deliverers) to claim victory in their fight against crime or addiction without threatening the continued funding of their organizations" (p. 79).

Estimates of the Drug Problem

Information on the drug problem in the United States is derived from five Indicators. Each indicator provides a different perspective on the problem, and they complement one another. Although the Indicators have recognized limitations and deficiencies that affect the quality of information and make specific estimates uncertain, the agencies that prepare them believe that the data can reliably portray general trends.

NNICC Narcotics Intelligence Estimates

The National Narcotics Intelligence Consumers Committee (NNICC) is a federal interagency mechanism for coordinating drug Intelligence collection requirements and producing joint intelligence estimates. NNICC issues periodic reports on the worldwide illicit drug situation. The reports contain estimates of illegal drug production and availability, and discuss the four major drug categories: marijuana, cocaine, opiates, and synthetic drugs. The report also contains Information on drug trafficking routes and methods and on the flow of drug-related money.

Estimates of Illegal drug quantities are difficult to make. Since the drugs are illegal, little reliable data exist. NNICC obtains drug production data for Individual countries from host country records, local contacts, informants, and sophisticated intelligence-gathering techniques. NNICC derives drug availability and consumption estimates from sample surveys, drug seizures, drug price and purity data, drug-related hospital emergencies, and other data.

National Survey on Drug Abuse

The National Survey on Drug Abuse (commonly referred to as the Household Survey) is funded by the National Institute on Drug Abuse (NIDA) and conducted under contract every two or three years. The survey provides data on incidence, prevalence, and trends of drug use for persons age twelve and older living in households. Results are based on interviews with persons randomly selected from the household population who record their responses on self-administered answer sheets. Household Survey data are used in conjunction with High School Senior Survey data to describe levels of drug use in specific segments of the population. These data may also be used in conjunction with Drug Abuse Warning Network data to describe long-term trends in drug abuse.

Survey limitations include the fact that the homeless and persons living in military installations, dormitories, and institutions, such as jails and hospitals, are not covered. Since the survey is voluntary and the questionnaires are self-administered, the results may be biased (and probably understate the scope of the drug problem).

High School Senior Survey

The High School Senior Survey, sponsored by the NIDA, is an annual survey of drug use among high school seniors. Information is collected from nearly seventeen thousand respondents in approximately one hundred thirty public and-private high schools. Primary uses of the data include: (1) assessing the prevalence and trends of drug use among high school seniors, and (2) gaining a better understanding of the lifestyles and value orientations associated with patterns of drug use, and (3) monitoring how these orientations are shifting over time.

The survey has several limitations. High school dropouts, who are associated with higher rates of drug use, are not part of the sampled universe. Chronic absentees, who may also have high rates of abuse, are less likely to be surveyed. Conscious or unconscious distortions in self-reporting the information can also bias results. In addition, new

trends in drug abuse, such as the use of "crack," may not be initially detected because the survey is designed to measure only those drugs abused at a significant level.

Drug Abuse Warning Network (DAWN)

DAWN, which is funded by NIDA is a large scale drug abuse data collection system designed as an early warning indicator of the nation's drug abuse problem. An episode report is submitted for each drug abuse patient who visits the emergency room of a hospital participating in DAWN and for each drug abuse death encountered by a participating medical examiner or coroner. In a single emergency room episode, a patient may "mention" having ingested more than one drug. DAWN records each drug a patient reports having used within four days prior to the hospital visit to the Drug Enforcement Administration (DEA). Data are collected from a nonrandom sample in selected metropolitan areas throughout the country representing approximately one-third of the U.S. population.

While there are standard definitions and data collection procedures, variations among individual reporters may occur. Incomplete reporting, turnover of reporting facilities and personnel, and reporting delays of up to one year (primarily for medical examiner data) are some of the system limitations. For hospital emergencies, NNICC, In Its last two publications, has used data from the DAWN Consistent Panel rather than from the Total Panel. The Consistent Panel includes only those hospitals reporting on a consistent basis (specifically, 90 percent of the time or more during each year). Data representing the total DAWN system were not used for trend analysis by NNICC because of reporting fluctuations. While medical examiner/coroner data are not subject to the same inconsistencies, reports are so small compared to the total DAWN system that it is not considered a valid trend indicator. (And medical examiner data for New York are considered incomplete and are not included.)

Retail Price/Purity

The price and purity levels of Illegal drugs at the retail (consumer) level are key values in the NNICC estimating process. The DEA gathers these data, which are used as an indicator of drug availability. Drug prices are developed from a computerized database and are derived primarily from reports on purchases of, and negotiations to purchase, illegal drugs by undercover federal, state, and local law enforcement officers. Purity levels for heroin and cocaine are determined through laboratory analysis, but are not applicable to marijuana and most synthetic drugs. A limited number of reports and lack of randomness are problems that have plagued these indicators in the past.

Drugs, Crime, and Violence

The current importance of drug abuse as an issue in the United States is due to the relationship between drugs and crime. Although a great deal of crime is committed by persons under the influence of alcohol—David Smith (1986, p. 118) reports that "over 60 percent of homicides involve alcohol use by both offender and victim, and 65 percent of aggressive sexual acts against women involve alcohol use by the offender"—public interest in the relationship between drug abuse and crime has clearly overshadowed the alcohol-crime nexus.

The outlawing of certain drugs not only makes those who possess these drugs criminals but also substantially inflates the cost of the substances to consumers. In order to pay these high prices, some abusers commit robbery and/or sell drugs.

(The business of drugs is discussed in chapter 6.) A substantial criminal population exists whose nondrug law violations are based only on the desire to secure drugs. However, many drug abusers, particularly those addicted to heroin, are criminals whose drug abuse is simply part of a pattern of hedonistic and antisocial behavior. George Vaillant (1970) suggests that no matter what their class origins, most persons who use narcotics "have a greater tendency than their socioeconomic peers to be delinquent" (p. 488).

There is undoubtedly a high correlation between heroin abuse and crime (see Gandossy, Williams, Cohen, and Harwood, 1980; Johnson et al. 1985: Nurco, Ball, Shaffer, and Hanlon, 1985; Inciardi, 1986; Wish and Johnson, 1986): a recent study found that more than half of the men arrested in twelve major cities tested positive for recent use of illicit drugs (Kerr. 1988b). However, we cannot be sure whether it is drug abuse that leads to crime or if criminals tend to abuse drugs. Or, perhaps the factors that lead to drug abuse and those that lead to crime are the same: "The relationship is not due to any causal connection, but rather to the fact that both criminals and drug-using behavior are the result of the same variables (McBnde and McCoy, 1981, p. 283: also Speckart and Anglin, 1985. 1987). Indeed, areas with high levels of delinquency and crime also have high levels of drug usage, while the reverse is also true. In their study. Carpenter, Glassner, Johnson, and Loughlin (1988) found that the most seriously delinquent adolescents also abused drugs, but crime and drug use appeared to be independent of one another—both apparently related to other causal variables.

The question of whether crime is a pre- or post-drug use phenomenon is actually an oversimplification. James Inciardi (1981) argues that the pursuit of some simple cause-and-effect relationship may be futile. His data found, for example, that among the males, there seems to be a clear progression from alcohol to crime, to drug abuse, to arrest, and then to heroin use. But upon closer inspection, the pattern is not altogether clear. At one level, for example, criminal activity can be viewed as predating ones drug-using career, since the median point of the first crime is slightly below that of first drug abuse, and is considerably before the onset of heroin use. But, at the same time, if alcohol intoxication at a median age of 16.6 years were to be considered substance abuse, then crime is nearly a phenomenon that succeeds substance abuse. Among the females, the description is even more complex. In the population of female heroin users, criminal activity occurred after both alcohol and other drug abuse and marijuana use, but before involvement with the more debilitating barbiturates and heroin. (p. 59)

This issue has serious policy implications. If drug abusers simply continue in crime after they have given up drug abuse, efforts to reduce crime by reducing drug abuse are doomed to fail. As James Q. Wilson (1975) points out, "some addicts who steal to support their habit come to regard crime as more profitable than normal employment. They would probably continue to steal to provide themselves with an income even after they no longer needed to use part of that income to buy heroin" (p. 137) or any other illegal substance. M. Douglas Anglin and George Speckart (1988) found, however, that "levels of criminality after the addiction career are near zero, a finding that is compatible with data presented by other authors and is illustrative of the 'maturing out' phase of the addiction career 'life cycle'" (p. 233).

The sequence of drug use and crime has produced contradictory findings. James Vorenberg and Irving Lukoff (1973) found that the criminal careers of a substantial segment of the heroin addicts they studied antedated the onset of heroin use, and that those whose criminality preceded heroin use tended to be more involved in violent criminal behavior. Anglin and Speckart (1988) report that between 60 and 75 percent of the addicts in their samples had arrest histories that preceded addiction. Paul Cushman, Jr. (1974) found, however, that the heroin addicts he studied were predominantly noncriminal before addiction and experienced "progressively increased rates of annual arrests after addiction started" (p. 43). (Of course, this could be the result of addicts being less adept at crime!) Bruce Johnson and his colleagues (1985) and Anglin and Speckart (1988) determined that the more frequent the drug use, the more serious the types of crime committed—for example, burglary and robbery instead of shoplifting and other larcenies. Whatever the relationship—addiction leading to crime or criminals becoming addicts—some researchers (McGlothlin, Anglin, and Wilson, 1978; Ball, Rosen, Friedman, and Nurco, 1979; Johnson, Lipton, and Wish, 1986a) have determined that the amount of criminality tends to be sharply reduced among persons who were once narcotic addicts but who no longer are addicted.

The issue of crime-drug abuse has typically been related to the abuse of heroin, not cocaine. During the time I worked as a parole officer in New York (1964-1978), offenders who had used cocaine were rare, while studies by the New York State Division of Parole indicated that those who had used heroin constituted a substantial majority of parole clientele in the New York City area. Almost two decades ago. Troy Duster (1970) stated that "cocaine usage is rare in the United States" (p. 42). However, between 1980 and 1986 there was a dramatic increase in the abuse of

The Worlds of Drugs and Drug Abuse

The worlds of drug abuse are as varied as the substances and the persons who abuse them. Between the persons who grow or process the substances and the ultimate consumer is a loosely organized chain of persons who make up the core of the business of drugs.

- Some ten thousand miles from the United States, an officer in full dress reviews his battle-ready troops in the hill country of northern Thailand, approximately 8 kilometers from the Burmese border. There are about six hundred men armed with M-16 rifles and another fifty with 30-caliber machine guns. The officer and his men belong to the armed forces of no recognized country; they are part of the Shan United Army (SUA), one of three major private militias in the Golden Triangle of Laos, Thailand, and Burma. Along with the Burmese Communist party and the Chinese irregular forces or Kuomington, the SUA is supported by trafficking in opium, from which is derived heroin destined for markets in the West.
- Shortly after dawn certain streets in a South Bronx neighborhood are already filling with young men whose furtive looks indicate that they are searching for their morning connection. Unshaved and wearing clothing that hardly protects them from the cold winter air, junkies are on the prowl for a fix—heroin.
- In a remote subtropical valley between the Andes and the jungles of Peru is Tingo Maria. This "Wild West" town of some twenty thousand persons has a grass runway used by jet aircraft to transport its most important product, coca paste, which is traded at the State Tourist Hotel and sometimes openly on the dusty streets. From Tingo Maria and dozens of other remote outposts in several countries of Latin America, the coca paste is shipped to cities in Colombia, where it is converted into cocaine destined for northern markets.
- Three stylishly dressed couples gather around a large mirror placed on a glass-top table in a fashionable home in southern California. Arrayed before them is a white powder that has been chopped with a razor blade to remove flakes and lumps and formed into six rows, one to two inches long and about one-eighth of an inch wide—six "lines of coke." Using rolled hundred-dollar bills, they suck the powder into their nostrils and wait for the "rush."
- On November 17, 1987, Mike Roark, the mayor of Charleston, West Virginia, known as "Mad Dog" for his relentless pursuit of drug dealers while a county prosecutor and assistant U.S. attorney, pleads guilty to drug conspiracy charges involving the distribution of cocaine.
- A sixteen-wheel vehicle hurtles through the night, its driver fighting the urge to sleep after ten hours on the road. Without taking his eyes off the road, he reaches into a coat pocket for his helpers, "speed" tablets (methamphetamine).

- At the dedication of a drug treatment program for adolescents, Kitty Dukakis, wife of the governor of Massachusetts, tells how she was addicted to prescribed amphetamines for twenty-six years (Bowd, 1987).
- A long double line of motorcycles moves down the open highway—a chapter of the Hells Angels is escorting their chief chemist to a meeting with a source of P2P, a primary ingredient in the manufacture of methamphetamine—"speed." The Angels have maintained a long-standing monopoly over the distribution of speed in the area.
- On the west coast of Colombia's Guajira Peninsula is the town of Riohacha. "Twice a year the town ... erupts. A bootlegged bottle of Johnny Walker Black Label goes for as little as $3, a weekend with a high-class prostitute for as much as $5,000. The streets are lined with Ford Mangers and Mercedes guarded by men carrying submachine guns. The whole city is an armed camp. Police either turn their backs or get killed .... The marijuana crop is in" (Michaels, 1980, p. 4).
- The blaring noise from a rented jukebox does not seem to bother any of the young men and women who alternate between keeping up with the rhythm and Inhaling deeply on a marijuana cigarette held with a pair of tweezers.
- On November 5, 1987, U.S. Court of Appeals Justice Douglas H. Ginsburg, President Ronald Reagan's nominee to the Supreme Court, reveals that he smoked marijuana as a college student in the 1960s—and on a few occasions while a law professor at Harvard University during the 1970s.
- Betty Ford, the wife of former President Gerald R. Ford, reveals that she was addicted to Valium and that this experience led her to found the Betty Ford Center for the treatment of chemical dependency.
- Russ Reed is the eighth generation off medical doctors in his family. Like his father, Reed tried every new psychoactive drug that came on the market. "Monday and Tuesdays I'd work my ass off," he said. "Wednesday and Thursday I'd have rounds. I was injecting myself at work, often right through my pants so that I didn't have to slow down to take my pants off" (Gonzales, 1988, p. 1).
- In 1987, after being identified as a key operative in the Iran arms-for-hostages debacle, Robert C. McFarlane, a former national security advisor to President Ronald Reagan, attempts suicide by taking an overdose of Valium.

cocaine by the same populations that traditionally had been the major consumers of heroin. David Smith (1986) reports that during these years cocaine use crossed social class lines and the age of onset dropped considerably.

Until recently it has been assumed that cocaine was not a criminogenic force toward income-generating crime because cocaine does not have the physiological addictive power of heroin and because

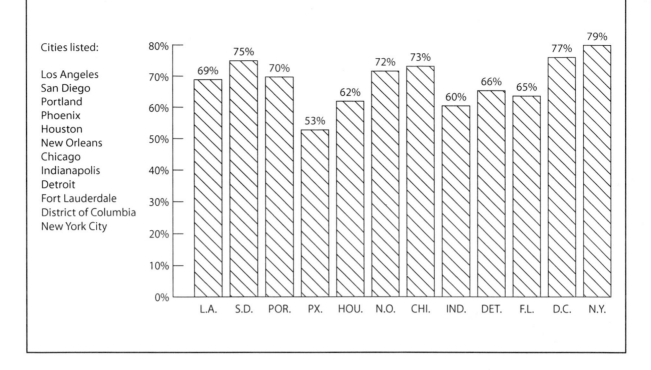

Figure 1. Percentage of male arrestees testing positive for any drug, including marijuana (June–November 1987).

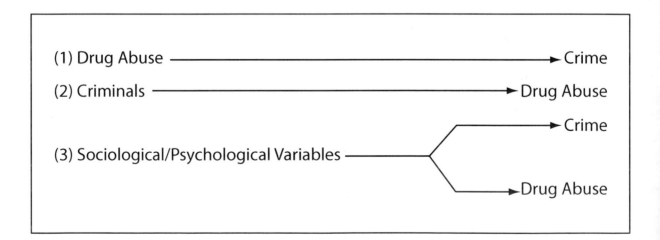

Figure 3. The Relationship Between Drugs and Crime: Three Possibilities.

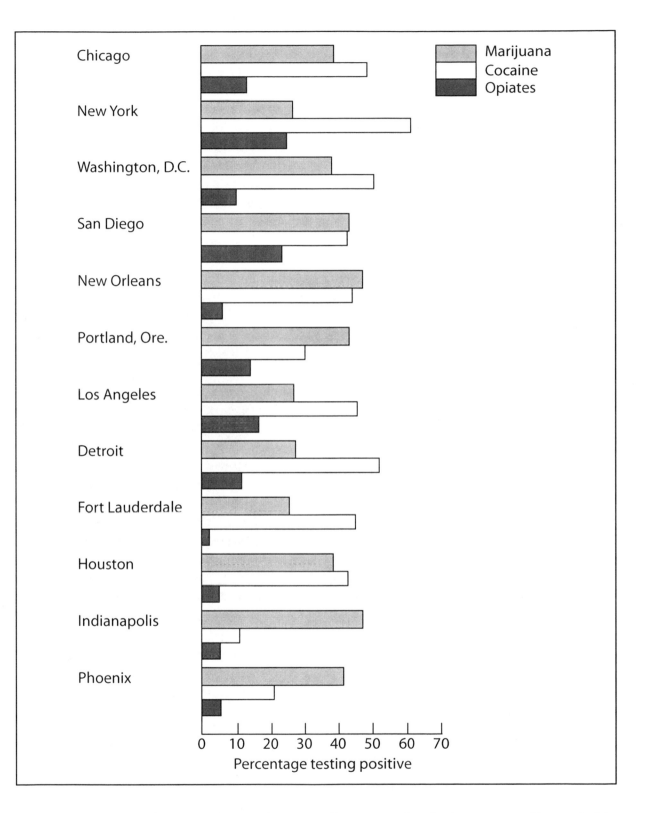

Figure 3. Percentage of arrestees in 12 U.S. metropolitan areas who, during one sampling period in 1987, tested positive for three major drugs.

cocaine users were viewed as unlikely to come from population groups with high crime rates. Cocaine was thought to be a drug of the middle and upper class. These assumptions appear to be unjustified. Weekly and daily cocaine use are associated with high levels of illegal income. (Collins, Hubbard, and Rachel, 1985, p. 759)

In testimony before the President's Commission on Organized Crime (1984, p. 94), Bruce Johnson reported that cocaine, not heroin, was clearly the "in" drug among young adults age eighteen to twenty-five in the low-income areas of New York City. This is a dramatic change from the drug scene of the late 1960s and early 1970s, when, Johnson said, heroin was the drug of choice. Furthermore, virtually all heroin abusers also use cocaine, many as frequently as heroin in a combination known as a "speedball." The use of these substances, he noted, is part of a lifestyle that also includes abuse of alcohol, marijuana, barbiturates, and amphetamines—and crime. The "crack" phenomenon—cocaine in a potent form that permits it to be smoked—has apparently led to an increase in the popularity of cocaine in neighborhoods that traditionally had a problem with heroin. In New York, "in the poorest neighborhoods of the city, heroin was the main addictive drug since its boom in popularity in the late 1960s. Today, there are still an estimated 250,000 heroin addicts in the city, but they are generally an aging group who began their habits more than a decade ago. No one knows how many crack users there are, but most experts agree that the drug is far more popular than heroin and is used by people of a wider age group" (Kerr, 1988f, p. 13).

More than two decades ago, Edwin Schur (1965) argued that narcotic addiction in the United States seems to reduce the inclination to engage in violent crime. (Schur excluded robbery as a violent crime—a questionable assertion from a legal point of view, though Schur is an attorney as well as a sociologist.) However, Johnson, Lipton, and Wish (1986a), in a more recent research effort, found that heroin abusers (not necessarily addicts), are at least as violent as, and perhaps more violent than, their nondrug- or nonheroin-using criminal counterparts. In fact, they report that "about half of the most violent criminals are heroin abusers" (1986b. p. 3). It is difficult to determine if this is simply a problem of changing definitions or of a changing drug population. While there is no evidence that crime results from the direct effects of heroin itself—indeed, the substance appears to have a pacifying effect—the irritability resulting from withdrawal symptoms has been known to lead to violence (Goldstein. 1985).

Other drugs, PCP and cocaine for example, may involve otherwise "'normal" persons in violent behavior. The Detroit medical examiner s office reports that "67 percent of that city's homicide victims had cocaine in their blood samples (Franklin, 1987), indicating that cocaine users either engage in dangerous behavior or expose themselves to places and/or situations where violence is likely to occur. And persons intent on committing violent crimes, such as robbery, may ingest alcohol or stimulants "for courage." Paul Goldstein (1985) notes that "the relationship between drugs and violence has been consistently documented in both the popular press and in social scientific research" (p. 494). Peter Kerr (1988f) reports that crack users are more likely to commit crimes against persons than against property, and that there has been an increase in child beating by crack-abusing parents.

The heroin distribution subculture, at every level—from wholesaling to street sale—is permeated with extreme levels of violence. Many drug abusers use more than one psychoactive chemical—polydrug abuse—thus expanding

Cocaine and Law Don't Mix

S.W., age thirty, had been practicing law for five years when he began using cocaine to help him unwind after many hours of work. It was 1976, a time when coke was "in" with many of his theatrical and advertising clients. S.W. went from monthly usage to being a "weekender." Eventually his habit increased to 2 ounces a week at a cost of $3,000 to $5,000, and his behavior changed dramatically. He had to leave meetings for a "snort," and his appearance deteriorated. He spent nights scouting the streets of Harlem for a connection, and his legal practice collapsed. He borrowed money to support his habit and eventually dipped into an escrow account. He was suspended from the bar for three years—his lawyer successfully argued that he suffered from a cocaine-induced mental illness. S.W. completed treatment and now works at Daytop Village, a drug rehabilitation center.

SOURCE: *Margolick 1988.*

the possible behavioral effects of the different combinations Insofar as the additional substance is alcohol and thus relatively inexpensive, the drug-crime nexus is mitigated, at least for income-generating crimes: a great deal of violent noneconomic crime is known to be linked to alcohol intoxication.

Drug Lifestyles and Subcultures

Different drug lifestyles may be linked to the use of particular substances or may be part of a larger subculture. Using participant observation, Patricia Adler (1985) provides an insider's look at a marijuana- and cocaine-smuggling subculture centered in the middle- and upper-class environs of the coastal communities of southern California. She states: "This subculture provides guidelines for their dealing and smuggling, outlining members' rules, roles, and reputation. Their social life is deviant as well, as evidenced by their abundant drug consumption, extravagant spending, uninhibited sexual mores, and focus on

immediate gratification" (p. 1). More recently, a new drug subculture developed around the use of crack: "The subcultural patterns include an argot of terms that describe the activities having to do with crack, the various crack combinations touted and paraphernalia needed for using, and the institution of base houses [where the substance is smoked] and crack houses [where the substance is purchased]" (Frank et al., 1987, p. 6). Blanche Frank and her colleagues (1987) point out that the development of this subculture is helping to glamorize and thereby spread the use of crack.

The abuse of drugs by medical doctors dates back to the latter part of the nineteenth century (Mattison, 1883). In 1964, Charles Winick wrote of the physician addict, a loner who does not knowingly associate with other addicts. Drug abuse is a significant problem for the medical profession, with the addiction rate for physicians estimated at anywhere from 30 to 100 times that of the population at large (Grosswirth, 1982), although this group does not seem to be part of any drug subculture.

Cocaine abusers do not appear to be a part of any clearly discernible subculture. Surveys of cocaine users have revealed that there is apparently no "typical" cocaine user (PCOC, 1986).

> Heavy cocaine users fit no easy stereotype of drug abuse. A large proportion are successful, well-educated, upwardly mobile professionals in their early twenties and thirties. They are stockbrokers and lawyers and architects with sufficient disposable income to sink into a diversion that even at "social" use levels can cost $100 or more an evening. Many are, for the most part, otherwise law-abiding citizens who would cringe at being labeled criminals, even though they know what they are doing is illegal. A majority are men, but a growing number are women. And, as cocaine prices fall, more and more are teenagers and others for whom the drug's exorbitant cost once kept it out ot reach. (National Institute on Drug Abuse, 1986, p. 1)

Probably the most studied drug subculture is that centering on the use of heroin, because heroin addiction is closely associated with street crime. Harold Finestone (1964) drew a portrait of the black heroin subculture in Chicago at the beginning of the 1950s. He found the stereotypical addict eschewing violence, using a deliberately colorful vocabulary, and disdaining work. (This contrasted with a small number of white addicts interviewed by Finestone whose adjustment placed a heavy stress on violence.) These addicts, who Finestone calls "cats," had a lifestyle that centered on achieving "kicks": any act tabooed by conventional society that "heightens and intensifies the present moment of experience and differentiates it as much as possible from the humdrum routine of daily life" (p. 284). To the cat, heroin abuse provided the ultimate kick.

"The addict lifestyle," says Marsha Rosenbaum (1981. pp. 14-15), "rotates around taking heroin for the purposes of alleviating withdrawal symptoms and/or getting high." A habit requires intravenous use three, four, or five times daily. "The addict's day," Rosenbaum notes, "often begins with withdrawal sickness .... In order to alleviate these symptoms, the addict knows that s/he must use heroin. The symptoms become more intense with time .... Therefore, if possible, the addict is out the door with the goal of buying heroin in order to feel well" (pp. 14-15). If the addict is also a dealer, he or she is able to start the day with a fix. Few addicts, however, have the ability to plan even for the immediate future—they rarely keep enough heroin in reserve to begin the day with a "wake-up fix." Without funds or drugs, the addict must begin the day "hustling" for money to get the first fix.

After a "connection" is made and the heroin purchased, a safe place must be found where the addict, often in the company of other addicts, can dissolve the substance in water—usually in a bottle cap—by heating it with a cigarette lighter or a match. The addict ties off a vein of his or her arm with a piece of rubber or other material, and the water–heroin solution is taken up into a hypodermic syringe and injected into the exposed vein. The addict typically allows the solution to mix with blood by bringing blood back and forth into the syringe—known as "booting"—an act that many users describe as more pleasurable and intense than sexual orgasm. The short-term heightened feeling of euphoria that follows ingestion—the "rush"—is often described in sexual terms as "orgasmic." As the rush subsides, the addict begins to experience the "high," a feeling of general well-being that lasts about four hours before the cycle needs to be repeated. Addicts often share their "works"—syringe and bottle cap—which are sources of transmitted diseases, particularly hepatitis and acquired immunodeficiency syndrome (AIDS). "This is the 'addict's cycle'—an existence almost literally from fix to fix—with the necessary heroin-related activities in between'" (Rosenbaum, 1981, p. 15).

A heroin user's addiction can be conceived of in terms of a "career" with a number of stages:

1. **Experimentation.** The individual experiments with a variety of substances such as alcohol, marijuana, and perhaps barbiturates and amphetamines and may snort or use heroin subcutaneously.

2. **Initiation.** The drug abuser is initiated into intravenous use of heroin, the first time often accompanied by unpleasant side-effects such as vomiting. Nevertheless, he or she learns to enjoy subsequent injections, and heroin use begins to be a center of existence.

3. **Commitment.** The user is now an addict and takes on the social identity associated with the drug subculture, orienting his or her life toward the maintenance of a heroin habit.

4. **Disjunction.** The addicts life is now characterized by crime, arrest, and imprisonment, interspersed with drug treatment programs in response to court direction (to avoid imprisonment), to reduce an expensive habit to manageable size, or to deal with severe physical ailments.

5. **Maturation.** At some point, usually as the addicts age is closer to forty than to twenty he or she typically begins to use drugs only sporadically, gives up drug use completely as a result of treatment, simply experiences spontaneous remission, or dies. There are relatively few addicts above the age of forty in the heroin-using population.

The heroin user recognizes the danger of addiction, but "it is typical of the early experience of the addict-to-be that he knows or knows of people who use narcotics and who get away with it." Users see themselves as indestructible: "the tendency of the ego to treat the self as exempt from the experience of personal disaster" (Duster, 1970, p. 192).

The stages in becoming a cocaine abuser are similar to those of the heroin abuser (D. Smith, 1986):

1. **Experimental use.** The individual begins his or her use out of curiosity in a social situation in which some friends offer a "taste" of cocaine. Most of his or her friends are nonusers, and the subject uses cocaine only when it is offered to enhance feelings. Relationships remain normal, and no significant health or financial problems appear. There may even be an improvement in work performance and social functioning—the person may become more gregarious.

2. **Compulsive use.** The subject begins to buy cocaine and gains more friends who are users. Solitary use of cocaine follows, and there is an increase in use to enhance moods and performance and to ward off depression. Social disruptions appear, particularly mood swings, as well as health problems due to a lack of good nutrition and sleep. Work performance steadily deteriorates, and the abuser avoids non-dmg- using friends. He or she begins to encounter financial problems relating to the support of a growing cocaine habit.

3. **Dysfunctional use.** The abuser is preoccupied with drug use and associates only with other cocaine-using friends. He or she may begin to deal in cocaine and/ or engage in other illegal or financially

damaging activities to support the drug dependence. Severe disruption of social life follows, including marital violence and divorce. Serious medical pathology appears with a risk of seizure and toxic psychosis, paranoia, delusions, and hallucinations; and there are chronic sleep and nutritional problems. The abuser experiences a deterioration in physical appearance, usually accompanied by a lack of concern with personal hygiene and dress. Compulsion, a loss of control, and an inability to stop despite adverse consequences lead to seeking treatment, often because of pressure from family, friends, and employer, and because of serious legal entanglements.

Cocaine in the form of crack appears to present a different progression; the speed with which this substance acts can lead to chronic habituation or addiction very quickly. For reasons that have not yet been determined, crack is more popular than heroin among women, leading to a significant increase in child neglect and abuse, as well as to increasing numbers of newborn babies with cocaine in their urine (Kerr, 1988f).

These depictions are not the inevitable outcome of heroin and cocaine use. As we shall discuss later, there are an unknown number of persons who use these substances for many years without the debilitating results experienced by many, if not most, drug abusers.

A Brief Introduction to the Science of Pharmacology

By Harold Doweiko

It is virtually impossible to discuss the effects of the various drugs of abuse without touching on a number of basic pharmacological concepts. Although a complete; understanding of the science of pharmacology can take years to attain, in this chapter we will discuss the impact that the different drugs of abuse might have on the user's body, and the pharmacological principles by which these effects take place.

A Basic Misconception

It is surprising how often people discuss the drugs of abuse as if they were somehow a special class of chemicals that are unique. In reality most of the drugs of abuse were pharmaceutical agents in the past, and of those that were not actual pharmaceuticals, many were investigated as possible medications at one point in time. Thus, they work in the same manner that the other pharmaceuticals do: by changing the biological function of target eels through chemical actions (Katzung, 1995). As is true for most of the pharmaceuticals in use today, the drugs of abuse strengthen/: weaken a potential that exists within, the cells of the body In the case of the drugs of abuse, the target cells are usually in the central nervous system.

The Prime Effect and Side Effects of Chemicals

It is often surprising for students to learn that it is virtually impossible to develop a mind-altering drug without unwanted side effects. This is "because the brain is so highly integrated, it is not possible to circumscribe mental functions without impairing a variety of other functions, typically causing generalized dysfunction of the brain and mind" (Breggin, 2008, p. 2).

Thus in order to achieve the prime effect of a compound, the user must endure the side effects of that compound as well. Some of the side effects will be relatively minor, whereas others might be life threatening. This rule is true both for pharmaceutical agents prescribed by a physician for a patient, and for drug abusers.

For example, a person might ingest a dose of aspirin to help them cope with the pain of a minor injury. Aspirin does this by inhibiting the production of a family of chemicals known as the prostaglandins, a subtype of which is produced at the site of the injury. This is the primary effect of the aspirin dose. However, aspirin also blocks the production of another subtype of prostaglandin used to regulate kidney and stomach function, possibly placing the user's life at risk from the unwanted inhibition of prostaglandin production in these organs.

Another example of the difference between the primary and side effects of a medication is seen in the patient who has developed a bacterial infection in the middle ear (a condition known as otitis media) who is prescribed an antibiotic such as amoxicillin. The desired effect is the elimination of the offending bacteria in the middle ear, but an unwanted side effect might also be the death of bacteria in the gastrointestinal tract, where they perform a useful function in the process of digestion. The point to keep in mind is that there are the desired primary effects and unwanted side effects, or what are also known as secondary effects, of every compound. The side effects can range in intensity from making the patient mildly uncomfortable to being life threatening.

The Method by Which a Compound is Administered

One factor that influences the intensity of the drug's primary and side effects is the manner in which it is administered. The specific form in which a compound is administered will have a major impact on (a) the speed with which that compound begins to have an effect on the body, (b) the way that the compound is distributed throughout the body, (c) the intensity of its effects, and (d) the speed with which the individual will begin to experience any side effects from the compound. Kamienski and Keogy (2006) identified 13 different ways that a compound could be introduced into the body. Fortunately, most of the drugs of abuse are administered either by the enteral or the parenteral route.

Enteral Forms of Drug Administration

Compounds administered by the enteral route enter the body by the gastrointestinal (GI) tract (T. N. M. Brody, 1994). Such compounds are usually administered in oral, sublingual, or rectal forms (A.J. Jenkins, 2007; B.R. Williams & Baer, 1994). The most common method of enteral drug administration is through the use of a tablet, which is essentially a selected dose of a compound mixed with a binding agent that acts to give it shape and hold its form until it enters the GI tract. In most cases the tablet is designed to be ingested whole, although in some cases it might be broken up to allow the patient to ingest a small dose, if desired. A number of compounds are administered in enteral form, including many pharmaceuticals, over-the-counter medications, and some illicit drugs.

Once in the GI tract the compound begins to break down and separate from the binding agent and is absorbed into the body.

Another common method of administration of an oral medication is the capsule. This is a modified form of tablet, with the medication being suspended in a solution and surrounded by a gelatin capsule. The capsule is designed to be swallowed whole, and once it reaches the GI tract it breaks down and the medication (and the solution in which it is suspended) is released, allowing the absorption of the desired compound. Some compounds are simply administered as liquids, such as children's medication(s). This allows for the titration of the dose according to a child's weight. An excellent example of a drug of abuse that is administered in liquid form is alcohol.

A number of compounds might be absorbed through the blood-rich tissues found under the tongue. A chemical that is administered in this manner is said to be administered sublingually, which is a variation of the oral form of drug administration. Some of the compounds administered sublingually include nitroglycerin and fentanyl. The sublingual method of drug administration avoids the danger of the "first pass metabolism" effect (discussed later in this chapter) (A.J. Jenkins, 2007). But in spite of this advantage, the sublingual form of drug administration is only rarely used.

While many compounds are rapidly absorbed rectally, this method of drug administration is uncommon in medical practice, and virtually unheard of by drug abusers (A.J. Jenkins, 2007). Thus methods of rectal drug administration will not be discussed further in this text.

Parenteral Forms of Drug Administration

The parenteral method of drug administration essentially involves the injection of a compound directly into the body. There are several advantages to parental forms of drug administration, including the fact that the drug(s) are not exposed to gastric juices, delays caused by the stomach-emptying process, or the danger of being mixed with food in the GI tract rather than being absorbed by the body. But the parenteral method of drug administration also presents dangers to the user, which will be discussed later.

Depending on the substance being discussed, parenteral administration might be the preferred method of administration, especially when a rapid onset of effects is desired. The subcutaneous method of drug administration involves the injection of a given amount of a compound (and the agent in which it is suspended) just under the skin. While this avoids the dangers of exposing the drug(s) to the digestive juices of the GI tract, compounds administered subcutaneously are only slowly absorbed. This is often a method by which illicit narcotics are first injected and is referred to as "skin popping" by injection drug addicts. While the onset of the drug's effects is slower than other forms of parental drug administration, subcutaneous drug administration methods allow for a reservoir of the drug to be established just under the skin.

A second method of parenteral drug administration involves the injection of a compound(s) into muscle tissue (IM injection). Muscle tissues have a good supply of blood, and many compounds injected into muscle tissue will be absorbed into the general circulation more rapidly than compounds injected just under the skin. This method of drug administration is used both for the administration of some pharmaceuticals in medical practice and sometimes by illicit drug abusers. Anabolic steroid abusers will often inject the drug(s) being abused into muscle tissue, for example; however, there are many compounds, such as the benzodiazepine chlordiazepoxide, that are poorly absorbed by muscle tissue and are thus rarely, if ever, administered by this route (DeVane, 2004).

A third method of parenteral drug administration is the intravenous (or IV) injection. In this process the compound(s) of choice are injected directly into a vein, thus being deposited directly into the general circulation (DeVane, 2004). This is a common method by which legitimate pharmaceuticals, and many drugs of abuse, are administered. One serious disadvantage of the intravenous method of drug administration is that it does not allow the body very much time to adapt to the foreign chemical, and thus the individual is at risk for a serious adverse reaction to that compound within seconds of when it was administered.

Although a compound might be administered via a parenteral method, that drug(s) will not have an instantaneous effect. The speed at which any drug will begin to have an effect depends on a number of factors, which will be discussed in the section titled Distribution, later in this chapter.

Other Forms of Drug Administration

There are a number of additional forms of drug administration, which will be discussed only briefly in this text. The transdermal method of drug administration involves a compound being slowly absorbed through the skin. This has the advantage of allowing a low, but relatively steady blood level of the compound(s) in question being established in the user's body. But this method of drug administration does not allow one to rapidly establish any significant blood level of a compound in the user's body. This can be seen in the fact that transdermal nicotine patches might require up to 24 hours before a sufficient level of nicotine is established in the user's blood to block nicotine withdrawal symptoms.

Another method of drug administration, one that is used more frequently by drug abusers than in medical practice, is the intranasal method. In this method of drug administration, the compound is "snorted," depositing it on to the blood-rich tissues in the sinuses. Both cocaine and heroin powder are occasionally abused in this manner. This allows for a relatively rapid absorption of the drug(s) in question, but the rate of absorption is slower than the intravenous route of administration, and absorption is rather erratic.

The process of "snorting" is similar to the process of inhalation, which is used both in medical practice and with certain compounds by drug abusers. The process of inhalation takes advantage of the fact that the circulatory system is separated from direct exposure to the air only by a layer of tissue less than l/100,000ths of an inch (0.64 micron) thick (Garrett, 1994). Many drug molecules are small enough to pass across this barrier relatively easily, entering the individual's circulation quickly. An example of this would be surgical anesthetic gasses. When smoked, many of the drugs of abuse become able to cross over this barrier as well, gaining access to the circulation. Some of these compounds include heroin and cocaine. Finally, in the case of some compounds, the process of inhalation is able to introduce small particles into the deep tissues of the lungs, where they are deposited. In a brief period of time, these particles are then broken down into small units until they are small enough to pass though the tissue barrier of the lungs into the circulation. This is the process that takes place when tobacco cigarettes are smoked, for example.

Each subform of inhalation takes advantage of the fact that the lungs offer a blood-rich, extremely large surface area, allowing for the rapid absorption of many compounds (A. J. Jenkins, 2007). But the amount of a given compound that actually is absorbed into the general circulation is highly variable for two reasons:

1. The individual must inhale the compound(s) at exactly the right point in the respiratory cycle to allow the drug molecules to reach the desired point in the lungs.
2. Some chemicals are able to pass through the tissues of the lung into the circulation only very slowly.

Marijuana is a good example of this problem, as the compounds in marijuana smoke are able to cross into the general circulation only slowly. The individual must hold his breath for as long as possible to allow as large a percentage of the compounds inhaled to cross into the circulation as might be accomplished before the person must exhale.

Bioavailability

To have an effect, a compound must enter the body in sufficient strength to achieve the desired effect. This is referred to as the bioavailability of a compound. Essentially the bioavailability of a compound is the concentration of unchanged chemical at the site of action (Bennett & Brown, 2003). The bioavailability of a compound, in turn, is affected by the factors of absorption, distribution, biotransformation, and elimination (A.J. Jenkins, 2007; Bennett & Brown, 2003). Each of these processes will be discussed in more detail in the following sections.

Absorption

Except for topical agents such as an antifungal cream, which are deposited directly on the site of action, most compounds must be absorbed into the body in order to have any effect (A.J. Jenkins, 2007). This involves the drug molecules moving from the site of entry, through various cell boundaries, to the circulatory system, where it is transported to the site of action. Compounds that are weakly acidic are usually absorbed through the stomach lining, whereas compounds that are a weak base are absorbed in the small intestine (A J. Jenkins, 2007; DeVane, 2004).

The human body is composed of layers of specialized cells, organized into specific patterns in order to carry out designated functions. The cells of the circulatory system are organized to form tubes (blood vessels) that contain the cells and fluids found in blood. Each layer of tissue that a compound must pass through in order to reach the circulatory system will slow absorption that much more. For example, as noted earlier

the circulation is separated from the air in the lungs by a single layer of tissue (the cell wall of the individual alveoli). Compounds that are able to cross this one cell layer are able to reach the general circulation in just a matter of seconds. In contrast to this, a compound that is ingested orally must pass through the layers of cells lining the GI tract and the blood vessels the surround it, before it reaches the circulation. Thus the oral method of drug administration is recognized as being much slower than inhalation, for example.

There are a number of specialized cellular transport mechanisms that the body uses to move necessary substances into/away from the circulatory system that drug molecules can take advantage of in order to move from the site of administration to the site of action. Without going into too much detail, it is possible to classify these cellular transport mechanisms as being either active or passive means of transport (A.J. Jenkins, 2007). The most common method by which drug molecules move across cell membranes, diffusion, is also a passive method of molecular transport. Active methods involve the drug molecule taking advantage of one of several natural molecular transport mechanisms that move essential molecules into or out of cells. Collectively, these different molecular transport mechanisms provide a system of active transport across the cell boundaries and into the interior of the body.

The process of drug absorption is variable, depending on a number of factors, the most important of which is the method of administration, as discussed earlier in this chapter. Another major variable is the rate of blood flow at the site of entry. For example, an intramuscular injection into the deltoid muscle of a person suffering from hypothermia will result in poor absorption, because the blood has been routed to the interior of the body to conserve body heat. Under these conditions, the muscle tissue will receive relatively little blood flow, and this will reduce the speed at which

FIGURE 1. The Process of Drug Absorption

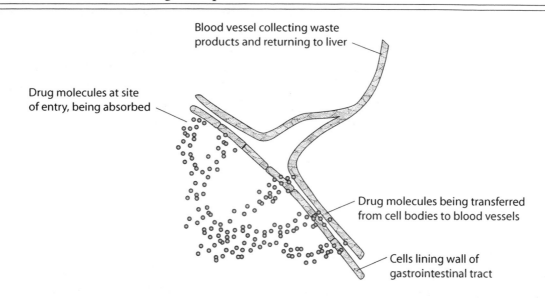

the drug molecules injected into muscle tissue(s) might be absorbed into the general circulation.

Yet another variable is the molecular characteristics of the compound itself. Some drug molecules are more easily absorbed than others. Also, if the compound is administered orally, a factor that affects absorption of that drug is whether or not it is ingested on an empty stomach (DeVane, 2004). Most compounds are better absorbed when ingested on an empty stomach, although some are better absorbed if ingested right after a meal (DeVane, 2004). Furthermore, one compound might best be absorbed if it does not have to compete with other drug molecules for admission into the body. All of these factors limit the absorption of the compound into the circulation. The next section addresses the second factor that influences the manner in which a given compound in the body, its distribution. The process of drug absorption is shown in Figure 1.

Distribution

The process of distribution refers to how the chemical molecules are transported within the body. This includes both the process of drug transport and the pattern of drug accumulation within the body. As a general rule, very little is known about drug distribution patterns in overdose situations (A. J. Jenkins, 2007). Although the process of distribution would seem relatively straightforward, in reality it is affected by factors such as the individual's age, sex, muscle/adipose tissue ratio, state of hydration, genetic heritage, and health. Because of such factors, there are significant interindividual differences in the distribution pattern of the same compound when the same dose is ingested (DeVane, 2004; A. J. Jenkins & Cone, 1998).

Transport

Once the drug molecules reach the general circulation, they can then be transported to the site of action. This would give the impression that the circulatory system exists just to provide a distribution system for drug molecules. In reality a drug molecule is a foreign substance that takes advantage of the body's own natural chemical distribution system to move from the site of entry to the site of action. There are several different methods by which this might be accomplished, depending on the chemical characteristics of the specific compound(s) in question.

Some chemicals are able to mix freely with the blood plasma, and as such are often referred to as water-soluble compounds. Such compounds, of which alcohol is a fine example, then are intermixed with the blood plasma and pumped through the body by the circulatory system. Because much of the human body is water, this provides a fine medium in which a compound might be suspended and pumped around the body. Again, depending on the chemical properties of the drug molecules, it might be possible for them to bind to one of the fat molecules that circulate through the body. Such compounds are called lipid-soluble compounds. The body uses lipids for a variety of purposes, including maintenance of cell walls, and any drug molecule that has attached itself to the lipid molecule will then be dragged along by that lipid as it circulates. Body tissues are constantly absorbing lipid molecules from the circulatory system as part of the cellular maintenance process. Compounds attached to the lipid molecules will then gain rapid access to body tissues because the human body organ ranges from 6 to 20% lipid molecules.

It is important to keep in mind some characteristics of molecular binding. First, as will be discussed in more detail later, drug molecular "binding" is usually not permanent. While the drug molecule is "bound" to the lipid molecule it is safe from elimination from the body, but it is also unable to achieve its desired effects. To become active again, it must detach from the lipid molecule. A compound that is 98% lipid soluble means that 98% of the drug molecules absorbed into the circulation are bound to blood lipids, leaving just 2% of the drug molecules to actually be biologically active. There are advantages and disadvantages to this characteristic of lipid binding. The process of lipid binding provides a drug reservoir within the body, as drug molecules detach from the lipid molecule over time. This allows new drug molecules to become active to replace those that have been biotransformed and eliminated from the body. But the lipid-bound drug molecules are unable to have an effect until they detach from the blood lipids.

In contrast to the rest of the body organs, which are 6-20% lipid molecules, 50% of the brain is actually lipid molecules (J.R. Cooper, Bloom, & Roth, 2002). So a compound that is lipid soluble will be concentrated in the brain tissues fairly rapidly. The ultra- short-acting and short- acting barbiturates are excellent examples of this process. Some forms of the parent barbiturate molecule are able to form bonds with blood lipids very rapidly, thus allowing them to have a rapid effect. This is what makes them so useful as a surgical anesthetic agent. In contrast to the lipid binding compounds, some drug molecules might bind to one of the protein molecules that circulates throughout the body in the circulation.[1] Different drug molecules differ in their ability to "bind" with protein or lipid molecules. The antidepressant amitriptyline is 95% protein bound, for example, whereas nicotine is only 5% protein bound (A.J. Jenkins, 2007). The antianxiety agent diazepam is 99% protein bound, and so its effects are actually caused by the 1% of the drug molecules that are unbound.

As with the process of lipid binding, some drug molecules form stronger bonds with the protein molecule than do others, and this is one factor that determines how long a given drug will remain in the body. Also, as is true for lipid-bound molecules, protein-bound drug molecules are unable to have any biological effect. So, it is the percentage of the drug molecules that are unattached from a blood protein/lipid that causes that compound's biological activity. The "bound" fraction provides a reservoir of drug molecules that will replace those molecules that are removed from the body by its natural defense mechanisms. It is important to keep in mind that drug molecules are foreign substances, and their presence in the body is tolerated by the body only until its natural elimination/defense mechanisms are able to latch onto and remove it. Thus there is a constant process of drug molecule replacement during the period of active dosing, as some molecules are eliminated from the body, and others break their bonds with the protein/lipid molecules and replace them.

Another point to keep in mind is that protein molecules can "bind" only to a limited number of drug molecules. Thus if an individual were to take an unusually large dose of a drug, or if the molecules of more than one compound were competing for the binding sites on the protein molecule, then those binding sites might become saturated, leaving a larger than normal percentage of the drug molecules free in the blood to have a biological effect. This is one of the mechanisms through which drugs might have a synergistic effect. This brings us to the process of Biotransformation.

Biotransformation

The biotransformation mechanisms in the human body evolved over millions of years to help the organism cope with potentially dangerous compounds found in food sources (Wynn, Oesterheld, Cozza, & Armstrong, 2009). These defensive detoxification systems are nonselective, eliminating poisons found in food with the same enthusiasm that they eliminate prescribed medications, because drug molecules are foreign to the body. In some cases, the body is able to simply filter the drug from the blood. Penicillin is an excellent example of such a compound. The penicillin molecules are filtered from the blood by the kidneys almost immediately without being altered. There are other compounds that are removed from the body unchanged. However, in the majority of cases the chemical structure of the drug(s) must be modified before they can be eliminated from the body.

This is accomplished through a process that was once referred to as detoxification or drug metabolism. However, because of the confusion over whether physicians were discussing the metabolic processes in the body or the process of breaking down a foreign chemical, the term biotransformation has gradually been gaining favor as the proper term when a pharmaceutical agent is being discussed, whereas the older term detoxification is applied to the drugs of abuse. Biotransformation is usually carried out in the liver, although on occasion other tissue(s) might also be involved. The microsomal endoplasmic reticulum of the liver produces a number of enzymes[2] that transform toxic molecules into a form that might be eliminated from the body. This is accomplished through one or more of the following mechanisms: oxidation, reduction, hydrolysis, and conjugation (Ciraulo, Shader, Greenblatt, & Creelman, 2006; Wynn et al. 2009). There are essentially two forms of biotransformation: (a) the zero-order biotransform at ion process and (b) the first-order Biotransformation process. In the zero-order biotransformation process, the biotransformation mechanism(s) quickly become saturated, and only a set amount of a compound can thus be biotransformed each hour (Bennett & Brown, 2003). Alcohol is an example of a compound that is biotransformed through a zero-order biotransformation process.[3] In the zero-order biotransformation process, the speed at which biotransformation progresses is relatively independent of the concentration of the drug molecules in the user's body.

In the first-order biotransformation process, a set percentage of the compound(s) in question is biotransformed each hour. Certain antibiotics are eliminated from the body in this manner, with a certain percentage being biotransformed each hour. The specifics of each subform of the process of biotransformation are quite complex and are best reserved for those readers who wish to pick up a pharmacology textbook to review the biochemistry involved in each phase of this process. It is enough for the reader to remember that there are four different subforms and two different pathways of biotransformation.

In both forms of biotransformation, the drug molecules are chemically altered only as rapidly as the enzymes involved in each step can do so. This takes place one atom at a time, at the rate at which the enzymes necessary for the biotransformation of that molecule can carry out their effect. In some cases, depending on the chemical characteristics of the drug(s) ingested, this process might involve several steps. For example, compounds that are highly lipid soluble require extensive biotransformation before they become less lipid soluble and are more easily eliminated from the body (A.J. Jenkins, 2007).

Technically, the compound that emerges at each step of the biotransformation process is referred to as a metabolite of the original compound. The original compound is referred to as the parent compound. Metabolites may have their own psychoactive effect on the user, a factor that must be considered by physicians when prescribing a pharmaceutical for a patent. If the parent compound had no or minimal biological effect, and its major impact is achieved by the metabolites of that compound, then the parent compound is referred to as a prodrug. Most compounds in use today are biologically active, and there are few that are used as prodrugs, but this is not always the case.

To add an element of confusion, normal variations in the individual's biological heritage, drug interactions, or various diseases can alter the speed at which some individuals can biotransform a compound. Sometimes the enzymes necessary for the biotransformation of one compound will increase the speed of the biotransformation of a second compound, reducing its effectiveness, for example. Furthermore, as a result of genetic variations some individuals are able to biotransform a given compound more rapidly than are others, making them rapid metabolizers of that compound. Also, by chance other people have a body that makes them slower at breaking down a given compound than is normal, making them a slow metabolizer of that compound. To date, there is no way to identify these individuals other than clinical experience obtained by giving the patient a drug and observing their reaction. Disease states, such as alcohol-induced liver damage, can also alter the liver's ability to biotransform many compounds, a situation that the attending physician must also consider when prescribing a pharmaceutical to treat an ill patient.

The First-Pass Metabolism Effect

The human digestive tract is designed not to let any chemical that is absorbed pass directly into the circulation, but to filter it first through the liver. This is called the first-pass metabolism effect (DeVane, 2004). By taking chemicals absorbed from the GI tract and passing them through the liver, any toxin in that food or drug might be identified and the biotransformation process started, hopefully before that compound can do any damage to the body itself. One consequence of the first-pass metabolism process is that the effectiveness of many orally administered compounds is limited. For example, much of an orally administered dose of morphine is biotransformed by the first-pass metabolism effect before it reaches the site of action, limiting its effectiveness as an analgesic unless injected into the body.

Collectively, the first-pass metabolism process, and the various subforms of biotransformation, work to prepare foreign chemicals for the last stage of pharmacokinetics, that of elimination.

Elimination

So closely intertwined are the processes of biotransformation and elimination that some pharmacologists consider them to be a single topic. The process of biotransformation changes the chemical structure of a compound so that the metabolites are more water soluble, so they can then be removed from the circulation by the organs involved in filtering the blood. This usually is carried out by the kidneys, although the lungs, sweat glands, and biliary tract might also be involved in the process of drug elimination (B. A. Wilson, Shannon, Shields, & Stang, 2007). For example, a small percentage of alcohol ingested will be eliminated through the sweat and breath when the person exhales, giving the intoxicated person a characteristic smell.

The process of drug elimination does not happen instantly. Rather, depending on the speed at which the process of biotransformation is carried out, it might take a period of time before the drug molecule(s) are transformed into a water-soluble metabolite that can be eliminated from the body. This brings us to another necessary concept to consider: the drug half-life.

The Drug Half-Life

The concept of a drug half-life provides a useful yardstick by which to make a rough estimate of a compound's effectiveness, duration of effect, and the length of time that it will remain in the body. But there are several different forms of drug half-life, depending on different aspects of the compound's actions in the body. We will discuss some of the more important of these half-life forms in this section.

The distribution half-life is the time that it takes a compound to work its way into the general circulation, once it is administered (Reiman, 1997). This information is important to physicians in overdose situations, where it is necessary to anticipate the long-term effects of compounds administered but that might not have reached the general circulation. It is also of importance in planning pharmacological interventions: If a patient is in acute pain, you would want to administer a compound that was able to reach the circulation as rapidly as possible, rather than a compound that is slowly absorbed. Patients in chronic pain might benefit more from a compound that is more slowly absorbed, providing more steady analgesia for their chronic discomfort.

Therapeutic half-life is a rough measure of the compound's duration of effect. The therapeutic half-life is the time necessary for the body to inactivate 50% of a compound. This may be complicated by compounds where the metabolites also have a biological action on the body. The therapeutic half-life usually is a reference to a single dose of a compound, and regular dosing of that compound can alter the therapeutic half-life by prolonging it.

Finally, there is the elimination half-life of a compound. This is the time that the body requires to eliminate 50% of a compound. Again, the elimination half-life is usually a reference to the time that it takes for 50% of a single dose of a compound to be eliminated from the body. In medical practice it is usually assumed that after the fifth dose, the individual will have achieved a steady state of a compound in her blood, although this is only a rough estimate and there are multiple factors that affect when a steady state is achieved. Furthermore, the concept of an elimination half-life is based on the assumption that the user has normal liver and kidney function. Patients with impaired liver or kidney function might require smaller than normal doses to achieve the same

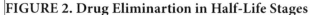

FIGURE 2. Drug Eliminartion in Half-Life Stages

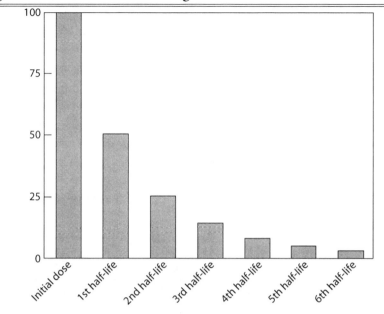

desired effect as a normal person, because the body will require more time to eliminate the compound.

The various half-lives of a compound are not the same. A compound might have a therapeutic half-life of minutes, for example, but an elimination half-life of hours. Several of the ultra-short-acting barbiturates[13] are excellent examples of how a compound might have a short duration of effect, but a prolonged elimination period. Furthermore, all half-life estimates are based on the assumption that the patient has used only one compound, If the patient is using multiple compounds, it becomes more difficult to estimate the drug half-lives, because multiple drugs would then compete for the processes of absorption, distribution, biotransformation, and elimination. For example, proteins found in the blood offer only a limited number of molecular binding locations, and if the patient is receiving multiple medications, the binding sites on the protein molecules might become saturated. This would force higher-than-normal levels of the drug to remain unbound and thus biologically active. This is one reason why

drug overdoses involving different agents might be lethal at doses that, independently, might not cause the user's death.

One popular misconception is that it takes only two elimination half-life periods to remove a compound from the body. In reality, fully 25% of the initial dose remains after the end of the second half-life period, and 12% is still in the body after three half-life periods. As a general rule, pharmacologists estimate that it will take five half-life periods before all of a single dose of a chemical is eliminated from the user's body, as illustrated in Figure 2.

Generally, compounds with longer half-life periods tend to remain biologically active for longer periods of time, whereas the reverse also is generally true. This is where the process of protein or lipid binding comes into play: Compounds with longer half-lives are more likely to become protein bound, with only a small percentage of the drug molecules actually being biologically active at any time. Those drug molecules that are still protein bound provide a reservoir of that drug, allowing new molecules to gradually be released back into the general circulation as the chemical bonds between the drug and the protein molecule become weaker and weaker until that molecule becomes "unbound" and it enters the circulation where it becomes biologically active.

Drug Interactions

In cases where a patient is receiving multiple medications, there is a very real danger of these compounds interacting in ways not anticipated by the user. Wynn et al. (2009) estimated that 5% of all hospitalizations in the United States were the result of adverse drug-drug interactions, and numerous less severe interactions result in consequences for the patient who does not require hospitalization. Serious drug-drug interactions result in an estimated 7000 deaths in this country alone. This is only an estimate, however, and many fatal drug-drug interactions probably are not reported, or the deaths are attributed to other conditions, according to the authors.

The Effective Dose

The concept of the effective dose (ED) is based on dose–response calculations in which scientists have calculated the approximate dose at which a given percentage of the population will respond to a given dose of a compound. For example, the dose at which 10% of the general population is expected to have the desired response would be identified as the ED_{10}, whereas the dose at which 50% of the general population is expected to have the desired response would be identified as the ED_{50}. Obviously, if you were a biochemist developing a new compound, you would want to find a dosage where as large a percentage of the general population as possible would achieve the desired response. However, as you increase the dose, you are more and more likely to (a) encounter the ceiling dose effect, and (b) develop toxic reactions.

The ceiling dose effect is just that: a dose above which additional drug molecules will not have any additional effect. Acetaminophen and ibuprofen, for example, are compounds with ceiling doses, and if the patient were to ingest a dose larger than this he would only be more likely to experience a toxic reaction.

The Lethal Dose and Therapeutic Index

This brings us to another useful concept: the lethal dose. Drugs are, by definition, foreign to the body, and although they might disrupt a body function(s) in a specific manner, they also present the risk of altering that body function so much that the user dies. For example, a hypothetical compound that suppressed respiration at a certain dose might be a useful pharmaceutical for certain forms of surgery. However, too large a dose would run the risk of the individual's respiration being suppressed permanently, hardly a desired response!

Drawing on the calculations as to how much radiation a person might be exposed to without becoming terminally ill, scientists have developed dose-response curves that estimate what percentage of the population would die as a result of being exposed to a certain dose of a chemical or toxin. This figure is then expressed in terms of the lethal dose (LD) ratio. A dose of a drug that would cause 1% of the population to die would be abbreviated as the LD01 and the dose that in theory would kill 25% of the population would be abbreviated as the LD25, etc. For example, as will be discussed in the next chapter, 1% of patients with a blood alcohol concentration of 0.350 mg/mL would be expected to die without medical help. Thus for alcohol, the LD01 would be 0.350 mg/mL of blood.

By comparing the effective dose and lethal dose ratios, it is possible to obtain a raw estimate of the therapeutic window or the therapeutic index of a compound. If you had a hypothetical chemotherapy compound used to treat cancer that had an ED_{99} of 100 mg and an LD_{001} (meaning only one death per thousand patients receiving this dose), that compound would be said to have a wide therapeutic window. In contrast, another hypothetical compound that caused 10% of the patients receiving it to die at a dose of 100 mg without medical intervention would be said to have a smaller therapeutic window. As should be obvious by now, you would want to use compounds with as large a therapeutic window as possible to reduce the risk to the user's life. Unfortunately, as will be discussed in the next few chapters, many of the drugs of abuse have very narrow "therapeutic" windows, with the result being that it is very easy to overdose on these compounds.

Therapeutic Threshold and Peak Effects

As the drug absorption process progresses following a single dose of a compound, the amount of a compound in the user's circulation will increase until it reaches the minimal level at which that compound might be effective. This is the therapeutic threshold for that compound. As the blood levels rise over time, the effects will continue to become stronger and stronger until the drug reaches its peak effect dose. Then, as the process of biotransformation proceeds, the effects of that compound will diminish until the blood levels of that compound fall below the therapeutic threshold. Scientists have learned to calculate dose-response curves for many compounds in order to estimate the potential for that compound to have an effect on the user after a single dose. For example, the period of peak effects varies from one compound to another. The peak effects of one of the ultra- short-acting barbiturates, for instance, might be achieved in a matter of seconds after the compound is injected into a vein, whereas a long-term barbiturate might take hours to achieve its peak effects. Further variables that affect absorption, distribution, biotransformation, and elimination will also impact on when a given compound reaches its peak effects.

The Site of Action

Essentially, the site of action is where the compound(s) introduced into the body carry out their main effects. For most of the psychoactive pharmaceuticals, and the various drugs of abuse, various neurons in the central nervous system (CNS)[4] will be the site of action. The CNS is, without question, the most complex organ system found in the human body. At its most fundamental level, the CNS is comprised of an estimated 100 billion neurons, each of which receives input from tens, hundreds, or perhaps thousands of other neurons. This is accomplished through the use of molecular neurotransmitters that are released by one neuron[5] with the goal of activating a receptor site on the next neuron in that neural chain.[6] It has been estimated that one mature human brain has more synaptic junctions than there are individual grains of sand on all of the beaches of the planet Earth (Stahl, 2008).

Although most of the CNS is squeezed into the confines of the skull, the individual neurons usually do not actually touch. Rather, they are separated by a microscopic space called the synapse. To communicate across the synaptic void, or synaptic gap, one neuron will release a cloud of chemical molecules that function as neurotransmitters. To date more than 150 compounds have been identified that function as a neurotransmitter within the brain, but the greater percentage of these neurotransmitters will remain outside of the scope of this text.[7]

The Process of Neurotransmission[8]

When a sufficient number of receptor sites in a given neuron are occupied by the right chemical messenger, a profound change is triggered in the postsynaptic neuron. There are two classes of neural responses to the reception of a neurotransmitter: the fast or inotropic responses. These usually involve the downstream neuron opening or closing a gated ion channel, which will alter the speed with which the downstream neuron can "fire." Another inotropic response might be for the downstream neuron to release a cloud of neurotransmitter molecules at select synaptic junctions in turn, passing the electrochemical message on to the next neuron in the chain. Longer-term responses, known as metabotropic responses, involve long-term alterations in the downstream neuron as it constantly adapts to the ever-changing input from upstream neurons. This includes the processes of: making or destroying synaptic junctions, reinforcing neural networks, urging axions to sprout, and the synthesis of various proteins, enzymes, and neurotransmitter receptors that regulate the function of the target neuron (Stahl, 2008).

To prevent premature or unnecessary neural activity, there is a "fail-safe" system built into the process of neurotransmission. A large percentage of the receptor sites must be occupied by neurotransmitter molecules at the same instant before the electrochemical potential of the downstream neuron is altered. For the sake of illustration, let us say that 70% of the receptor sites must be occupied by neurotransmitter molecules at the same instant before neurotransmission occurs.[9] If a lower number of receptor sites are occupied, say by stray neurotransmitter molecules that have

"leaked" into the synaptic junction from other sites, then the receptor site is not activated.

Cotransmission

When neurotransmitters were first discovered, scientists believed that each neuron utilized just one neurotransmitter type. But in the last years of the 20th century, scientists began to uncover evidence that neurons both transmit and receive secondary neurotransmitter molecules, which often have far different characteristics from those of the primary neurotransmitter. The process of releasing both types of neurotransmitter is called cotransmission, and this helps to explain why many drugs that affect the CNS have such wide-reaching, secondary or side effects. For example, some neurons that utilize serotonin as the primary neurotransmitter might also release small amounts of norepinephrine during the process of neurotransmission.

The Receptor Site

This is usually a large protein molecule(s) in the cell wall (Bennett & Brown, 2003; Olson, 2006). To understand how a receptor site works, imagine the analogy of slipping a key into a lock. The structure of the neurotransmitter molecule fits into the receptor site much as a key does into a lock, although on a molecular scale. But by co-incidence, some natural and artificial chemicals closely mimic the shape of the molecular "key," or neurotransmitter molecule, that activates the "lock" (receptor site). The closer that the drug molecule matches the natural neurotransmitter molecule, the stronger that compound's effects will be on the neuron.[10] The drugs of abuse fall into one of two groups: (a) those that cause the target neuron(s) to increase the rate at which they fire, or (b) those that cause the target neuron(s) to decrease the rate at which they fire. By achieving either effect, the drug(s) of abuse alter the normal function of the CNS.

Neurotransmitter Reuptake/Destruction

Once a neurotransmitter has been released, there is a danger that it will "leak" from the synaptic junction, float into other synaptic junctions, and activate other receptor sites than the one it was intended to reach. To prevent this, many neurons utilize what are known as molecular reuptake pumps that absorb as many of the just-released neurotransmitter molecules as possible for reuse. In the case of those neurons that utilize serotonin mentioned earlier, the norepinephrine molecules that are also released seem to activate the reuptake pumps on both the upstream and downstream neurons, allowing for those molecules to be recycled to the greatest degree possible. But many neurotransmitters are also broken down after release by one of a number of specific enzymes designed for this purpose. Thus if the neurotransmitter should escape the reuptake process, the enzymes will hopefully destroy them before they cause false signals in the neural net.

Up-Regulation/Down-Regulation

The individual neurons of the CNS are not passive participants in the process of information transfer, but are constantly rewiring themselves to allow for greater/reduced sensitivity to the neurotransmitters being thrown at them. If a receptor site is constantly exposed to high levels of a given neurotransmitter, it might decrease the number of receptor sites available to those molecules (down-regulate) (Bennett & Brown, 2003). This is accomplished by the neuron absorbing, or inactivating, some of the receptor sites, making that neuron less sensitive to that neurotransmitter. The analogy of somebody turning down the

sound on a car radio would not be entirely out of place here.

But if the neuron is not being stimulated enough by the neurotransmitter molecules at the synapse, then that neuron might build new receptor sites, to give the limited number of neurotransmitter molecules the largest possible number of "targets" to hit (bind at). This is the process known as up-regulation (Bennett & Brown, 2003). The analogy of somebody using a directional microphone as opposed to a regular microphone might be useful in explaining this concept.

Tolerance/Cross-Tolerance

Tolerance to a compound is defined as "a shortened duration and decreased intensity of drug effects after repeated administration" (Ghoneim, 2004b, p. 1279). Technically, this process is also known as neuroadaptation, especially when the compound has been prescribed by a physician, but many people still use the older term tolerance for both prescribed and illicit use of a compound.[11]

Because the molecules of the drugs of abuse alter the normal function of the brain, it attempts to chemically alter the influence of that compound at a neural level (Breggin, 2008; Cruz, Bajo, Schweitzer, & Roberto, 2008). One mechanism of neuroadaptation is the alteration of the number of receptor sites in the neural wall through either up-regulation or down-regulation of the number of receptor sites. This process helps to explain both the phenomena of tolerance/neuroadaptation to a compound, as well as that of "cross-tolerance" to related compounds. As the neurons adapt to the continued use of the compound(s) in question, the subjective experience will be one of a reduced reaction to the effects of a given dose of a compound. To overcome neuroadaptation (or tolerance), the user must often increase the dosage, possibly to dangerous levels.

However, multiple compounds might affect the body through similar mechanisms, and thus the adaptive changes made for one chemical might also help the brain adjust to the effects of other, similar chemicals. This is referred to as cross-tolerance. Alcohol provides a good example: The person who drinks frequently might find that benzodiaze pines do not provide the same degree of sedation as for the nondrinker, because they are cross-tolerant to the effects of the latter compounds.

Another process that is often seen with frequent, heavy use of a compound is the process of metabolic tolerance. Through this process, the body becomes more proficient in the process of biotransformation, at least for a limited period. This is commonly seen in the early stages of alcohol dependence, for example, where drinkers will report that they must use more alcohol to achieve the same level of intoxication once achieved with a lower level of alcohol intake (T. Nelson, 2000). Unfortunately, the liver can maintain this extra effort at alcohol biotransformation for only a limited period before it starts to break down, resulting in the phenomenon of lower tolerance to alcohol often found later in the drinker's life.

Behavioral tolerance reflects the behavioral outcome of the brain's efforts to maintain normal function in spite of the presence of foreign molecules. Individuals' behavior appears almost normal in spite of the presence of a compound in their body. Again, using alcohol as an example, even law enforcement or health care professionals are shocked to discover that the individual who appeared to be mildly intoxicated was in reality significantly over the legal blood alcohol level.

Drug Agonists/Antagonists

Essentially, a drug agonist is a compound that activates a receptor site by being able to mimic the actions of a natural neurotransmitter or enhancing its actions (B.A. Wilson et al. 2007). The more closely a chemical molecule resembles that of natural chemical the more normally will that receptor site be activated.[12] For the drugs of abuse, the receptor sites are the individual neurons of the brain, and the more closely the molecule resembles that of a naturally occurring neurotransmitter, the stronger the drug's effect will be on the neuron. The analogy of a "skeleton" key for a lock would not be out of place here: The narcotic analgesic family of compounds use binding sites normally utilized by the brain for pain perception. However, the narcotics are not perfect matches for the receptor site.

Some compounds are able to fit into the receptor site without activating it. Such compounds are called antagonists (or, antagonists). The drug Narcan (used to treat narcotic overdoses) functions as an opioid antagonist, blocking the opioid receptor sites without activating them and thus preventing the narcotic molecules from reaching the receptor sites in the brain. The analogy of a key that was broken off just beyond the handle might not be out of place here. There are also compounds that are partial agonists. This means that the drug molecules are able to activate the receptor site very weakly if at all, while preventing other drug molecules the opportunity to bind at that receptor site. Again, using the lock-and-key analogy, imagine the night watchman with a ring full of keys, who is forced to go through key after key to find the right one for a specific lock. Some of the keys might match some of the tumblers in the lock, but only one will match the specific combination necessary to open that lock.

Potency

Essentially, a neuropharmaceutical's potency is the ratio between the size of a dose and the behavioral response (Ghoneim, 2004b). Imagine that you had two hypothetical compounds with the same side-effect profiles, which impacted at the same receptor site and had the same mechanism of action to accomplish the same effect. One compound requires that you take an oral dose of 1000 mg to achieve a certain effect, whereas the second compound will achieve the same goal with an oral dose of just 100 mg. The latter compound would be said to be more potent than the former and is often the preferred compound. For example, as will be discussed in the chapter on narcotic analgesics, a standard conversion formula is that it takes 10 mg of morphine to achieve the same degree of analgesia that 4 mg of heroin can induce. Thus heroin is said to be more potent than morphine, although the pharmacology of both compounds will be discussed in Chapter 14.

The Blood-Brain Barrier

The human brain is an energy-intensive organ, and 20% of the blood pumped with each heartbeat is sent to the brain to supply it with needed nutrients and oxygen. But the capillaries involved in cerebral blood flow differ from those found elsewhere in the body in that the endothelial cells are tightly joined together around the capillaries. This forms part of the blood-brain barrier (or BBB), which is composed of the tightly knit endothelial cells and a thin layer of tissue contributed by the astrocytes of the brain, which separate the brain from direct contact with the circulatory system.

Although it is referred to as a "barrier," the BBB is better thought of as a selective screen. Specialized cellular transport mechanisms, each one adapted to allow one type of water-soluble molecule such as glucose, iron, and certain vitamins, to pass through the BBB into the neurons beyond. Lipids are also able to pass through the endothelial cells by first binding with, and slowly passing through the cell walls of the endothelial

cells to reach the brain. In the process, compounds that are lipid soluble are also admitted into the brain in spite of the BBB.

But all of this is a reflection of normal conditions. If the BBB were to be damaged as a result of trauma or infection, then it would lose its ability to filter out many unwanted compounds, and the individual might experience an atypical response to some compounds. The BBB is thus an important element of the individual's health.

Summary

Although the field of pharmacology, and the subspecialty of neuropharmacology, are each worthy of a lifetime of study by themselves, it is not possible to do justice to either topic in this text. However, some of the basic concepts necessary to better understand how the drugs of abuse might exert their effects, including how such compounds are administered, absorbed, distributed, and biotransformed/eliminated from the body, were discussed. Also discussed were concepts such as the drug agonist, the antagonist (or antagonist), and the mixed agonist/antagonist were introduced. A brief overview of the blood-brain barrier, and its function, was provided, and the concepts of tolerance and cross-tolerance to a compound(s) were reviewed. These basic concepts should provide a foundation on which the student might begin to build an understanding of the drugs of abuse, and the mechanism(s) by which they work.

Notes

1. The most common of which is albumin. Sometimes, compounds are referred to as albumin bound, rather than protein bound. Technically, drug molecules that are more acidic tend to bind to albumin, whereas those that are

more basic tend to bind to the alpha 1-acid glycoprotein molecules in the blood.

2. The most common of which is the P-450 metabolic process, or the microsomal P-450 pathway.

3. Although, technically, alcohol's biotransformation at extremely high doses does not follow the zero-order biotransformation cycle exactly. But alcohol's deviation(s) from the zero-order biotransformation cycle is best reserved for toxicology texts.

4. Although the CNS is by itself worthy of a lifetime of study, for the purposes of this text the beauty and complexities of the CNS must be compressed into a few short paragraphs. Those who wish to learn more about the CNS are advised to seek a good neuroanatomy, neuropsychology, or neurology textbook.

5. Called the "upstream" neuron.

6. Called the "downstream" or "postsynaptic" neuron.

7. I bet you thought that I was going to name them all, didn't you?

8. Admittedly, this is a very simplified summary of the neurotrans mission cascade, but it should be sufficient for the purposes of this text. There are a number of very good books on neuroanatomy that provide a detailed description of this process, if you should wish to pursue this area for further study.

9. The number of receptor sites that must be occupied before the neurotransmission cascade is initiated is called the affinity of the compound to the receptor sites.

10. Technically, this is called the sensitivity of the compound for the receptor site.

11. In this text the term tolerance will be used when illicit drugs are being discussed, and the term neuroadaptation will be used when discussing prescription substances.

12. Which is referred to as the ligand in professional literature.

Depressants

By Howard Abadinsky

This category of drugs—depressants—includes alcohol, barbiturates, sedatives/tranquilizers, and the narcotics. The latter may be natural (opium derivatives such as morphine and codeine), semisynthetic (such as heroin), or synthetic (such as methadone and Demerol).[1] Depressants are typically addicting, and studies have indicated the possibility of a relationship between certain chemical deficiencies and the propensity for addiction to depressants.

Endorphins

During the 1970s a number of scientists, working independently, discovered material and analgesics in brain and body tissues generally referred to as endorphins, a contraction of the term endogenous morphine. Three families of endorphins (enkephalins, dynorphins, and beta-endorphins) have many of the characteristics of morphine, and the body contains receptor sites that are programmed to receive these neurotransmitters. When they reach the receptor sites in the. central nervous, system (CNS), endorphins relieve pain. Pain is the result of a trauma experienced by the body, information about which is detected by sensors that send impulses along the nervous system, through neurons and across synapses as they move toward the brain. The subsequent release of endorphins in the brain inhibits pain impulses. Eventually, endorphins are destroyed by enzymes.

When people stub a toe or injure a finger, they usually grit their teeth and clench their fists, activities that apparently cause the release of these naturally occurring opiates that reduce sensations of pain. The athlete's ability to overcome pain during competition and the soldier's ability to perform heroic feats while severely wounded can be explained by the endorphin-receptor phenomenon, as can success in treating pain with

---

[1] In contrast to depressants, which act centrally on the brain, analgesics such as acetaminophen (e.g., Tylenol, Panadol, Anacin-3), ibuprofen (e.g., Nuprin, Mediprin, Advil), and aspirin relieve pain via localized action. They are not addictive (Brody 1988).

Howard Abadinsky, *Drug Use and Abuse: A Comprehensive Introduction*, pp. 93-95, 106-112. Copyright © 2008 by Cengage Learning, Inc. Reprinted with permission.

acupuncture (Snyder 1977,1989; Davis 1984; J. Goldberg 1988).[2] These receptor sites are programmed to receive endorphins, but they are also receptive to external chemicals such as opiates.

These opioid receptors are found in the brain's reward pathways and are distributed widely throughout the nervous system and in the nerves that supply the extremities, the skin, the blood vessels, and most internal organs. These receptors are found along pain pathways and, when activated, interrupt the pain pathway to the brain, diminishing the perception of pain (A. Goldstein 2001).

Endorphins also enable the organism (including many animals) to deal with psychological stress by curbing an autonomic overreaction and producing calm: They slow breathing, reduce blood pressure, and lower the level of motor activity (Davis 1984). A "deficiency in an endorphin system that ordinarily would support feelings of pleasure and reinforcement might lead to feelings of inadequacy and sadness" (Levinthal 1988: 149), a phenomenon that would make the use of depressants essentially a form of self-medication.[3] As was noted in Chapter 3, the use of psychoactive substances does not automatically produce a pleasurable response. However, people who are at risk for addiction may suffer from an endorphin deficiency. For such people, addiction would be the result of a genetically acquired deficiency or of a temporary or permanent impairment of the body's ability to produce endorphins. "This point of view would help account for the puzzling variability from individual to individual in the addictive power of opiate drugs. If an endorphin deficiency exists, however, the question would still remain as to what precipitating circumstances would lead to such a deficiency and whether these circumstances were environmental, inherited genetically, or a product of both" (Levinthal 1988: 154).

The ingestion of large amounts of heroin or some other opiate can also cause this deficiency (Snyder 1977). Thus, an abstaining addict would be unusually sensitive to feelings of pain or stress and would be inclined to use narcotic drugs again. In other words, receptors become increasingly dependent on external depressants, which in turn further reduce the production of endorphins, leaving the receptors increasingly dependent on substances from the outside. "If the opiate drug is later withdrawn, the receptors are now left without a supply from any source at all, and the symptoms of withdrawal are a consequence of this physiological dilemma" (Levinthal 1988: 156).

Stress And Addiction

Depressants such as heroin inhibit stress hormones (such as Cortisol and adrenalin) and stress-related neurotransmitters. A person who is having difficulties dealing with stress and is exposed to opiates is likely to find them rewarding and thus become addicted. In the absence of stress, many people who take heroin over long periods of time do so without becoming addicted, and hospital patients who self-administer morphine for pain do not increase their intake over time, nor do they suffer from a morphine craving when the pain subsides and they no longer have access to the drug (Peele 1985; E. Rosenthal 1993). One study found that only four out of more than 12,000 patients who were given opioids for acute pain became addicted to the drugs. Even long-term morphine use has limited potential for addiction. In a study of thirty-eight

---

[2] In one study, treating drug abusers with acupuncture was not found to be beneficial (Latessa and Moon 1992). Another study found it effective in detoxification treatment (Brewington, Smith, and Lipton 1994).

[3] Mark Gold (1994) disputes the self-medication thesis.

chronic pain patients, most of whom received opioids for four to seven years, only two patients actually became addicted, and both had a prior history of drug abuse (National Institute on Drug Abuse data).

Drug addicts who are trying to remain off drugs can often resist the cravings brought on by seeing reminders (cues) of their former drug life. For months they can walk past the street corner where they used to buy drugs and not succumb. But then there is a sudden relapse that addicts explain with statements such as "Well, things weren't going well at my job" or "I broke up with my girlfriend." Sometimes the problem is as simple as a delayed welfare check. That they often relapse, apparently in response to what most people would consider mild stressors, suggests that addicts are perhaps more sensitive than nonaddicts to stress. This hypersensitivity "may exist before drug abusers start taking drugs and may contribute to their initial drug use, or it could result from the effects of chronic drug use on the brain, or its existence could be due to a combination of both" (Jeanne Kreek quoted in Stocker 1999: 12). Chronic use of heroin, however, may increase hypersensitivity to stress and trigger a cycle of continued drug use when the effects of heroin wear off.

Research has shown that during withdrawal the level of stress hormones rises in the blood, and stress-related neurotransmitters are released in the brain. These chemicals trigger emotions that are perceived as highly unpleasant, driving the addict to take more drugs. Because the effects of heroin last only four to six hours, addicts often experience withdrawal three or four times a day. This constant switching on and off of the stress systems of the body heightens whatever hypersensitivity these systems might have had before the person started taking drugs. The result is that these stress chemicals are on a sort of hair-trigger release, surging at the slightest provocation (Kreek in Stocker 1999).

The body reacts to stress by secreting two types of chemical messengers: hormones in the blood and neurotransmitters in the brain. Some of the hormones travel throughout the body, altering the metabolism of food so that the brain and muscles have sufficient stores of metabolic fuel for activities, such as fighting or fleeing, that help the person to cope with the source of the stress. In the brain the neurotransmitters trigger emotions, such as aggression or anxiety, that prompt the person to take action.

Normally, stress hormones are released in small amounts throughout the day, but when the body is under stress, the level of these hormones increases dramatically. Endorphins inhibit these stress hormones, thereby inhibiting stressful emotions. Heroin and morphine inhibit the stress hormone cycle and presumably the release of stress-related neurotransmitters just as endorphins do; Thus, when people take heroin or morphine, the drugs add to the inhibition already being provided by the endorphins.

Barbiturates

There are about 2,500 derivatives of barbituric acid and dozens of brand names. Lawfully produced barbiturates are found in tablet or capsule form; illegal barbiturates may be found in liquid form for intravenous use because barbiturates are poorly soluble in water. Classified as sedative/hypnotics, they include amobarbital (e.g., Amytal), pentobarbital (e.g., Nembutal), pheno-barbital (e.g., Luminal), secobarbital (e.g., Seconal), and the combination amobarbital-secobarbital (e.g., Tuinal).

Effects of Barbiturates

"Barbiturates depress the sensory cortex, decrease motor activity, alter cerebellar function, and produce drowsiness, sedation, and hypnosis" (Physicians Desk Reference 1987: 1163). They inhibit seizure activity and can induce unconsciousness in the form of sleep or surgical anesthesia. Unlike opiates, barbiturates do not decrease reaction to pain and may actually increase it. They can produce a variety of alterations in the CNS, ranging from mild sedation to hypnosis and deep coma. In high enough dosage they can induce anesthesia, and an overdose can be fatal. Although they are CNS depressants, in some people they produce excitation (Physicians Desk Reference 1988). The user's expectations can have a marked influence on the drug's effect: "For instance, the person who takes 200 mg of secobarbital and expects to fall asleep will usually sleep, if provided with a suitable environment. Another individual, who takes the same amount of secobarbital and expects to have a good time in a stimulating environment, may experience a state of paradoxical stimulation or disinhibition euphoria" (Wesson and Smith 1977: 28).

Barbiturates are often used for their intoxicating effects. Some people take them in addition to alcohol or as a substitute. Heavy users of other drugs sometimes turn to them if their usual drugs are not available or to counteract the effects of large doses of stimulants such as amphetamines or cocaine. Barbiturates are known generally on the street as "downers" or "barbs." Many are named for the colors of their brand-name versions: blues or blue heavens (Amytal), yellow jackets (Nembutal), red birds or red devils (Seconal), and rainbows or reds and blues (Tuinal).

A small dose (e.g., 50 mg or less) may relieve anxiety arid tension. A somewhat larger dose (e.g., 100 to 200 mg) will, in a tranquil setting, usually induce sleep. An equivalent dose in a social setting, however, can produce effects similar to those of drunkenness—a "high" feeling, slurred speech, staggering, slowed reactions, loss of inhibition, and intense emotions often expressed in an extreme and unpredictable manner. High doses characteristically produce slow, shallow, and irregular breathing and can result in death from respiratory arrest. Barbiturate use during pregnancy has been associated with birth defects.

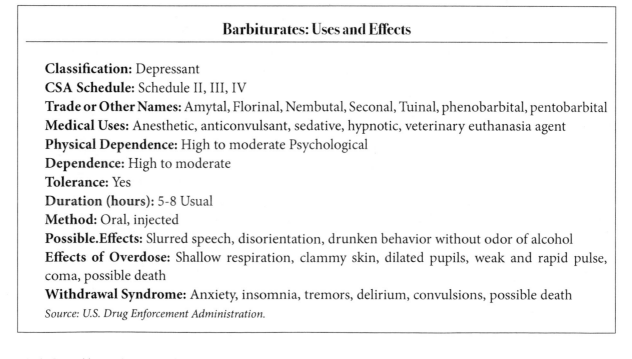

Barbiturates: Uses and Effects

Classification: Depressant
CSA Schedule: Schedule II, III, IV
Trade or Other Names: Amytal, Florinal, Nembutal, Seconal, Tuinal, phenobarbital, pentobarbital
Medical Uses: Anesthetic, anticonvulsant, sedative, hypnotic, veterinary euthanasia agent
Physical Dependence: High to moderate Psychological
Dependence: High to moderate
Tolerance: Yes
Duration (hours): 5-8 Usual
Method: Oral, injected
Possible.Effects: Slurred speech, disorientation, drunken behavior without odor of alcohol
Effects of Overdose: Shallow respiration, clammy skin, dilated pupils, weak and rapid pulse, coma, possible death
Withdrawal Syndrome: Anxiety, insomnia, tremors, delirium, convulsions, possible death
Source: U.S. Drug Enforcement Administration.

Barbiturates are classified according to the speed with which they are metabolized (broken down chemically) in the liver and eliminated by the kidneys: slow, intermediate, fast, and ultrafast. In low doses, barbiturates may actually increase the reaction to painful stimuli. The fast-acting barbiturates, particularly Nembutal (pentobarbital sodium)j Amytal (amobarbital sodium), Seconal (secobarbital sodium), and Tuinal (secobarbital sodium and amobarbital sodium combined), are most likely to be abused (O'Brien and Cohen 1984). Exactly how barbiturates cause their neurophysiological effects is not fully understood, but the substance impairs the postsynaptic action of excitatory neurotransmitters (McKim 1991). Barbiturates serve as a positive reinforcer for laboratory animals.

Tolerance for Barbiturates

As with opiates, tolerance develops to barbiturates; but in contrast to opiates there is a fatal dosage level, and the margin between an intoxicating dosage and a fatal dosage becomes smaller with continued use. "Tolerance to a fatal dosage, however, does not increase more than twofold. As this occurs, the margin between an intoxicating dosage and a fatal dosage becomes smaller" {Physicians Desk Reference 1988: 537). Drinking alcohol can further reduce that margin because alcohol "enhances the absorption and produces an additive CNS depression." When under the influence of small amounts of barbiturates or a combination of alcohol and barbiturates, a "person may 'forget' that he has already taken barbiturates and continue to ingest them until he reaches a lethal dose." Such overdoses often appear, incorrectly, to be suicidal (Wesson and Smith 1977: 24).

Barbiturate Withdrawal

Withdrawal symptoms range from the mild—muscle twitching, tremors, weakness, dizziness, visual distortion, nausea, vomiting, and insomnia—to the major—delirium, convulsions, and possibly death (Physicians Desk Reference 1987).

Medical Use of Barbiturates

Barbiturates are used primarily as sedatives for the treatment of insomnia and as anticonvulsants to help prevent or mitigate epileptic seizures. The ultrafast barbiturates—the best-known being sodium pentothal—are used to induce unconsciousness in a few minutes. At relatively high dosages, they are used as anesthetics for minor surgery and to induce anesthesia before the administration of slow-acting barbiturates.

Because of the risks associated with barbiturate abuse and because new and safer drugs such as the tranquilizers/benzodiazepines are now available, barbiturates are less frequently prescribed than in the past. Nonetheless, they are still available both by prescription and illegally.

Dangers of Barbiturate Use

The disinhibition euphoria that can follow intake is what makes barbiturates appealing as intoxicants (Wesson and Smith 1977). Intoxication results in slurred speech, unsteady gait, confusion, poor judgment, and a marked impairment of motor skills. Unlike opiates, barbiturates make it dangerous to operate a motor vehicle. With continuous intoxication at high doses the user typically neglects his or her appearance, bathing infrequently and becoming unkempt and dirty as well as irritable and aggressive (McKim 1991). Like opiates, barbiturates are addicting, with both psychological and physiological dependence. High doses characteristically produce slow, shallow, and irregular breathing and can result in death from respiratory arrest. "Following a large overdose of secobarbital or phenobarbital (short-acting barbiturates), an individual may be in coma for several days" (Wesson and Smith 1977: 20).

Taking barbiturates with other CNS depressants, for example, alcohol; tranquilizers such opioids as heroin, morphine, meperidine (Demerol), codeine, or methadone; or antihistamines (found in cold, cough, and allergy remedies), can be extremely dangerous, even lethal. Over the long term, high dosage produces chronic inebriation; the impairment of memory and judgment; hostility, depression, or mood swings; chronic fatigue; and stimulation of preexisting emotional disorders, which can result in paranoia or thoughts of suicide. The prescribing of barbiturates has declined notably since the safer benzodiazepine tranquilizers (discussed below) were introduced.

Benzodiazepines

Benzodiazepines (ben-zo-di-az-a-pins), which are minor tranquilizers or sedatives—referred to pharmacologically as sedative-hypnotics—art among the most widely prescribed of all drugs. One of earliest, Valium (diazepam), was approved by the Food and Drug Administration in 1963 to treat anxiety. Others now include Librium (chlordiazepoxide) and Equanil and Miltown (meprobamate). Prozac is a more recent and more widely prescribed selective serotonin reuptake inhibitor (SSRI), and the newer and longer-acting Klonopin is believed to have fewer withdrawal problems because it is metabolized more slowly and leaves the body gradually. The full extent of the nonmedical use of sedatives is not known, although it appears that their abuse often occurs in combination with other controlled substances. They produce effects that are subjectively similar to those of alcohol and barbiturates, but unlike these other depressants, benzodiazepines have few effects outside the CNS (McKim 1991). Major

or antipsychotic tranquilizers such as Thorazine (chlorpromazine) do not produce euphoria and therefore are rarely used nonmedically.

Effects of Tranquilizers

Minor tranquilizers or SSRIs are absorbed into the bloodstream and affect the CNS, slowing down physical, mental and emotional responses. The CNS contains benzodiazepine receptors that (through a complex process involving GABA receptors) inhibit the brain's limbic system, which regulates emotions (Smith and Wesson 1994). Although it has yet to be discovered, scientists believe that the body produces its own benzodiazepine-like substance that controls anxiety.

Medical Use of Benzodiazepines

Minor tranquilizers are usually prescribed for anxiety or sleep problems. They can be used to treat panic disorders and muscle spasms. Sometimes referred to as "sleeping pills," these CNS depressants have largely replaced barbiturates, which reportedly have a significantly greater potential for abuse and risk for fatal overdose. In laboratory animals benzodiazepines have proven to be less effective reinforcers than barbiturates (National Institute on Drug Abuse 1991). Benzodiazepines have an upper limit of effectiveness; after a certain point, increasing the dosage will not increase the effect, and overdoses are rarely fatal (McKim 1991): "Even when a benzodiazepine is taken in an overdose of 50-100 times the usual therapeutic dose, fatalities from repertory depression is rare" (Smith and Wesson 1994: 180).

Valium is often prescribed to relieve stress, because it produces a sense of calm and well-being. It is also addictive. Benzodiazepines are not effective for treating anxiety beyond four months, and Valium can generate intense and severe secondary anxiety. Therefore, if the underlying cause of the anxiety is not treated, benzodiazepines may worsen the condition and increase the risk of suicide (Miller and Gold 1990). Valium has a very long half-life (twenty-four to forty-eight hours), which means that even after it is discontinued, it stays in the system, metabolizing slowly (Bluhm 1987). A benzodiazepine known as Versed is ten times more potent than Valium and is used to induce "twilight sleep" for surgery patients who need to be relaxed but conscious.

Tolerance for Benzodiazepines

When benzodiazepines are used as sleeping pills, tolerance develops rapidly, and effectiveness may wear off after three nights. Because of tolerance, even if the dosage is increased, benzodiazepines are not effective for treating anxiety beyond four months.

Withdrawal front Benzodiazepines

Repeated use leads to dependence, and discontinuing tranquilizers can produce withdrawal symptoms, although it is unclear in what proportion of users. Symptoms include anxiety, insomnia, agitation, anorexia, tremor, muscle twitching, nausea/vomiting, hypersensitivity to sensory stimuli and other perceptual disturbances, and depersonalization. Discontinuing use after prolonged exposure to high doses can produce hallucinations, delirium, grand mal convulsions, and, on rare occasions, death (National Institute on Drug Abuse 1987; Smith and Wesson 1994). Valium withdrawal symptoms may first appear after seven to ten days and may be quite serious and even life-threatening (Bluhm 1987). Someone using minor tranquilizers under medical supervision for more than two or three weeks is usually withdrawn gradually over a period of months.

Dangers of Tranquilizer Use

Common short-term effects of tranquilizer use include drowsiness, dizziness, confusion, and mood swings. Common long-term effects include lethargy, irritability, nausea, loss of sexual interest, increased appetite, and weight gain. Regular use of minor tranquilizers can produce both psychological and physical dependence. Combining minor tranquilizers with alcohol, painkillers, or drugs containing antihistamines, such as cough, cold, and allergy medications, can result in unconsciousness and failure to breathe. A life-endangering CNS depression can result when benzodiazepines are used in conjunction with alcohol. In some people benzodiazepines can induce hostility and even aggression (McKim 1991). Valium overdose is the second leading cause of drug-related emergency room admissions in the United States. Some tranquilizers block receptors for the neurotransmitter dopamine, which can lead to symptoms of Parkinson's disease. In 2005 it was revealed that babies born to women who take SSRIs late in pregnancy often exhibit jitteriness, irritability, and serious respiratory problems. Although the symptoms were generally mild, some babies required hospitalization and intensive care (Associated Press 2005).

Methaqualone

Such drugs as glutethimide (Doriden), methyprylon (Noludar), ethchlorvynol (Placidyl), and methaqualone (found in Mandrax) were introduced as barbiturate substitutes in the belief that they would be safer. It was soon-found, however, that they shared problems similar to those of barbiturates, including abuse leading to overdose and interaction with other CNS depressants. The caution that is necessary in using barbiturates therefore applies to these other sedative/hypnotics as well.

Methaqualone was first synthesized in 1951 in India, where it was introduced as an antimalarial drug but proved to be ineffective. At the same time its sedating effects caused it to be introduced in Great Britain as a safe, non-barbiturate "sleeping pill." The substance subsequently found its way into street abuse, and similar patterns occurred in Germany and Japan. In 1965 methaqualone was introduced into the United States as the prescription drugs Sopors and Quaalude without any restrictions—it was not listed as a scheduled (controlled) drug. By the early 1970s "ludes" and "sopors" were part of the drug culture. Physicians were overprescribing the drugs for anxiety and insomnia, believing that they were safer than barbiturates. Street sales were primarily diversions from legitimate sources.

Eight years after methaqualone was first introduced into the United States, the drug's serious dangers had become evident, and in 1973 it was placed on the DEA's Schedule II list. Although the drug is chemically unrelated to barbiturates, methaqualone intoxication is similar to barbiturate intoxication. Addiction develops rapidly, and an overdose can be fatal. However, though similar to barbiturates in its effect, methaqualone produces an even greater loss of motor coordination, which is why it is sometimes referred to as a "wall-banger." Methaqualone is now illegally manufactured in Colombia and smuggled into the United States.

Downers

Alcohol

By Darryl S. Inaba William E. Cohen

Whether it is bojalwwa, a homebrewed beer-like drink from Botswana; mosto, a grape wine from Argentina; arrack, a traditional drink distilled from fermented molasses in India; or pontikka, distilled spirits from Finland, alcohol consumption is a worldwide phenomenon.

"Russia is a drinking culture. Refusing to drink is unacceptable unless you give a plausible excuse, such as explaining that health or religious reasons prevent you from imbibing."
—Sergei Ivanchuk on the
Russian business culture
Website: Executive Planet, 2006

"A pragmatic race, the Japanese appear to have decided long ago that the only reason for drinking alcohol is to become intoxicated and therefore drink only when they wish to be drunk."
—William Gibson,
Tokyo Pastoral, 1982

"To drink in the French style, moderately and with meals, being afraid for one's health, is to limit too much the favors of Bacchus, that god. In any case, getting drunk is almost the only pleasure revealed to us by the passing of the years."
—Anonymous, 1991

"Everyone thinks that Australians drink just beer and during the day that's pretty much true; when you go out in the afternoon, you have a beer. But at night, like nightclub hours, you drink hard alcohol, that's it."
—Australian bartender, 2002

Darryl S. Inaba & William E. Cohen. *Uppers, Downers, All Arounders: Physical and Mental Effects of Psychoactive Drugs*, pp. 209-243. Copyright © 2007 by CNS Productions, Inc. Reprinted with permission.

Worldwide:

- the majority of people in most countries, except Islamic countries, drink alcoholic beverages;
- China's alcohol consumption has doubled;
- India's alcohol consumption has increased 50%;
- 23% of English boys and 27% of English girls 15 to 16 years old were drunk three times or more in the past month; and
- Russian men consume the equivalent of six to seven bottles of vodka per capita per year.

Unfortunately:

- 75,000 alcoholics were homeless in Japan (there are about 100,000 homeless in Japan);
- more than 2 million people died due to alcohol; and
- approximately 10% of all diseases and injuries were a direct result of alcohol abuse.

In the United States:
- last month about 126 million Americans (52% of those 12 or older) had at least 1 beer, 1 glass of wine, or 1 cocktail; 16 million of this group are considered heavy drinkers (5 or more drinks in one sitting at least five times in the past month);
- more than two-thirds of the 11 million college students (at four-year colleges) had 1 drink, and more than two-thirds of those drinkers had 5 or more drinks on at least one occasion;
- about 6.2% of eighth-grade .students, 18.5% of tenth-grade students, and 30.0% of twelfth-grade students had been drunk;
- yesterday about $250 million was spent at bars, restaurants, and liquor stores for alcoholic drinks; and
- champagne toasts were made to 7,500 brides and grooms.

Unfortunately:

- 25% to 30% of hospital admissions were due to direct or indirect medical complications from alcohol;
- about half of the murder victims and half of the murderers were drinking alcohol at the time of the crime;
- more than half of the rapes that occurred involved alcohol;
- about half of American adults have a close family member who has or has had alcoholism;
- some 2.7 million crime victims reported that the offender had been drinking alcohol prior to committing the crime; and
- every year alcohol abuse and addiction cost businesses, the judicial system, medical facilities, and the United States more than $184 billion, or $638 for every man, woman, and child.

(Bellandi, 2003; Dawson & Grant, 1998; Harwood et al, 2000; Internal Revenue Service, 2006; Johnston, O'Malley, Bachman, et al., 2006A&B; National Institute on Alcohol Abuse and Alcoholism [NIAAA], 2000; Nelson, Naimi, Brewer, et al, 2005; Substance Abuse and Mental Health Services Administration [SAMHSA], 2005 & 2006; U.S. Department of Justice, 1998; World Health Organization [WHO], 2005)

History

A few years ago, archeologists uncovered evidence of the use of a fermented rice, honey, and fruit alcoholic beverage in Jiahu, China, dating back to 7000 B.C. (McGovern, Zhang, Tang, et al, 2004). Other excavators have also found a recipe for beer along with alcohol residues in clay pots in Mesopotamia and Iran dating from 5400 to 3500 B.C. Alcohol is the oldest known and at present the most widely used psychoactive drug in the world. It has presumably been present since airborne yeast spores started fermenting plants into alcohol about 1.5 billion years ago.

Our ancient ancestors' discovery of this first psychoactive drug probably occurred by accident when a bunch of grapes or a batch of plums was left standing in the sun, allowing the fruit sugar to ferment into alcohol. Perhaps some wild honey that had fermented was found, diluted with water, and sampled. This early alcoholic beverage would later be called mead. People were most likely drawn to the taste and the mood-altering effects. Curiosity was followed by experimentation as thirsty farmers discovered that the starch in potatoes, rice, corn, fruit, and grains could also be fermented into alcohol (beer or wine). Further experimentation found the value of alcohol as a medicine and as a solvent for other therapeutic substances.

The desire for ready access to the pleasurable effects as well as the health benefits of beer and wine led humans to search out and grow the raw ingredients for alcohol. Some historians believe that about 10,000 years ago the first civilized settlements were created to ensure a regular supply of grain for food and beer, grapes for wine, and poppies for opium (Keller, 1984).

The use of alcohol is documented in almost all civilized societies throughout history, in myths, religions, rituals, stories, songs, hieroglyphs, sacred writings, and commercial sales records written on clay tablets. The Babylonian Epic of Gilgamesh says that wine grapes were given to the earth as a memorial to fallen gods. The Bible contains more than 150 references to wine, some positive, some negative.

> "God give you of the dew of the sky, of the fatness of the earth, and plenty of grain and new wine."
> —Genesis 27:28

> "And don't get drunk with wine, which leads to reckless actions, but he filled with the Spirit: speaking to one another in psalms, hymns, and spiritual songs, singing and making music to the Lord in your heart."
> —Ephesians 5:18-19

The Legal Drug

Historically, the acceptability of alcohol has been intertwined with cultural, social, and financial imperatives. It has been used as a reward for pyramid workers, as a food (grain-rich beer) for peasants, as a solvent for opium in the eighteenth-century cure-all known as laudanum, as a sacrament for Jewish and Christian religious ceremonies, as a water substitute for contaminated wells, as a social lubricant for all classes, as a tranquilizer for the anxious, and as a source of taxes for the ruling class.

Because beer, wine, and liquor were so widely available and legal in most societies (except in Muslim-governed countries) and because they were promoted by custom and advertising, many people did not think of alcohol as a drug (though that attitude has almost disappeared over the past few decades). Whether it's been used for those desirable reasons or as the focus of prohibition forces, alcohol will continue to be the object of both desire and vilification, depending on moral attitude, social acceptability, and the politics of the prevailing government.

Almost every country has had periods in its history in which alcohol use was restricted or even banned completely. Those prohibitions were usually rescinded (Langton, 1995).

- The Chinese Canon of History, written about 650 B.C., recognized that complete

- prohibition was almost impossible because men loved their beer (Keller, 1984).
- Many Buddhist sects in India prohibited alcohol starting in 500 B.C. and continuing to this day.
- In sub-Saharan Africa, the idea of banning alcohol was usually avoided because home-brewed beers had great nutritional value.
- The Gin Epidemic in England in the 1700s emphasized that poverty, unrestricted use, and industrial despair coupled with the higher concentration of distilled alcohol soon led to abuse and, for many, addiction. The unrestricted sale of gin (20 million gallons per year in England) and the resulting problems of illness, public inebriation, absenteeism from work, and death led to increased taxes and severe restrictions on its manufacture just a few decades after its use was promoted by the government (O'Brien & Chafetz, 1991).
- In colonial America alcohol was a part of everyday life. The Pilgrims on the Mayflower regarded it as an "essential victual"; the founding fathers realized that the cultivation, manufacture, sale, and taxation of whiskey and rum could finance the American Revolution (and the slave trade).
- There were attempts at temperance and treatment by such groups as the Washington Temperance Society in the 1840s, the Oxford Group in the 1920s, and Alcoholics Anonymous in the 1930s, the latter of which believed in the concept of recovering from alcohol abuse and addiction through personal spiritual change (Alcoholics Anonymous, 1934, 1976; Miller et al, 1998; Nace, 2005).
- Official prohibition of alcohol by the U.S. government started in 1920, but widespread flouting of the law, criminalization of the manufacturing and distribution system, and pressure by those who wanted to drink, including the Wet Party, led to the repeal of Prohibition 13 years later.

One reason why many restrictions, and even Prohibition, have been overturned is the value of alcohol as a major source of excise taxes as well as a commodity. Currently, the federal government collects $13.50 per proof gallon that's shipped from distilleries while state governments collect up to $6.50 per gallon.

Because alcohol has played a central economic and social role since colonial times in America (and even farther back in other countries' cultures), contemporary society's view of the heavy drinker is more forgiving than its view of a cocaine, heroin, LSD, or even marijuana user.

Alcoholic Beverages

The Chemistry Of Alcohol

There are hundreds of different alcohols. Some are made naturally through fermentation while most that are used in dustrially are synthesized. Some of the more familiar alcohols include:

- ethyl alcohol (ethanol, grain alcohol), the main psychoactive component in all alcoholic beverages;
- methyl alcohol (methanol or wood alcohol), a toxic industrial solvent;
- isopropyl alcohol (propanol or rubbing alcohol), used in shaving lotion, shellac, antifreeze, antiseptics, and lacquer; and
- butyl alcohol (butanol), used in many industrial processes.

Ethyl alcohol is the least toxic of the alcohols. Few people drink pure ethyl alcohol because it is too strong and fiery tasting. By convention any beverage with an alcohol content greater than 2% is considered an alcoholic beverage.

Alcoholic beverages also include trace amounts of other alcohols, such as amyl, butyl, and propyl alcohol, that result from the production process and storage (e.g., in wooden barrels). Other components produced during fermentation, known as congeners, contribute to the distinctive tastes, aromas, and colors of the various alcoholic beverages. Congeners include acids, aldehydes, esters, ketones, phenols, and tannins. Beer and vodka have a relatively low concentration of congeners while aged whiskeys and brandy have a relatively high concentration. It is thought that congeners may contribute to the severity of hangovers and other toxic problems of drinking, though the main culprit is the ethyl alcohol.

When airborne yeast feeds on the sugars in honey or any watery mishmash of overripe fruit, berries, vegetables, or grain, the resulting fermentation process results in ethyl alcohol and carbon dioxide (Figure 5-1). Elephants, bears, deer, birds, and insects have been observed in a state of intoxication, exhibiting unsteady and erratic behavior after eating fermented plant matter.

Types Of Alcoholic Beverages

The principal categories of alcoholic beverages are beer, wine, and distilled spirits.

- Beer is produced when grain ferments.
- Wine is produced when fruit ferments.
- Distilled spirits with different concentrations of alcohol are made from fermented grains, tubers (e.g., potatoes), vegetables, and other plants. They can also be distilled from wine or other fermented beverages.

Some examples of fermented plant matter are Mexican pulque made from cactus, Russian kvass made from cereal or bread, Asian kumiss made from mare's milk, and even California garlic wine.

The actual consumption of beer vs. wine vs. distilled alcohol depends very much on the culture of a country. For example, Germans drink six times as much beer per capita as they do wine; the French drink eight times more wine per capita than do Americans.

Beer

Beer brewing and bread making were probably started about 8000 B.C. in neolithic times. The raw ingredients (usually grain) were produced in cultivated fields. Some of the first written records concerning beer were found in Mesopotamian ruins dating back to 5400 to 3500 B.C. It seems the Mesopotamians taught the Greeks how to brew beer, and the Europeans in turn learned it from the Greeks.

Beer is produced by first allowing cereal grains, usually barley, to sprout in water, where an enzyme called amylase is released. After the barley malt is crushed, the amylase helps convert the starches into sugar. This crushed malt is boiled into a liquid mash, which is then filtered, mixed with hops (an aromatic herb first used around A.D. 1000-1500) and yeast, and allowed to ferment. Beer includes ale, stout, porter, malt liquor, lager, and bock beer. The differences among beers have to do with the type of grain used, the fermentation time, and whether they are top-fermenting beers (those that .rise in the vat) or bottom-fermenting beers. Top-fermenting beers are more flavorful and include ales, stouts, porters, and wheat beers. Bottom-fermenting beers include the most popular pale lager beers (e.g., Budweiser® and Coors®). Traditional home-brewed beers are dark and full of sediment, minerals, vitamins (especially B vitamins), and amino acids and thus have appreciable food value, unlike modern commercial beers that are highly filtered.

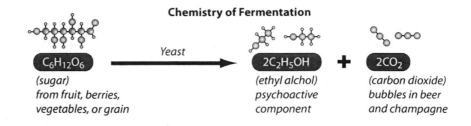

FIGURE 1. Yeast feeds on sugar and excretes alcohol and carbon dioxide.

The alcohol content of most lager beers is 4% to 5%; ales, 5% to 6%; ice beers, 5% to 7%; malt liquors, 6% to 9%; while light beers are only 3.4% to 4.2% alcohol.

Wine

In some early cultures, beer was the alcoholic beverage of the common people and wine was the drink of the priests and nobles possibly because vineyards were more difficult to establish and cultivate. In Egypt, however, pharaohs did have beer entombed with them in their pyramids to sustain them on their afterlife journeys and to offer a gift to the gods. Ancient Greek and Roman cultures seem to have preferred wine; the ruling classes kept the best vintages for themselves. These cultures also cultivated vineyards in many of their colonies. After the fall of the Roman Empire, many monasteries in Germany, France, Austria, and Italy carried on the cultivation of grapes and even hybridized new species.

Wines are usually made from grapes, though some are made from berries, other fruits (e.g., peaches and plums), and even starchy grains (e.g., Japanese sake rice wine). Generally, grapes with a high sugar content are preferred. A disease-resistant hybrid of Vitas vinifera grafted onto several American species was heavily planted worldwide particularly in the temperate climates of France, Italy, Spain, Argentina, California, and New York. Wine had a short shelf life until the 1860s, when Louis Pasteur showed that heating it would halt microbial activity and keep the wine from turning into vinegar (pasteurization).

Grapes are crushed to extract their juices. Either the grapes contain their own yeast, or yeast is added and fermentation begins. The kind of wine produced depends on the variety and the ripeness of the grapes, the quality of the soil, the climate, the weather, and the balance between acidity and sugar. White wines typically are aged from six to 12 months, red wines from two to four years.

European wines contain 8% to 12% alcohol, whereas U.S. wines have a 12% to 14% alcohol content. Wines with an alcohol content higher than 14% are called fortified wines because they have had pure alcohol or brandy added during or after fermentation; their final alcohol content is 17% to 21%. Wine coolers, which are usually diluted with juice, contain an average of 6% alcohol.

Distilled Spirits (liquor)

The alcoholic content of naturally fermented wine is limited to about 14% by volume. Recently, new fermentation techniques and more-resistant yeasts have allowed alcohol concentrations to reach 16% and even slightly higher. At higher levels the concentration of alcohol becomes too toxic and kills off the fermenting yeast, thus halting the conversion of sugar into alcohol. Outside of Asia, drinks with greater than 14% alcohol weren't available until about A.D. 800, when the Arabs discovered distillation. Distillation is the

TABLE 1. Consumption Of Beer & Wine In Europe & The United States

	Liters per Capita Beer	Wine
Germany	131	22
England	103	13
United States	95	20
France	40	60
Italy	103	59

Source: Eurocare, 2005

process of liquid separation by evaporation and condensation. A liquid can be separated from solid particles or from another liquid with a different boiling point. This eventually led to the production of distilled spirits such as brandies, whiskeys, vodka, and gin.

Brandy is distilled from wine, rum from sugar cane or molasses, whiskey and gin from grains, and vodka from potatoes. Distilled spirits can be produced from many other plants, including figs and dates in the Middle East and agave plants in Mexico (to make mescal and tequila).

One result of the invention of distilled beverages was that eventually it became much easier to get drunk. Initially, distilled alcohol was used more for medical reasons. Alcoholism eventually exploded in Europe and other countries due to the increased manufacture of distilled spirits and the desire for excise tax revenues. Similarly, alcoholism became a major social problem in colonial America with the manufacture of increasing amounts of corn whiskey and rum that was easier and more profitable to transport and market than bushels of corn. Grains and other sugar-producing commodities could be reduced in volume into more potent, portable, and higher-priced commodities. Rum was so popular that the second publicly funded building in New

Amsterdam (New York) was a rum distillery on Staten Island.

Absorption, Distributions & Metabolism

Absorption & Distributions

When beer, wine, or other alcoholic beverage is drunk, it is partially metabolized by digestive juices in the mouth and the stomach. Because alcohol is readily soluble in water and doesn't need to be digested, it immediately begins absorption and distribution. Absorption of alcohol into the bloodstream takes place at various sites along the gastrointestinal tract, including the stomach, the small intestines, and the colon. In men 10% to 20% of the alcohol is absorbed by the stomach; in women there is very little absorption there. Most of the alcohol enters the capillaries in the walls of the small intestines through passive diffusion (movement from an area of higher concentration of alcohol to an area of lower concentration without an energy expenditure).

Given the same body weight, women and men differ in their processing of alcohol. Women have higher blood alcohol concentrations than men do from the same amount of alcohol. A woman who weighs the same as a man and drinks the same number of drinks as a man absorbs about 30% more alcohol into the bloodstream and feels its psychoactive effects faster and more intensely (NIAAA, 1999).

This difference between women's and men's reactions to alcohol results from three possible explanations:

- Women have a lower percentage of body water than men of comparable size, so there is less water to dilute the alcohol.
- Women have less alcohol dehydrogenase enzyme in the stomach to break down al-

cohol, so less alcohol is metabolized before getting into the blood.

- Finally, changes in gonadal hormone levels during menstruation affect the rate of alcohol metabolism. Women absorb more alcohol during the premenstrual period than at other times (NIAAA, 1997; Register, Cline & Shively, 2002).

Thus chronic alcohol use causes greater physical damage to women than to men—female alcoholics have death rates 50% to 100% higher than male alcoholics (Blume & Zilberrnan, 2005; NIAAA, 2000).

The alcohol is absorbed into the bloodstream and partially metabolized by the liver (first-pass metabolism) and then quickly distributed throughout the body. Because alcohol molecules are small, water-and lipid-soluble, and move easily through capillary walls by passive diffusion, they can enter any organ or tissue. If the drinker is pregnant, the alcohol will cross the placental barrier into the fetal circulatory system. Once alcohol passes through the blood/brain barrier, psychoactive effects begin to occur.

The highest levels of blood alcohol concentration occur 30 to 90 minutes after drinking. How quickly the effects are felt is determined by the rate of absorption. Absorption is influenced by an individual's weight and body fat, body chemistry, and such factors as emotional state (e.g., fear, stress, fatigue, or anger), health status, and even environmental temperature.

Other factors that speed absorption in both men and women are:

- increasing the amount drunk or the drinking rate;
- drinking on an empty stomach;
- using high alcohol concentrations in drinks, up to a maximum of 95% with Everclear®;

- drinking carbonated drinks, such as champagne, sparkling wines, soft drinks, and tonic mixers; and
- warming the alcohol (e.g., hot toddies, hot sake).

Factors that slow absorption are:

- eating before or while drinking (especially eating meat, milk, cheese, and fatty foods)
- diluting drinks with ice, water, or juice.

Metabolism

Because the body treats alcohol as a toxin or poison, elimination begins as soon as it is ingested. Approximately 2% to 10% of the alcohol is eliminated directly without being metabolized (a small amount is exhaled while additional amounts are excreted through sweat, saliva, and urine). The remaining 90% to 98% of alcohol is neutralized through metabolism (mainly oxidation) by the liver and then by excretion through the kidneys and the lungs (Jones & Pounder, 1998).

Alcohol is metabolized in the liver, first by alcohol dehydrogenase (ADH) into acetaldehyde, which is very toxic to the body and especially the liver, and then by acetaldehyde dehydrogenase (ALDH) into acetic acid, which is finally oxidized into carbon dioxide (CO_2) and water (H_2O) (Figure 5-2).

The varying availability and the metabolic efficiency of ADH and ALDH, due in part to hereditary factors, account for some of the variation in people's reactions to alcohol (Bosron, Ehrig & Li, 1993; Lin & Anthenelli, 2005; Prescott, 2002).

For example, it is suspected that the high rate of alcoholism and the high rate of cirrhosis of the liver in American Indians are due to disruptions in the ALDH and ADH systems as well as a tradition of binge-drinking patterns (Foulks, 2005). Besides ALDH irregularities, drugs such as aspirin also inhibit metabolism of alcohol and lead to higher blood alcohol concentration in both men and women (Schuckit, Edenberg, Kalmijn, et al., 2001).

> "We get drunk and we have fun. We have a good time. That's what we're about. And I'm healthy. I'm in better shape than any of you guys, well maybe not on the inside. My stomach's kind of messed up a little bit. I can't drink liquor that good. I did take blood tests. I get my results on Friday ... I forgot."
>
> —25-year-old male alcohol abuser

Blood Alcohol Concentration (BAC)

Though absorption of alcohol is quite variable, metabolism occurs at a relatively defined continuous rate. About 1 oz. of pure alcohol (1.5 drinks) is eliminated from the body every three hours. Thus we can estimate the amount of alcohol that will be circulating through the body and the brain and how long it will take that amount to be metabolized and eliminated. Due to heredity, however, each person's biochemical makeup can have a strong effect on metabolism and elimination. The actual reaction and level of impairment can vary widely, depending on a person's drinking history, behavioral tolerance, mood, and a dozen other factors. Physical impairment is greater in a rising BAC. From the moment of ingestion, it takes 15 to 20 minutes for alcohol to reach the brain via the intestines and begin to cause impairment. It takes 30 to 90 minutes after ingestion to reach maximum blood alcohol concentration (NIAAA, 1997).

This BAC table (Table 5-3) measures the concentration of alcohol in an average drinker's blood. (Other versions of BAC tables give slightly lower levels than this one; the differences are minimal.) In all 50 states as of August 2005, legal

TABLE 2. Percentage Of Alcohol By Volume

WINE

Unfortified (red, white)	12-14%
Fortified (sherry, port)	17-21%
Champagne	12%
Vermouth	18%
Wine cooler	6%

BEER

Regular beer	4-5%
Light beer	3.4-4.2%
Malt liquor	6-9%
Ale	5-6%
Ice beer	5-6%
Low-alcohol beer	1.5%
Nonalcoholic beer	0.5%

MALT BEVERAGES

Hard lemonade, Bacardi Silver,® Smirnoff Ice®	5-6%

LIQUORS & WHISKEYS

Bourbon, whiskey, Scotch, vodka, gin, brandy, rum	40-50%
Overproof rum	75%
Tequila, cognac, Drambui®	40%
Amaretto,® Kahlua®	26%
Everclear®	95%

Note: To calculate the proof of a product, double the alcohol content (e.g., 40% alcohol = 80 proof; 100% alcohol = 200 proof).

intoxication is defined as 0.08 whether or not the driver can function. Some think it should be 0.05 for safety. For truck drivers the legal limit is 0.04; for pilots it is 0.02. The unit of measurement for BAC is weight by volume (e.g., milligrams per deciliter), but it can also be expressed as a percentage (e.g., 10% alcohol by volume). In Europe most countries set the limit at just 0.025. England allows .04, Norway just 0.10, and Australia 0.05.

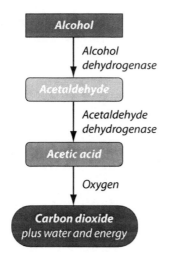

FIGURE 2. Metabolism is accomplished in several stages involving oxidation. First the enzyme alcohol dehydrogenase (ADH), found in the stomach and the liver, acts on the ethyl alcohol (C_2H_5OH) to form ac-etaldehyde (CH_3CHO), a highly toxic substance. Acetaldehyde is then quickly altered by a second enzyme, acetaldehyde dehydrogenase (ALDH), that oxidizes it into acetic acid (CH_3COOH). Acetic acid is then further oxidized to carbon dioxide ($CO2$) and water (H_2O).

For example, if a 200 lb. male has 5 drinks in 2 hours, his blood alcohol would be 0.108 minus the timetable factor of 0.030, so his BAC would be about 0.078 and he would be legally sober enough to drive. If his 200 lb. female companion has 5 drinks in 2 hours, her blood alcohol level would be 0.126 minus the timetable factor of 0.030, so her BAC would be 0.096; not only would she be quite a bit more intoxicated than her companion even though they weighed the same and drank the same amount over tiie same period of time but she would also be legally impaired in all states.

Desired Effects, Side Effects & Health Consequences

"Little by little alcohol became my friend. It would give me confidence and it would give me that buzz, and I would get that euphoric feeling that you feel when you've got alcohol."

—43-year-old man

"Escape, absolutely escape. It's all about running away, numbing your feelings because you can't, I can't, accept life on life's terms."

—35-year-old woman

Levels Of Use

The effects of any drug depend on the dosage. The same substance can be a poison, a powerful prescription medication, or an over-the-counter medicine, depending on the dose and the frequency of use. Alcohol is no exception and, as with other psychoactive drugs, there are escalating patterns of use.

Abstention (nonuse)

"My brother experimented with Puerto Rican rum on New Year's Eve when he was 15. He threw up on me on the way to the toilet. That took care of his drinking for five years and mine forever."

—54-year-old nondrinker

Experimentation (use for curiosity with no subsequent drug-seeking behavior)

"When you're a little boy, your dad says, 'Go get me a beer.' You pop it open for him, and he lets you take a sip every once in a while as long as Mom's not looking. It tasted good. When you're 10 or 12, you don't really know what alcohol is, you just experience it every once in awhile."

—33-year-old drinker

Social/Recreational Use (sporadic infrequent drug-seeking behavior with no established pattern)

"We know which dorm has the drinkers, so when we feel like a bit of a party and a few drinks, that's where we go. They're more serious about their drinking; they like forties [40 oz. malt liquor bottles or cans], but I can take it or leave it."

—20-year-old college sophomore

Habituation (established pattern of use with no major negative consequences)

"I think the pleasure left. This was the only way I knew how to have fun. This was the only way I knew how to feel better. But it didn't work, and it took me a while to realize that it had become a habit."

—36-year-old recovering alcoholic

Abuse (continued use despite negative consequences)

"I always got Bs, and then my grades dropped down to Ds, and then I started failing my classes, and I skipped school, and I got suspended all the time for that when I got caught. I'd skip school and I'd go get high, or we'd just skip it because we were always high."

—15-year-old high school dropout in treatment

Addiction (compulsion to use, inability to stop use, major life dysfunction with continued use)

"I would have the shakes, just really sick. I mean my body could not take alcohol at all. I would be sick in the morning like for days. It was hard to go to work and hard to take care of my children, hard to do my daily chores. It took me a long time to get well in the morning until I realized there was a magical cure. I could start drinking Bloody Marys."

—33-year-old recovering alcoholic

The effects of alcohol depend on the amount used, the frequency of use, and the duration of use:

- low-to-moderate-dose use (up to one drink a day for women and two drinks a day for men) can occur with experimentation, social/recreational use, and even habituation;
- high-dose use can occur at any level of drinking; and
- chronic high-dose use occurs with abuse and addiction (alcoholism).

TABLE 3. Approximate Blood Alcohol Concentration For Different Body Weights

No. of Drinks	1	2	3	4	5	6	7	8	9	10
Male										
100 lbs.	0.043	0.087	0.130	0.174	0.217	0.261	0.304	0.348	0.391	0.435
125 lbs.	0.034	0.069	0.103	0.139	0.173	0.209	0.242	0.287	0.312	0.346
150 lbs.	0.029	0.058	0.087	0.116	0.145	0.174	0.203	0.232	0.261	0.290
175 lbs.	0.025	0.050	0.075	0.100	0.125	0.150	0.175	0.200	0.225	0.250
200 lbs.	0.022	0.043	0.065	0.087	0.108	0.130	0.152	0.174	0.195	0.217
225 lbs.	0.019	0.039	0.058	0.078	0.097	0.117	0.136	0.156	0.175	0.195
250 lbs.	0.017	0.035	0.052	0.070	0.087	0.105	0.122	0.139	0.156	0.173
Female										
100 lbs.	0.050	0.101	0.152	0.203	0.253	0.304	0.355	0.406	0.456	0.507
125 lbs.	0.040	0.080	0.120	0.162	0.202	0.244	0.282	0.324	0.364	0.404
150 lbs.	0.034	0.068	0.101	0.135	0.169	0.203	0.237	0.271	0.304	0.338
175 lbs.	0.029	0.058	0.087	0.117	0.146	0.175	0.204	0.233	0.262	0.292
200 lbs.	0.026	0.050	0.076	0.101	0.126	0.152	0.177	0.203	0.227	0.253

If a person drinks over a period of time, the alcohol is metabolized at a rate of 0.015 per hour. Use the following table to factor in the time since the first drink.

TIMETABLE FACTORS

Hours since first drink	1	2	3	4	5
Subtract from BAC	0.015	0.030	0.045	0.060	0.075

Source: O'Brien & Chafetz, 1991

Low-To-Moderate-Dose Episodes

Most studies show that:

- small amounts of alcohol and even infrequent mild intoxication episodes generally do not have negative health consequences for men, even over extended periods of time;
- however, low-level alcohol use is generally not safe for people who are pregnant;
- have certain pre-existing physical or mental health problems that are aggravated by alcohol;
- are allergic to alcohol, ni-trosamines, or other congeners and additives;
- have a high genetic/environmental susceptibility to addiction;
- have a history of abuse and addiction problems with alcohol or other drugs; and
- are at risk for breast cancer.

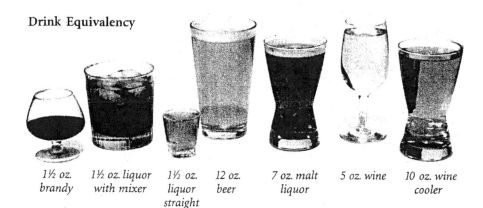

Drink Equivalency

1½ oz. brandy | 1½ oz. liquor with mixer | 1½ oz. liquor straight | 12 oz. beer | 7 oz. malt liquor | 5 oz. wine | 10 oz. wine cooler

FIGURE 3. One drink is defined as 1.5 oz. brandy; 1.5) oz. liquor (with or without mixer), 12 oz. lager beer, 7 oz. malt liquor, 5 oz. wine, or 10 oz. wine cooler. There is slightly more than 0.5 oz. of pure alcohol in the average alcoholic beverage. © 1995 CNS Productions, Inc.

Each person has a different definition of moderate drinking. We define it as drinking that doesn't cause problems for the drinker or for those around him or her. Drinkers begin to have pathological consequences from alcohol, however, when they have more than two drinks per day in men and one drink per day in women. Severe effects, especially long-term health and social consequences, usually result from high-dose use episodes and frequent high-dose (chronic) use.

Low-to-Moderate-Dose Use: Physical Effects

Therapeutic Uses. Alcohol is used as a solvent for other medications because it is water-and lipid-soluble. It is used as a topical disinfectant, as a body rub to reduce fever because it evaporates so quickly, and as a pain reliever for certain nerve-related pain; it is occasionally used to prevent premature labor (Woodward, 2003). Systemi-cally, ethanol is used to treat methanol and ethylene glycol poisoning.

Desired Effects. Some people who drink alcoholic beverages think that they taste good, quench the thirst, and relax muscle tension. Consumed in low doses before meals, alcoholic beverages activate gastric juices, improve stomach motility, and stimulate the appetite. They produce a feeling of warmth because vessels dilate and increase blood flow to subcutaneous tissues (Woodward, 2003). Red wines made from muscadine grapes and others high in antioxidants have an anti-inflammatory effect on the circulatory system (Greenspan, Bauer, Pollock, et al., 2005). In general, light-to-moderate use of alcohol (1 to 2 drinks per day for men and 1 or less for women [Puddey & Beilin, 2006]) has been shown to reduce the incidence of heart disease and plaque formation whether the cause is:

- the anti-inflammatory effect;
- an increase in high-density lipoproteins, particularly HDL_3;
- a different interaction with lipoproteins; or
- simply the decrease in tension that a drink can induce.

The doses must be low enough to not cause liver damage, induce other adverse health effects, or trigger heavier drinking (Mukamal, Conigrave, Mittle-man, et al., 2003; NIAAA, 2000). This is especially true in women who are more susceptible to the adverse effects of alcohol than men. Of course any beneficial effects may also be obtained through exercise, low-fat diet, stress-reduction techniques, and an aspirin a day. (Upon autopsy many end-stage alcoholics have clean blood vessels, but they also have cirrhotic livers, flabby hearts, and damaged brains.)

One or two drinks decrease the chance of gallstones in men and women. In postmenopausal women alcohol seems to slow bone loss because of its effect on estrogen. Women who drink in moderation seem to have a higher bone mass than women who don't drink (Turner & Sibonga, 2001).

Researchers at Columbia University found in a study of 677 stroke victims that those who have one or two drinks per day have a lower risk of stroke because alcohol keeps blood platelets from clumping (Sacco, Elkind, Boden-Albala, et al., 1999). But, again, because heavy drinking actually increases the risk of stroke, and even moderate drinking has unwanted side effects, and because no benefit is shown in recommending moderate drinking to abstainers, using alcohol as a stroke-preventive measure should be done only in consultation with a physician.

Sleep. Alcohol is often used by people to get to sleep, particularly if anxiety is causing insomnia. In fact, alcohol does decrease the time it takes to fall asleep, but it also seems to disturb the second half of the sleep period especially if consumed within an hour of bedtime (Landolt et al, 1996; Vitiello, 1997). It interferes with rapid eye movement (REM) and dreaming—both essential to feeling fully rested. Disturbances in sleep patterns can also decrease daytime alertness and impair performance (Roehrs & Roth, 2001). Chronic drinking also puts one at a higher risk for experiencing obstructive sleep apnea, a disorder whereby the upper breathing passage (pharynx) narrows or closes during sleep, causing the person to wake up, often a number of times during a sleep period, thus leading to severe fatigue as well as neurological and cardiac problems. Alcoholics not only have an increased risk of sleep apnea but they seem to aggravate their disease .by drinking (Brower, 2001; Dawson, Bigby, Poceta, et al, 1993; Miller et al, 1988).

Low-to-Moderate-Dose Use: Psychological Effects

The mental and emotional effects depend more on the environment (setting) in which the drug is used, along with the mood and the general psychological makeup of the user (set) .

In general, alcohol affects people psychologically by lowering inhibitions, increasing self-confidence, and promoting sociability. It calms, relaxes, sedates, and reduces tension.

> "I started out drinking when I was about 15 out of peer pressure, but it made me forget about everything. It felt like a whole new way of life. I was happy, I was gregarious, I was outgoing—more extroverted I guess. I love dancing, and I thought I was Ginger Rogers in that I thought I could do anything."
>
> —42-year-old recovering alcoholic

Unfortunately, for someone who is lonely, depressed, angry, or suicidal, the depressant and disinhibiting effects of alcohol can deepen negative emotions, including verbal or physical aggressiveness and even violence. Low-to-moderate doses in both men and women can also result in vehicular crashes and legal conflicts. Disinhibition can also promote high-risk sexual activity leading to unwanted pregnancies and sexually transmitted diseases (STDs).

"When I used, my behavior was really dangerous, I'd do things that normal people wouldn't do. I was very promiscuous; I had a lot of unsafe sex. I contracted hepatitis C. I don't know if I'm HIV. I get tested periodically but I'm, like, very high risk. I've also had numerous STDs."

—37-year-old female recovering alcoholic

Neurotransmitters Affected by Alcohol

The psychological effects of alcohol are caused by its alteration of neurochemistry in the higher centers of the cortex that control reasoning and judgment and the lower centers of the limbic system that rule mood and emotion. Most psychoactive drugs affect just a few types of receptors or neurotransmitters (e.g., anandamide for marijuana; norepinephrine, epinephrine, and dopamine for cocaine). Alcohol, on the other hand, interacts with receptors, neurotransmitters, cell membranes, intracellular signaling enzymes, and even genes.

- Alcohol initially elevates mood by causing the release of serotonin (a key mood neurotransmitter), then depletes it with excess use; serotonin scarcity causes depression.
- Dopamine release at multiple levels of alcohol use gives a surge of pleasure in the mesolimbic dopaminergic reward pathway as does norepinephrine release. Dopamine Dl, D2, and most recently D3 receptors are involved (Heidbreder, Andreoli, Marcon, et al., 2004).
- Met-enkephalin release by drinking reduces pain.
- Glutamate release causes a certain pleasurable stimulation thus reinforcing the drinking.

- The alcohol-induced release of endorphins and anandamides also enhances the reinforcing effect (Colombo, Serra, Vacca, et al., 2005).
- In addition, alcohol reduces excitatory neurotransmission at the NMDA receptors (a subtype of glutumate receptors), inhibiting their reactions and affecting memory and movement (Stahl, 2000).
- Most important, alcohol causes GABA (the major inhibitory neurotransmitter in the brain) to enhance neurotransmission at the GABA-A receptor thus lowering psychological inhibitions and eventually slowing down all of the brain processes (Boehm, Valenzuela & Harris, 2005; Koob, 2004).

"I always had to use alcohol to be able to socialize, if I go to the party and I'm not drinking, I wouldn't be able to function. I felt like I couldn 't dance right or everybody was looking at me, just really uncomfortable. One or two drinks, that'd loosen me up and then I'd keep going 'til I got to a level that I wanted to be at. Where I thought that I was acceptable."

—43-year-old recovering alcoholic

Low-to-Moderate-Dose Use: Sexual Effects

Alcohol's physical effects on sexual functioning are closely related to blood alcohol levels. In low doses alcohol usually increases desire in males and females, often heightening the intensity of orgasm in females while slightly decreasing erectile ability and delaying ejaculation in males (Blume & Zilberman, 2005).

"It's no mystery why guys in college fraternities, many of whom don't have all that much money, still come up with plenty of money to have outrageous amounts of alcohol and let any woman in for free. The whole point is they're setting up an environment whereby people are going to get more drunk. Women's inhibitions and a guy's inhibitions are going to get lowered."

—23-year-old college peer counselor

More than any other psychoactive drug, alcohol has insinuated itself into the lore, culture, and mythology of sexual and romantic behavior: a singles' bar to look for a date, a glass of wine before sex, or champagne to celebrate an anniversary. Almost half of a group of 90,000 college students at a number of two-and four-year institutions believed that alcohol facilitates sexual opportunities (Presley, 1997). Whether it does so because of actual psychological and physiological changes or because of heightened expectations is still open to question.

The acceptability of using alcohol in sexual situations extends to high school students. A survey done for the U.S. Surgeon General found that 18% of high school females and 39% of high school males say it is acceptable for a boy to force sex if the girl is stoned or drunk (U.S. Surgeon General, 1992).

High-Dose Episodes

High-Dose Use: Physical Effects of Intoxication

For many the purpose of drinking is to get intoxicated, often with a disregard for physical consequences. In fact, intoxication is a combination of psychological mood, expectation, mental/physical tolerance, and past drinking experience as well as the physiological changes caused by elevated blood alcohol levels. Up to a certain point, some of the effects of intoxication can be partially masked by experienced drinkers (behavioral tolerance).

In surveys and research, binge drinking is defined as consuming five or more drinks at one sitting for males and four or more for females. About 44% of college students say they are binge drinkers, and 21% (of the total) say they binge frequently (Wechsler, Lee, Kuo, et al, 2002). Adults between 21 and 25 went on drinking binges an average of 18 times in the past year, while those between 18 and 20 did it 15 times (Bellandi, 2003). Underage binge drinking has increased almost 50% since 1993. Many who are defined as "bingers" say that five drinks won't get them drunk but will raise their BAC over 0.08 and make them liable for a DUI (driving under the influence) arrest.

Heavy drinking is defined as five or more drinks in one sitting at least five times a month. Any person who binge drinks (whether sporadically or frequently) is more likely to have hangovers, experience injuries, aggravate medical conditions, damage property, and have trouble with authorities.

After enough drinks are consumed, the depressant effects of the alcohol take over. Expectation, setting, and the mood of the drinker cease to have a strong influence. Blood pressure is lowered, motor reflexes are slowed, digestion and absorption of nutrients become poor, body heat is lost as blood vessels dilate, and sexual performance is diminished. In fact, every system in the body is strongly affected. Slurred speech, staggering, loss of balance, and lowered alertness are all physical signs of an increased state of intoxication (Figure 5-4).

High-Dose Use: Mental & Emotional Effects

"When a man drinks wine he begins to be better pleased with himself and the more he drinks the more he is filled full of brave hopes, and conceit of his power, and at last the string of his tongue is loosened, and fancying himself wise, he is brimming over with lawlessness, and has no more fear or respect, and is ready to do or say anything."

—Athenian Stranger in *The Laws by Plato* 360 B.C.

High-dose alcohol use depresses other functions of the central and peripheral nervous systems. Initial relaxation and lowered inhibitions at low doses often become mental confusion, mood swings, loss of judgment, and emotional turbulence at higher doses. At a BAC above 0.12, a drinker may demonstrate slurred speech and, beyond that level, progressive mental confusion and loss of emotional control. Heavy alcohol consumption before sleep, as with light-to-moderate consumption, may also interfere with the REM, or dreaming sleep, essential to feeling fully rested. Chronic alcoholics may suffer from fatigue during the day and insomnia at night as well as nightmares, bed wetting, and snoring.

High-Dose Use: Alcohol Poisoning (overdose)

If truly large amounts of alcohol are drunk too quickly, severe alcohol poisoning occurs, with depression of the central nervous system (CNS) possibly leading to respiratory and cardiac failure, then to unconsciousness (passing out), coma, and death. Some clinicians use a BAC level of 0.40 as the threshold for alcohol poisoning, although lower levels can be deadly to novice drinkers. When other depressants, including sedative-hypnotics or opiates, are used, the danger is greatly increased because metabolism of .alcohol takes precedence over metabolism of other substances thus delaying neutralization and elimination of those other drugs.

Blood alcohol concentration levels of 0.20 or greater, especially in individ-" uals who have low tolerance, can result in severely depressed respiration and vomiting while semiconscious. The vomit can be aspirated or swallowed, blocking air passages to the lungs, resulting in asphyxiation and death. This can also cause infections in the lungs.

"A freshman died from alcohol poisoning during a pledge incident, and we have had two other students die in the past going through their rite of passage of 21 drinks on their twenty-first birthday. I think there's a myth with this age group that alcohol is so accepted that it is not harmful and that you may get a hangover but you'll wake up in the morning, but that's not always the case."

—Shauna Quinn, drug and alcohol counselor, California State University, Chico

High-Dose Use: Blackouts

About one-third of all drinkers report experiencing at least one blackout; the percentage more than doubles for alcohol-dependent individuals (Schuckit, 2000). During blackouts a person seems to be acting normally and is awake and conscious but afterward cannot recall anything that was said or done. Sometimes even a small amount of alcohol may trigger a blackout, which is caused by an alcohol-induced electrochemical disruption of the brain. Blackouts are often early indications of alcoholism. They are different from passing out or losing consciousness during a drinking episode. A drinker can also have only partial recall of events, which is known as a brownout

A possible indicator of susceptibility to blackouts and brownouts and therefore a marker for alcoholism can be seen on an electroencephalogram (EEG). The marker is a dampening of the P3 or P300 brain wave that affects cognition, decision-making, and processing of short-term memory. This dampening is found in alcoholics and their young sons but generally not in individuals without a drinking problem (Begleiter, 1980; Blum, Braverman, Holder, et al, 2000). Other researchers found that auditory-cued P300 amplitude waves are also reduced in alcoholics, particularly in those with anxiety disorders (Enoch, White, Harris, et al, 2001).

"With alcohol I was out of control because I would drink to the point where I didn't know what I was doing, which made it easier for the man to do whatever he wanted and my not realizing it until the next day or the next morning when I woke up and didn't have any recollection of what had happened."

—32-year-old female recovering binge drinker

High-Dose Use: Hangovers

The causes of hangovers are not clearly understood. Additives (congeners) in alcoholic beverages are thought to be partly responsible although even pure alcohol can cause a hangover. Irritation of the stomach lining by alcohol may contribute to intestinal symptoms. Low blood sugar, dehydration, and tissue degradation may also play their parts. Symptoms vary according to individuals, but it is evident that the greater the

Level of Impairment vs. Blood Alcohol Concentration

.00 Blood Alcohol Concentration
Lowered inhibitions, relaxation
Some loss of muscular coordinatiion
Decreased alertness
Reduced social inhibitions
Impaired ability to drive
Further loss of coordination
Slowed reaction time
Clumsiness, exaggerated emotioins
Unsteadiness standing or walking
Hostile behavior
Exaggerated emotions
Slurred speech
Severe intoxication
Inability to walk without help
Confused speech
Incapacitation, loss of feeling
Difficulty in rousing
Life-threatening unconsciousness
Coma
Death from lung and heart failure

.50 Blood Alcohol Concentration

FIGURE 4. As consumption increases, the amount of alcohol absorbed increases and therefore the effects increase but at different rates depending on the physical and mental makeup of the drinker.

quantity of alcohol consumed, the more severe the aftereffects (Swift & Davidson, 1998).

The effects of a hangover can be most severe many hours after alcohol has been completely eliminated from the system. Typical effects include nausea, occasional vomiting, headache, thirst, dizziness, mood disturbances, abbreviated sleep, sensitivity to light and noise, dry mouth, inability to concentrate, and a general depressed feeling (Finnegan, Schulze, Smallwood, et al., 2005). Hangovers can occur with any stage of drinking, from experimentation to addiction.

More-severe withdrawal symptoms usually occur with chronic high-dose users.

Some research shows that those with a high genetic susceptibility to alcoholism suffer more-severe hangover and withdrawal symptoms and often continue drinking to find relief (NIAAA, 1998; Piasecki, Sher, Slutske, et al, 2005; Span & Earleywine, 1999).

High-Dose Use: Sobering Up

A person can control the amount of alcohol in the blood by controlling the amount drunk and the rate at which it is drunk. But the elimination of alcohol from the system is a constant. The body metabolizes alcohol at the rate of 0.25 oz. to 0.33 oz. of pure alcohol per hour. Until the alcohol has been eliminated and until hormones, enzymes, body fluids, and bodily systems come into equilibrium, hangover symptoms will persist. An analgesic may lessen the headache pain, and fruit juice can help hydrate the body and correct low blood sugar, but neither coffee, nor exercise, nor a cold shower cures a hangover. Feeling better comes only with rest and sufficient recovery time. One danger of using too much acetaminophen (e.g., Tylenol®) to relieve a hangover-induced headache while alcohol is still in the system is the chance of liver damage.

Chronic High-Dose Use

The effects of long-term alcohol abuse not only on physical health but also on neurochemistry and cellular function are more wide-ranging and profound than for most other psychoactive drugs.

"In the past year due to my alcoholism and drug addiction, I have had two overdoses. I have been in 2 North—that is the mental ward of the hospital.

I have set myself on fire, passed out with a cigarette in my hand, and have fallen down all over the place, receiving various broken bones. The last time my husband saw me, I was near death."

—43-year-old recovering alcoholic

Digestive System & Liver Disease

The main impact of alcohol on the digestive system is caused by its direct effects on organs and tissues. Because roughly 80% of the alcohol drunk passes through the liver and must' be metabolized, high-dose and chronic drinking inevitably compromise this crucial organ. When the liver becomes damaged due to fatty liver, hepatitis, or cirrhosis, its ability to metabolize alcohol decreases, allowing the alcohol to travel to other organs in its original toxic form. Even persistent moderate drinking can damage the liver. For example, fatty liver—the accumulation of fatty acids in the liver—can occur after just a few days of heavy drinking. Abstention will eliminate much of the accumulated fat. About 20% of alcoholics and heavy drinkers develop fatty liver (Mann, Smart, Govoni, et al, 2003).

Unfortunately, as the heavy drinking continues, the problems become more severe. In the United States, approximately 10% to 35% of heavy drinkers develop alcoholic hepatitis and 10% to 15% develop cirrhosis (Mann, Smart & Govoni, 2003).

"Until I am clean and sober long enough for them to do more testing on me and to do another liver panel, I do not know how much damage has been done."

—34-year-old female practicing alcoholic

Alcoholic hepatitis causes inflammation of the liver, areas of fibrosis (formation of scarlike tissue), necrosis (cell death), and damaged membranes. Although alcoholic hepatitis often follows a prolonged bout of heavy drinking, it usually takes months or years of heavy drinking to develop this condition, which is manifested by jaundice, liver enlargement, tenderness, and pain. It is a serious condition that can be arrested only by abstinence from alcohol, and even then the scarring of the liver and the collateral damage remains (Saitz & O'Malley, 1997). (It is important to remember that alcoholic hepatitis is not directly related to hepatitis A, B, or C.) Continued heavy drinking by those with alcoholic hepatitis will lead to cirrhosis in 50% to 80% of the cases (Kinney, 2005).

Cirrhosis occurs when alcohol kills too many liver cells and causes scarring. It is the most advanced form of liver disease caused by drinking and is the leading cause of death among alcoholics. Approximately 12,000 Americans die each year from cirrhosis due to alcohol Consumption (Centers for Disease Control & Prevention [CDC], 2006). The damaging effects of alcohol to tissues occur not only because alcohol itself is toxic but also because the metabolic process produces metabolites, such as free radicals and acetaldehyde, that are even more toxic than the alcohol itself (Haber, 2003; Kurose, Higuchi, Kato, et al, 1996). Cirrhosis is even less amenable to treatment and cannot be reversed, although abstinence, diet, and medications can often arrest the progression of the disease.

"I was sick to my stomach and I threw up and little did I know because it was dark that it was blood and I turned on the light and I had a little garbage can there by the bed and the damn thing filled up. There was an artery in my liver that had just exploded I guess, and they said when that happens it's a gusher. And so after they put me out, they said, 'You've got cirrhosis very bad.' Well they put me on the transplant list. I didn't know it at the time but you have to be sober for a year before they'll even consider transplanting your liver."

—65-year-old recovering alcoholic

Over the years liver cirrhosis rates have gone up and down with the rise and fall of alcohol consumption. With the dramatic increase in hepatitis C, however, many more nonalcohol-related cases of cirrhosis will be altering the statistics.

It is estimated that alcoholic cirrhosis is a major contributing factor in about 80% of all cases of cirrhosis in the United States (Nidus Information Services, 2002). The prevalence of cirrhosis in the United States also varies by age, gender, and ethnic group. For example, in one study by the National Institute on Alcohol Abuse and Alcoholism (NIAAA), Hispanic men showed the highest cirrhosis mortality rates followed by Black men, White men, Hispanic women, Black women, and White women. A majority of the Hispanic men were of Mexican ancestry (Singh & Hoyert, 2000). About 2.5 times more men than women of all races die from cirrhosis (mostly because more men drink than women).

The drinking habits of various cultures worldwide have a strong effect on the incidence of cirrhosis. Heavy-drinking countries such as France and Germany have rates of cirrhosis two to three times higher than the United States (Table 5-5).

A problem with estimates about drinking rates is that in many coun-. tries, particularly poorer ones, large amounts of alcohol production and consumption go unreported. The World Health Organization (WHO) reports that in a country such as Kenya about 80% of alcohol consumption is not officially reported. In the Russian Federation, one-half to four-fifths of the consumption goes unreported, while in Slovenia 50% is unreported (WHO, 2005). In comparing the increase in drinking, the WHO report found that the largest increases in consumption were among developing countries and those in transition, such as former Soviet bloc countries.

Other Digestive Organs

While lower doses of alcohol can aid digestion, moderate-to-higher doses stimulate the production of stomach acid and delay the emptying time of the stomach. Excessive amounts of alcohol can cause acid stomach and diarrhea.

> "So I was, oh, six hours into my drinking; I was in the bathroom by the toilet all night long. I couldn't leave. Every minute I was throwing up; and when I couldn't throw up, I was dry heaving. And at the end when I wasn't throwing up anymore, I wanted to drink again."
>
> —43-year-old female recovering alcoholic

Gastritis (stomach inflammation) is common among heavy drinkers as are inflammation and irritation of the esophagus, small intestine, and pancreas (pancreatitis). Inflammation of the pancreas is often caused by blockage of pancreatic ducts and overproduction of digestive enzymes. Other serious disorders, including ulcers, stomach hemorrhage, gastrointestinal bleeding, and the risk of cancer, are also linked to heavy drinking.

Pure alcohol contains calories (about 150 per drink) but almost no vitamins, minerals, or proteins. Heavy drinkers receive half their energy but little nutritional value from their drinking. As a result, alcoholics may suffer from primary malnutrition, including vitamin Bj deficiency leading to beriberi, heart disease, peripheral

TABLE 4. Rates Of Cirrhosis Of The Liver In The United States

Year	Rate of Cirrhosis per 100,000
1911	17.0
1932	8 .0 (end of Prohibition)
1973	14.9
2004	9.0 (26,549 deaths)

Source: Grant, 1985; National Center for Health Statistics, 2005; Saadatmand, Stinson, Grant, et al, 2000

nerve degeneration, pellagra, scurvy, and anemia (caused by iron deficiency). In addition, because heavy drinking irritates and inflames the stomach and the intestines, alcoholics may suffer from secondary malnutrition (especially from distilled alcohol drinks) as a result of faulty digestion and absorption of nutrients even if they eat a well-balanced diet.

Another problem with alcohol is its effect on the body's sugar supply. Alcohol can cause hypoglycemia (too little sugar [glucose]) in drinkers who are not getting sufficient nutrition and have depleted their own stores of glucose. The liver is kept busy metabolizing the alcohol, so it cannot use other nutrients to manufacture more glucose. Blood sugar levels can drop precipitously, causing symptoms of weakness, tremor, sweating, nervousness, and hunger. If the levels drop too low, coma is possible, particularly for those with liver damage or for diabetics who are insulin dependent. If there is sufficient nutrition, alcohol use can cause the opposite effect—hyperglycemia (too much sugar)—in susceptible individuals. This condition is of particular danger to diabetics who have problems controlling their blood sugar in the first place (Kinney, 2005).

TABLE 5. Worldwide Per-Capita Use Of Alcohol Vs, Incidence Of Chronic Liver Disease

	Alcohol in Liters of Pure Ethanol				Cirrhosis Rate per 100,000		
	Total	Beer	Spirits	Wine	Overall Rate	Men	Women
Germany	13.77	8.01	2.50	3.26	15.4	22.6	9.0
France	14.37	2.45	3.01	8.91	12.1	17.8	7.2
Greece	12.54	2.43	4.23	5.88	3.4	5.4	1.6
Spain	11.06	3.86	2.86	4.34	12.2	19.1	6.2
Italy	10.21	1.41	1.06	7.74	13.9	19.6	9.0
Australia	10.57	6.07	1.72	2.78	4.6	7.0	2.4
United Kingdom	10.00	6.34	1.72	1.94	6.4	8.3	4.7
United States	8.91	5.36	2.43	1.12	7.7	10.9	4.8
Japan	5.97	3.21	2.62	0.14	7.2	11.2	3.5
Kazakhstan	7.72	0.47	7.09	0.16	23.9	33.2	16.8
Israel	1.75	0.81	0.42	0.52	4.9	7.3	2.9

Source: WHO, 2005

Cardiovascular Disease

Though many headlines tout the positive cardiovascular effect of light-to-moderate drinking, chronic heavy drinking is related to a variety of heart diseases, including hypertension (high blood pressure) and cardiac arrhythmias (abnormal irregular heart rhythms). Heavy drinking increases the risk of hypertension by a factor of 2 or 3 (He, 2001). Coronary diseases occur in alcohol-dependent people at a rate up to six times normal (Schuckit, 2000). One form of irregular heart rhythm is called holiday heart syndrome because it appears in patients from Sundays through Tuesdays or around holidays after a large amount of alcohol has been consumed.

Because acetaldehyde, a metabolite of alcohol, damages striated heart muscles directly, cardiomyopathy—an enlarged, flabby, and inefficient heart—is found in some chronic heavy drinkers. The heart of a heavy drinker can be twice the size of a normal heart. This condition is also known as alcoholic heart muscle disease {AHMD). Full-blown AHMD is found in only a small percentage (2%) of heavy drinkers, but the great majority (80%) have some heart muscle abnormalities.

Heavy drinking increases the risk of stroke and other intracranial bleeding within 24 hours of a drinking binge (Brust, 2003). The exact mechanism for many of the cardiovascular problems is not definitely known, but the connection is clear.

Nervous System

Physiologically, alcohol limits the brain's ability to use glucose and oxygen thus killing brain cells as well as inhibiting message transmission. Low-to-moderate use does not seem to cause permanent functional loss, whereas chronic high-dose use causes direct damage to nerve cells that can have far-reaching consequences in susceptible individuals. Alcohol-induced malnutrition, not just the direct toxic effects, can also injure brain cells and disrupt brain chemistry.

Both physical brain damage and impaired mental abilities have been linked to advanced alcoholism. Brain atrophy (loss of brain tissue) has been documented in 50% to 100% of alcoholics at autopsy. Breathing and heart rate irregularities caused by damage to the brain's autonomic nervous system have also been traced to brain atrophy. Dementia (deterioration of intellectual ability, faulty memory, disorientation, and diminished problem-solving ability) is a further consequence of prolonged heavy drinking. Abnormalities in the corpus callosum are much greater in older long-term drinkers, aggravating the effects of the alcohol abuse (Pfefferbaum, Adalsteinsson & Sullivan, 2005).

One of the more serious diseases due to brain damage caused by chronic alcoholism and thiamine (vitamin B]) deficiency is Wernicke's encephalopathy, whose symptoms include delirium, imbalance, visual problems, and impaired ability to coordinate movements particularly in the lower extremities (ataxia). The other serious condition that involves thiamine deficiency is Korsakoff's psychosis. Its symptoms include disorientation, memory failure, and repetition of false memories (confabulation). Most alcoholics suffering from Wernicke's encephalopathy develop Korsakoff's psychosis (Johnson & Ait-Daoud, 2005; Martin, Singleton & Hiller-Sturmhofel, 2003).

> "Exactly what I have is called atrophy of the cerebellum, which is the back part of the brain that goes into your spinal cord that has to do with coordination and balance. My drinking for probably 20 years has caused it to shrink."
>
> —Ex-drinker with Wernicke's encephalopathy

Hippocrates wrote about the association between alcohol and seizures/ epilepsy more than 2,000 years ago. The prevalence of epilepsy is up to 10 times greater in those with alcoholism (Devantag, Mandich, Zaiotti, et al., 1983). Although the seizures could be caused by head trauma due to drunkenness or other causes, the direct damage to neurological systems as well as the adrenaline storm caused by withdrawal is strongly implicated.

Sexual Desire & the Reproductive System

Female. Although light drinking lowers inhibitions, prolonged use decreases desire and the intensity of orgasm. In one study of female chronic alcoholics, 36% said they had orgasms less than 5% of the time. Chronic alcohol abuse can inhibit ovulation, decrease the gonadal mass, delay menstruation, and cause sexual dysfunction (Blume & Zilberman, 2005). Heavy drinking also raises the chances of infertility and spontaneous abortion (Emanuele, Wezeman & Emanuele, 2002).

Male. Though low-to-moderate levels of alcohol can lower inhibitions and enhance the psychological aspects of sexual activity, the depressant effects soon take over. Chronic use causes effects beyond a temporary inability to perform. Researchers in one study of 66 alcoholics found an erectile dysfunction rate of 71% vs. just 7% for abstainers (Muthusami & Chinnaswamy, 2005). Long-term alcohol abuse impairs gonadal functions and causes a decrease in testosterone (male hormone) levels. Decreased testosterone causes an increase in estrogen (a female hormone) that can lead to male breast enlargement, testicular atrophy, low sperm count, loss of body hair, and loss of sexual desire. When resuming sexual activity, a recovering alcoholic may experience excessive anxiety; dysfunction can be intensified by one or two bad performances.

One of the most long-lasting effects of alcohol abuse is an inability to experience normal sexual relationships because, before recovery, romance usually occurred in bars or at parties where alcohol was readily available.

> "I don't really remember making love with a woman when I was sober. It was usually when I had a couple of drinks in me or if I was that fargone, then I would probably go with the woman or bring the woman home, and I would go to bed with her, and I would probably fall asleep."
>
> —43-year-old recovering alcoholic

Cancer

Breast Cancer. The association between heavier drinking (three or more drinks per day) and breast cancer is clear. The evidence concerning the correlation between drinking small amounts of alcohol and the incidence of breast cancer is less compelling. In one study of 1,200 women with breast cancer, there was an association between moderate alcohol use and breast cancer (even amounts as low as one drink per day increased the risk by 50%. In fact, 25% of all breast cancer was associated with even brief use of alcohol (Bowlin, 1997). Other studies, however, have found only small increases in the incidence of breast cancer (Ellison, Zhang, McLennan, et al, 2001; Terry, Zhang, Kabat, et al, 2005; Zhang, Lee, Manson, et al, 2007).

Other Cancers. The risk of mouth, throat, larynx, and esophageal cancer are 6 times greater for heavy alcohol users, 7 times greater for smokers, and an astonishing 38 times greater for those who smoke and drink alcohol (Blot, 1992). Liver cancer is also a risk in those with longstanding cirrhosis. Some studies give different rates of cancer in heavy drinkers, but the increase is there in all Cases (Bagnardi, Blangiardo, Vecchia, et al, 2001).

Systemic Problems

Musculoskeletal System. Alcohol leeches minerals from the body, causing a much greater risk of a fracture of the femur, wrist, vertebrae, and ribs. The unbalancing of electrolytes by chronic or acute use, along with direct toxic effects, can cause myopathy (painful swollen muscles).

Dermatologic Complications. The reddish complexion and other skin conditions of chronic alcoholics is caused by a number of factors: the dilation of blood vessels near the skin, malnutrition, jaundice, thinning of the skin, and liver problems all add to the alcoholic's appearance. Other infections and conditions potentiated by the toxic effects of alcohol include acne rosacea, psoriasis, eczema, and facial edema.

Immune System. Heavy drinking may disrupt white blood cells and in other ways weaken the immune system, resulting in greater susceptibility to infections. Excessive drinking has been linked to cancer as well as such infectious diseases as respiratory infections, tuberculosis, and pneumonia.

Chronic High-Dose Use: Mental/Emotional Effects

With chronic high-dose use, almost any mental, emotional, or psychiatric symptom is a possibility, including memory problems, hallucinations, paranoia, severe depression, insomnia, and intense anxiety. These symptoms, particularly amnesia and blackouts, become more common as alcohol abuse progresses. The inability to learn problem-solving techniques that help one cope with life is a long-lasting effect of alcoholism (and most addictions).

"It's like I'm a 30-year-old woman stuck with these 12-year-old issues and I don't know what to do with them, not because I'm not willing or not because I don't have my intellectual mind but it's what is going on inside of my heart and my feelings, not knowing what to do with my feelings and then just pushing it all down."

—30-year-old female recovering alcoholic

Alcohol and memory problems go hand-in-hand. Alcohol damages activity in the frontal lobes and the hippocampus, making it difficult to concentrate and get information into the brain. Alcohol also damages the memory centers, so heavy drinkers have trouble retaining information not just getting it into the brain.

Mortality

Heavy drinking shortens the alcoholic's life span (e.g., 4 years from alcohol-induced cancer, 4 years from heart disease, and 9 to 22 years from liver disease (NIAAA, 2000; Vaillant, 1995). Overall, if people continue heavy drinking, they are likely to die 15 years earlier than the general population (Moos, Brennan & Mertens, 1994).

Addiction (alcohol dependence, or alcoholism)

- 10% to 12% of the 140 million adult drinkers in the United States have developed alcoholism.
- The incidence of alcoholism in men is approximately two to three times greater than in women (14% of male drinkers vs. 6% of female drinkers).

- The onset of alcoholism usually occurs at a younger age in men than in women.
- In terms of consumption, 20% of drinkers consume 80% of all alcohol (Greenfield & Rogers, 1999).

Classification

Early Classifications

Over the years there have been many attempts to classify different types of alcoholism. The purpose of classification is to develop a framework by which an illness or a condition can be studied systematically rather than relying strictly on experience (Hasin, 2003).

One of the earliest attempts at imposing scientific reasoning on drinking patterns was attempted by Dr. Benjamin Rush, physician, medical educator, patriot, reformer, and the first U.S. Surgeon General. He published the first American treatise on alcoholism in 1804—An Inquiry into the Effects of Ardent Spirits on the Human Body and Mind. It was a compendium of current attitudes toward alcohol abuse.

At about the same time, Dr. Thomas Trotter in An Essay, Medical, Philosophical and Chemical, on Drunkenness and Its Effects on the Human Body expounded, in scientific terms, his thesis that drunkenness was a disease produced by a remote cause that disrupts health.

According to scientific literature from the nineteenth and early-twentieth centuries, researchers developed dozens of classifications of alcoholics (e.g., acute, periodic, and chronic oenomania; habitual inebriate; continuous and explosive inebriate; and dipsomaniac, among others).

It wasn't until the 1930s that scientific progress on the study of alcoholism really accelerated with the experiences of the newly created Alcoholics

Anonymous and the founding of Yale's Laboratory of Applied Psychology (Trice, 1995). Researchers Yandell Henderson, Howard Haggard, Leon Green-berg, and later E. M. Jellinek made the study of alcoholism scientifically respectable, aided by their founding of the Quarterly Journal of Studies on Alcoholism and the Yale Center of Alcohol Studies.

E. M. Jellinek

In 1941 psychiatrist Karl Bowman and biometrist E. M. Jellinek presented an integration of 24 classifications of alcoholism that had appeared over the years in scientific literature, reducing alcoholics into four types:

- primary or true alcoholics: immediate liking for alcohol and rapid development of an uncontrollable need;
- steady endogenous symptomatic drinkers: alcoholism is secondary to a major psychiatric disorder;
- intermittent endogenous symptomatic drinkers: periodic binge drinking, again often with a psychiatric disorder; and
- stammtisch drinkers: drinkers in whom alcoholism is precipitated by outside causes, often start as social drinkers.

Twenty years later Jellinek, in his landmark book The Disease Concept of Alcoholism, proposed five types of alcoholism: alpha, beta, gamma, delta, and epsilon. Gamma and delta alcoholics were considered true alcoholics (Jellinek, 1961).

- Gamma alcoholics have a high psychological vulnerability but also a high physiological vulnerability; they develop tissue tolerance rapidly, they lose control quickly, and their progression to uncontrolled use is marked.

- Delta alcoholics have strong socio-cultural and economic influences along with a high physiological vulnerability; they also acquire tissue dependence rapidly, and it's hard for them to abstain. Their progression to alcoholism is much slower than that of gamma alcoholics. (Babor, 1996; Jellinek, 1961)

Modern Classifications

As valuable as Jellinek's classification was, the scientific basis for alcoholism wasn't as clear-cut as with other illnesses and conditions. Four developments starting in the 1950s led to a deeper understanding of alcoholism as a biological phenomenon.

- First was the discovery of the nucleus accumbens, the area of the brain that gives a surge of pleasure and a desire to repeat the action when stimulated by an experience, by electricity, or by psychoactive drugs (Olds, 1956; Olds & Milner, 1954).
- Next was the discovery of endogenous neurotransmitters, starting in the 1970s, that showed that drugs worked by influencing existing neurological pathways and receptor sites in the central nervous system, including the reward pathway that researchers had hinted at in the 1950s and 1960s (Goldstein, 2001).
- In the 1980s and 1990s, genetic research tools developed insights into hereditary influences on addiction; in 1990 the first gene (DRD_2A} allele) that seemed to have an influence on vulnerability to alcoholism was discovered (Blum, Braverman, Holder, et al., 2000; Noble, Blum, Montgomery, et al, 1991).
- In the 1990s and 2000s, imaging techniques visualized the actual reaction of the brain

to drugs (Gatley, Volkow, Wang, et al, 2005; Volkow, Wang & Doria, 1995).

These developments moved the classification of alcoholism and addiction away from qualitative classification toward a more quantifiable and empirical basis.

Type I & Type II Alcoholics. These studies were based on an extensive study of Swedish adoptees and their biological or adoptive parents by Dr. C. Robert Cloninger and colleagues. Type I alcoholism (also called milieu-limited) was defined as a later-onset syndrome that can affect both men and women. It requires the presence of a genetic and environmental predisposition, it can be moderate or severe, and it takes years of drinking to trigger it (much like Jellinek's delta alcoholic). Type II alcoholism (also called male-limited) mostly affects sons of male alcoholics, is moderately severe, is primarily genetic, and is only mildly influenced by environmental factors (Bohman, Sigvardson & Cloninger, 1981; Cloninger, Bohman & Sigvardson, 1996).

Type A & Type B Alcoholics. Dr. T. F. Babor and his research colleagues at the University of Connecticut School of Medicine introduced the A/B typologies in 1992. They are similar to Dr. C. Robert Cloninger's type I/II typologies. Type A, like type I, is a later onset of alcoholism with less family history of alcoholism and less severe dependence. Type B, like type II, refers to a more severe alcoholism with an earlier onset, more-impulsive behavior and conduct problems or disorders, more co-occurring mental disorders, and more-severe dependence (Babor, Dolinsky, Meyer, et al., 1992).

The Disease Concept of Alcoholism

Much of the current research in the treatment of alcoholism is based on the disease concept. The idea of alcoholism as a disease goes back thousands of years but only recently has the concept become widely accepted.

TABLE 6. Some Alcohol-Related Causes Of Death

Diseases (directly caused by alcohol)	Diseases (indirectly caused by alcohol)	Injuries/Adverse Effects (indirectly caused by alcohol)
Alcoholic psychoses	Tuberculosis	Boating accidents
Alcoholism (dependence)	Cancer of the lips, mouth, and pharynx	Motor vehicle, bicycle, other road
Alcohol abuse	Cancer of the larynx, esophagus, stomach,	accidents
Nerve degeneration	and liver	Airplane accidents
Heart disease	Diabetes	Falls
Alcoholic gastritis	Hypertension	Fire accidents
Fatty liver	Stroke	Drowning
Hepatitis	Pancreatitis	Suicides, self-inflicted injuries
Cirrhosis	Diseases of stomach, esophagus, and	Homicides or shootings
Other liver damage	duodenum	Choking on food
Alcohol poisoning	Cirrhosis of bile tract	Domestic violence
Seizure activity		Rapes or date rapes

- In 1972 the National Council on Alcoholism developed Criteria for the Diagnosis of Alcoholism, Signs and Symptoms and defined it as a "chronic progressive disease, incurable but treatable."
- In 1980 the American Psychiatric Association (APA) made Substance Use Disorders a separate major diagnostic category in its Diagnostic and Statistical Manual of Mental Disorders, also known as DSM.
- The Natural History of Alcoholism published in 1983 by Dr. George Vaillant, professor of psychiatry at Harvard Medical School, was based mostly on a long-term study of two groups of men (college students vs. inner-city young men). His major conclusions were that poverty and pre-existing psychological problems were not predictors of the development of alcoholism. The predictors of alcoholism were much more likely to be a family history of alcoholism and/or an environment with a high rate of alcoholism.
- In 1994 remission and substance-induced conditions were defined in DSM-IV.
- The latest edition of the APA manual, DSM-IV-TR, lists alcohol dependence and alcohol abuse under Alcohol Use Disorders. Under Alcohol-Induced Disorders it lists alcohol intoxication, alcohol withdrawal, delirium, and 10 other conditions (American Psychiatric Association, 2000).

Both the World Health Organization and the American Medical Association view alcoholism as a specific disease entity. In 1992 a medical panel from the American Society of Addiction Medicine and the National Council on Alcoholism and Drug Dependence defined alcoholism as follows:

"Alcoholism is a primary chronic disease with genetic, psychosocial, and environmental factors influencing its development and manifestation. The disease is often progressive and fatal. It is characterized by impaired control over drinking, preoccupation with the drug (alcohol), use of alcohol despite adverse consequences, and distortions in thinking, most notably denial. Each of these symptoms may be continuous or periodic." (Morse, Flavin, et al, 1992)

> "I don't consider myself an alcoholic. I have five drinks a day—and that's an average. It's always three and sometimes it's a lot more but it's never interfered with my work. I haven't been to the doctor for 15 years. But since it's never interfered with my work, I see nothing wrong with sitting down and having a drink."
>
> —41-year-old avowed habitual drinker

Heredity, Environment & Psychoactive Drugs

Instead of focusing on typologies, it is useful to look at alcoholism and addiction as continuums of severity that depend, to varying degrees, on genetic predisposition, environmental influences (family, workplace), and the actual use of alcohol and other psychoactive drugs themselves, which can alter the body's neurochemistry and instill an intense vulnerability to craving (see Chapter 2).

Heredity

> "Women who drink wine excessively give birth to children who drink excessively of wine."
>
> —Aristotle, 350 B.C.

As early as the fourth century B.C., the philosopher Aristotle wrote about the tendency of alcohol abuse to run in families, but not until the past 40 years has the scientific basis for this belief been explored.

"I think that there are genes that impact a variety of different characteristics that increase or decrease your risk for alcoholism. We already know the genes related to the alcohol-metabolizing enzymes; some very good laboratories are closing in on some of the genes likely to contribute to disinhibition. Other laboratories are certainly actively searching forgenes that might indirectly increase your risk for alcoholism through psychiatric disorders, such as schizophrenia and bipolar disorder. And our group and others are searching for the genes that are contributing to the low response to alcohol, which indirectly increases your risk for alcoholism in a heavy drinking society (Schuckit, Edenberg, Kalmijn, et al, 2001). Obviously there are going to be a whole slew of genes that contribute to the alcoholism risk but altogether they're explaining a very important part of the picture, probably 60% of the risk."

—Marc Schuckit, M.D., professor of psychiatry, University of California Medical School, San Diego, CA

Family studies, twin studies, animal studies, and adoption studies show strong genetic influences particularly in severe alcoholism (Anthenelli & Schuckit, 2003; Blum, Braverman, Holder, et al, 2000; Knop, Goodwin, Teasdale, et al, 1984; Li, Lumeng, McBride, et al., 1986; Lin & Anthenelli, 2005; Woodward, 2003). A Study that assessed alcohol-related disorders among 3,516 twins in Virginia concluded that the genetic influence was 48% to 58% of the various influences, a rate much higher than postulated in the past (Prescott & Kendler, 1999).

It is widely theorized that several genes have an influence on one's susceptibility to alcoholism and other drug addictions. A person could have one, several, or all of the genes that make someone susceptible to addiction not just a single gene such as the dopamine DRD_2 A_1 allele receptor gene (Blum, Braverman, Holder, et al, 2000) (see Chapter 2). The drinker could have a defective $ALDH_2$ gene that encodes aldehyde dehydrogenase, a key liver enzyme that helps metabolize alcohol. The defective gene is more prevalent in Asians. Because the defective gene means less enzyme to rid the body of alcohol, its presence acts as a preventive to alcoholism because the person becomes uncomfortable or ill after even a few drinks. In addition about half of all Japanese, along with some other Asian populations (e.g., Chinese), are born with a more efficient ADH (alcohol dehydrogenase), called atypical ADH, and a less efficient form of $ALDH_2$, known as KM $ALDH_1$ Thus, when they drink even small amounts of alcohol, the toxic acetaldehyde builds up (up to 10 times the normal amount) and causes a flushing reaction due to vasodilation. Tachycardia and headaches also occur. At higher doses edema (water retention), hypotension, and vomiting ensue (Goedde, Harada & Agarwal, 1979; Teng, 1981; Woodward, 2003; Yokoyama, Yokoyama, Yokoyama, et al, 2005). Though Asians have a higher rate of abstention and a lower rate of alcoholism, Asian Americans' rate of alcoholism is higher, showing that environmental and cultural influences can overcome some biological propensities (Lee, 1987). Other genes being studied include the HT-TLPR, which alters the function of serotonin transporters and seems to affect the stress response, anxiety, and dysphoria—factors that can lead to relapse (Oroszi & Goldman, 2004).

Other markers for a strong genetic influence are a tendency to have blackouts, a greater initial tolerance to alcohol, an impaired decisionmaking area of the brain, a major shift in personality while drinking, an impaired ability to learn from mistakes, retrograde amnesia, and a low level of response (LR) to alcohol. LR is one of the stronger markers. One study of adolescents (average age 12.9 years) showed that a low level of response correlated with a higher level of drinking even at an early age (Schuckit, Smith, Beltran, et al., 2005).

"When I was younger, I was always surrounded by alcohol and drugs. My mom became an alcoholic, my sister used, and so did my two stepbrothers and stepsister. My stepdad also used to grow [marijuana]. So I was kind of around it a lot."

—19-year-old recovering alcoholic

There also seems to be a hereditary link to the physical consequences of alcoholism, especially cirrhosis and alcoholic psychosis (Reed, Pagte, Viken, et al., 1996).

Environment

For other people the environmental factors are the overwhelming influences: child abuse; alcohol-or other drug-abusing parents, friends, and/or relatives; chaotic familial relations; peer pressure; and extreme stress. Easy access to alcohol, a permissive societal view of drinking, unsafe living conditions, poor nutrition, and limited access to healthcare and drug recovery programs are also influential.

"I remember holidays, it being pretty disgusting; my father would be pretty intoxicated. And I remember the Tooth Fairy, the Easter Bunny, and Santa Claus all smelling the same way."

—25-year-old recovering alcoholic

Sexual, physical, and emotional abuse at a young age are the most powerful environmental factors in raising a person's susceptibility to alcohol/drug abuse. In one study of 275 women and 556 men receiving detoxification services, 20% of the men and 50% of the women said that they had been subject to physical or sexual abuse (Brems, Johnson, Neal, et al., 2004). Abuse is also a powerful factor in the development of behavioral addictions.

Alcohol & Other Drugs

Once the genetic and environmental factors have determined susceptibility, the toxic effects of alcohol and other drugs that change neurochem-istry come into play.

"After a while it got to the point where I didn't care what it tasted like. I just wanted that buzz to keep going. The brain was craving alcohol. It was the hard liquor and the higher volume of alcohol involved with it, I think. To this day I still like the taste of Jack Daniels® and I watch myself real close."

—32-year-old recovering alcoholic

Often, long after the reasons for seeking the rush or escape have faded, the craving remains. In the end what is important varies with the point of view of the person involved.

- To a researcher or scientist, classification and a systematic view of alcoholism are important.
- To a psychiatrist, counselor, or social worker, the environmental factors and

the neurochemical effects of addiction are important because they lead to strategies to counteract craving and regain control.

- To the problem drinker or alcoholic, any help, knowledge, or techniques that will keep them sober up and lessen the craving are important.

"Most alcohol-dependent people or drug-dependent people, when terrible crises occur, they can stop. Their trouble, however, is staying stopped. So when they go back to use, whether it's the first or the thirtieth time they use, you can bet money that one of those times they won't be able to stop and problems are going to develop dramatically."

—Marc Schuckit, M.D., professor of psychiatry, University of California Medical School, San Diego, CA

Tolerance, Tissue Dependence & Withdrawal

"Exposure of the brain to alcohol initiates a process of adaptation that works to counteract the altered brain function resulting from initial exposure to alcohol. This adaptation or change in brain function is responsible for the processes called alcohol tolerance,' alcohol dependence, 'and alcohol withdrawal syndrome." Tenth Special Report to Congress on Alcohol and Alcoholism (NIAAA, 1000)

Tolerance

Tolerance is a process through which the brain defends itself against the effects of alcohol.

Dispositional (metabolic) tolerance, pharmacodynamic tolerance, behavioral tolerance, and acute tolerance are four ways the body tries to adapt to the effects of alcohol. The result of tolerance is that the chronic drinker is able to handle larger and larger amounts of alcohol. It also indicates the body's growing dependence (tissue dependence) as it attempts to maintain its normal physiological balance in the face of alcohol's toxic effects. The rate at which tolerance develops varies widely among drinkers.

"Well, I started drinking one beer and then I went on to two. A week later I went on to a six-pack, and then through the years I went on to two six-packs, and then I ended up drinking tequila. I used to drink a fifth of tequila two years after I got addicted to the alcohol."

—38-year-old female recovering alcoholic

Dispositional (metabolic) tolerance means the body changes so that it metabolizes alcohol more efficiently. As a person drinks over a period of time, the liver adapts to create more enzymes to process the alcohol and its metabolite acetaldehyde (Tabakoff, Cornell & Hoffman, 1992; Woodward, 2003). This accelerated process eliminates alcohol more quickly from the body. It also accelerates the elimination of other prescription drugs, lessening their effectiveness. In addition, because liver cells are being destroyed by drinking and by the natural aging process, the liver eventually becomes less able to metabolize the alcohol, a process called reverse tolerance. A heavy drinker who could handle a fifth of whiskey at the age of 30 can become totally incapacitated by a two glasses of wine or less at the age of 50.

Pharmacodynamic tolerance means brain neurons and other cells become more resistant to the effects of alcohol by increasing the number of receptor sites needed to produce an effect or by creating other cellular changes that make tissues less responsive to alcohol (e.g., GABA becomes less sensitive to ethanol) (Boehm, Valenzuela, Harris, et al, 2005).

Behavioral tolerance means drinkers learn how to "handle their liquor" by modifying their behavior or by trying to act in such a way that they hope others won't notice they are inebriated. (Vogel-Sprott, Rawana & Webster, 1984).

Acute tolerance also develops from high-dose alcohol use. This rapid tolerance starts to develop with the first drink and is the body's method of providing instant protection from the poisonous effects of ethanol.

Select tolerance means that tolerance does not develop equally to all the effects of alcohol, so while a person may learn how to walk steadily with a 0.14 BAC, he might have trouble threading a needle.

Withdrawal

"Your body is going through so many changes, you can hardly breathe; you're shaking. A hangover, yeah, you might be sick for a couple of hours. That's different than withdrawals; but with withdrawals, it will kill you."

—32-year-old female recovering alcoholic

As mentioned, hangovers can occur with any level of drinking from experimentation to addiction. More severe withdrawal symptoms occur with chronic high-dose use.

"I hurt so much when I sobered up that I said, 'the heck with this.' I said, 'if that's going to kill the pain, I'll go back to drinking,' and I really thought about it several times, and it was a war within myself whether to drink or not drink."

—65-year-old recovering alcoholic

Although a majority of patients develop significant symptoms of withdrawal when they come in for detoxification and treatment for their alcoholism (Saitz & O'Malley, 1997), 85% to 95% of those experiencing withdrawal will have only the more minor symptoms, not the life-threatening ones (Schuckit, 1996). The presence of true withdrawal symptoms is one important indication that the drinker has developed a dependence on alcohol.

The alcoholic coming into treatment will often try to explain away what he or she is feeling as a hangover instead of accepting it as true withdrawal.

Various classic experiments have shown that minor withdrawal symptoms will develop for people who drink heavily for 7 to 34 days whereas major withdrawal symptoms will probably develop after 48 to 87 consecutive days of heavy drinking (Isbell, Fraser, Wikler, et al., 1955). Many withdrawal symptoms involve the autonomic nervous system.

Minor symptoms of withdrawal include rapid pulse, sweating, increased body temperature, hand tremors, anxiety, depression, insomnia, and nausea or vomiting.

Major symptoms of withdrawal include tachycardia; transient visual, tactile, or auditory hallucinations and illusions; psychomotor agitation; grand mal seizures; and delirium tremens.

"I was very sick—very nauseous, pains in my stomach, headaches, shaking filled with sheer terror. I've never known fear like that in my life. This has been the hardest thing I've had to do, but the alternative is worse."

—34-year-old recovering alcoholic

Because the main symptoms of severe withdrawal can combine with complications, such as malnutrition or liver problems, medical care for a chronic alcohol abuser must be considered in any course of treatment.

In less than 1% of serious cases of alcohol withdrawal, full-blown delirium tremens, called "the DTs," occurs. The DTs usually begins 48 to 96 hours after the last drink in a long period of heavy drinking and can last for 3 to 5 sometimes up to 10 days, although some cases have lasted up to 50 days (Mayo-Smith, 2003). The dramatic symptoms can include trembling over the whole body, grand mal seizures, disorientation, insomnia, and delirium, and severe auditory, visual, and tactile hallucinations. The DTs are a serious condition requiring hospitalization. Untreated, the mortality rate ranges from 10% to 20%.

Neurotransmitters & Withdrawal. At first, alcohol increases the effectiveness of GABA, blocking the actions of the brain's energy chemicals and thus making the person drowsy and depressing other body functions. Over time the brain compensates by creating an excess of energy chemicals and decreasing (down regulating) the number of GABA receptors, resulting in hyperarousal. During withdrawal the rebound excess of energy chemicals causes anxiety, increased muscular activity, tachycardia, hypertension, and occasionally seizures. The brain becomes less able to control the hyperactivity (Blum & Payne, 1991). Current research also explores the role of serotonin in the alcohol withdrawal process. A 30% reduction in the availability of brainstem serotonin transporters was found in chronic alcoholics, which correlates with their self-reported ratings of depression and anxiety during withdrawal (Gorwood, Lanfumey & Hamon, 2004; Heinz, Ragan, Jones, etal., 1998).

Kindling. With many long-term heavy drinkers, a process called kindling occurs: repeated bouts of drinking and withdrawal actually intensify subsequent withdrawal symptoms and can cause seizures. The theory is that the repeated presence of alcohol actually alters brain chemistry, impairing the body's natural defenses against damage from alcohol (Becker, 1998). Kindling is also known as inverse tolerance.

Directions In Research

As it becomes more evident that the cause of alcoholism is a combination of heredity, environment, and the toxic effects of alcohol, research has divided itself along those lines.

Research into heredity has focused on identifying the genes that make a user more susceptible to addiction (e.g., DRD_2A_1 allele, $ALDH_2$).

"If you are going to have a way to intervene therapeutically, what you

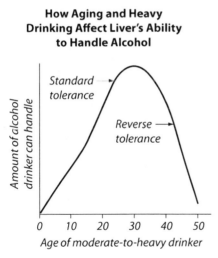

How Aging and Heavy Drinking Affect Liver's Ability to Handle Alcohol

Standard tolerance

Reverse tolerance

Amount of alcohol drinker can handle

0   10   20   30   40   50

Age of moderate-to-heavy drinker

FIGURE 5. **This graph shows the decrease in liver capacity to process alcohol as a person ages. As the liver is taxed and poisoned by the alcohol, its capacity is diminished to the point where an older chronic drinker can get tipsy on just one drink.**

want to know is which are the most importantgenes and which are the most important proteins and enzymes that are carrying out the mission of those genes because those are the ideal targets for new medications. I can imagine a day in the future when we will be able to sort out the different kinds of alcoholic subjects, and well learn that some of them have problems with one transmitter system, others have a problem with a different transmitter system, but the treatment designed for those patients will be designed to meet their specific needs."

—Ivan Diamond, M.D, director, Ernest Gallo Clinic and Research Center

Research into environmental causes of alcoholism has focused on identifying which changes in the addict's surroundings will decrease the use of alcohol and other drugs. Studies on raising the drinking age, reducing child abuse in the home, limiting sale of alcohol, and lowering stress in everyday life are reported every month in dozens of professional medical and sociological journals worldwide.

Research into drug-caused physiological and psychological changes that occur with chronic and high-dose use also keeps many researchers occupied. Studying the impacts on the immune system, on the development of dispositional and pharmacodynamic tolerance, on the beneficial cardiovascular effects, and on the learning disabilities in drug-affected infants all show promise in developing treatment for alcoholism.

In addition, research into various drugs that could reduce the craving for alcohol is intense. The CB1 receptors, which are sensitive to cannabinoids, have been found to help modulate the reinforcing effects of alcohol and other abused drugs (Thanos, Dimitrakakis, Rice, et al., 2005).

Other Problems With Alcohol

These issues with alcohol—polydrug abuse, mental problems, alcohol use during pregnancy, aggression and violence, and drunk driving and associated injuries and suicide—can occur at almost any level of use although high-dose chronic use and alcoholism are involved most often.

Polydrug Abuse

Most illicit-drug users also drink alcohol, and most alcohol abusers use other drugs. In one European study of 600 adolescent drug users, 80% used both marijuana and alcohol (Redzic, Licanin & Krosnjar, 2003). In the United States, the figure for alcohol and illicit-drug use among a group in treatment is 96%. Among all heavy drinkers, 32.2% were also current illicit-drug users (SAMHSA, 2006). Some 80% to 95% of alcoholics smoke cigarettes, while 70% are heavy smokers (NIAAA, 1998). The reasons for using alcohol and another drug vary:

- Alcohol and tobacco are widely used to facilitate social situations.
- Alcohol and marijuana can be used together to rapidly increase relaxation.
- Alcohol taken before using cocaine will prolong and intensify the cocaine's effects by creating the metabolite cocaethylene, which also seems to intensify a predisposition to violence.
- Alcohol can be used to come down off a three-day methamphetamine run.
- Sedative-hypnotics or opioids can be used to get loaded if alcohol is unavailable.

- Compulsive gamblers drink while gambling or gamble while drinking.

"I used downers just to come down off the alcohol because I was so shaky. And then I would try using amphetamines just to lift me up so I wouldn't drink so much. But what I would do was stay awake longer and drink more, so that didn't work."

—40-year-old recovering polydrug abuser

Polydrug abuse has become so common that treatment centers often have to treat simultaneous addictions. Although the emotional roots of addiction are similar no matter what drug is used, the physiological and psychological changes that each drug causes, particularly during withdrawal, often have to be treated differently. For example, if a client has a serious alcohol and benzodiazepine problem, the clinic has to be extremely careful detoxifying the client because it can't use a benzodiazepine to try to control alcohol withdrawal symptoms.

Although 70% of alcoholics are heavy smokers (more than one pack a day) compared with 25% of the general population, the converse is not as dramatic: smokers are only slightly more likely to drink alcohol compared with nonsmokers (SAMHSA, 2006). But there is a strong link between alcohol and early use of tobacco. Adolescents who smoke are three times more likely to begin using alcohol (Shiftman & Balabanis, 1995).

Alcohol & Mental Problems

Alcohol is most often used to change one's mood or mental state. The mood could be mild anxiety,

confusion, boredom, or sadness. The mental state could be symptoms of a preexisting mental illness such as major depression or a personality disorder (Petrakis, Gonzalez, Rosenheck, et al., 2002). For example, a study of adults with panic disorder showed that the subjects reported significantly less anxiety and fewer panic attacks when drinking. Unfortunately, the use of alcohol to control the symptoms resulted in a higher rate of alcohol-use disorders among those with panic disorder (Kushner, Abrams, Thuras, et al., 2005).

An association has been found between drinking and certain mental illnesses. In a study of alcohol-dependent men and women, 4% also had an independent bipolar disorder-four times the rate for the general public (Schuckit, Tipp, Bucholz, et al., 1997). Whether the relationship is causal or associative, it is the subject of much debate among professionals in the mental health community and those in the chemical dependency treatment community. In the two major studies about dual diagnosis, the incidence of major depression among those diagnosed with alcohol dependence was about 28% and the incidence of anxiety was 37%, which is much, much higher than for the general population (5.3% and 16.4%, respectively) (Kessler, Nelson & McGonagle, 1996; Regier, Farmer, Rae, et al., 1990).

"I would pick up some beer to put me out of it. I didn't like the effect that regular psychiatric drugs, such as antidepressants, had on my brain and I'd rather just put myself out with the booze."

—Patient with major depression and an alcohol problem

On the other hand, if alcohol is used to excess, drinking or withdrawal can induce symptoms of mental illness. For example, a person who uses alcohol to escape sadness might advance to depression though chronic drinking (Miller, Klamen, Hoffman, et al., 1995). In one study depressed subjects with a history of alcoholism showed higher lifetime aggression and impulsivity and were more likely to report a history of childhood abuse, suicide attempts, and tobacco smoking (Oquendo, Galfalvy, Grunebaum, et al., 2005). Some of the reasons for mental problems are that heavy drinking disrupts opioid peptides, dopamine, serotonin, and GABA, neurotransmitters that trigger feelings of well-being in the mesolim-bic/dopaminergic reward pathway. In addition, heavy drinking raises the levels of neurochemicals that cause tension and depression (Koob, 1999). The brain tries to compensate for the depletion of neurotransmitters by releasing corticotropin-releasing factor, a stress chemical that unfortunately can induce depression. Alcohol-induced mental problems, particularly if they are adult onset, will abate as the brain chemistry rebalances itself (Dammann, Wiesbeck & Klapp, 2005).

> "The problems did get worse when I was drinking. That was one reason why I never figured out I was a manic-depressive. I figured I was depressed because I was drunk all the time."
>
> —Alcoholic with bipolar illness

Any psychiatric diagnosis must always take into account the possibility of drug-induced symptoms, so the professional must often wait weeks or months for the user's brain chemistry and cognition to stabilize before making an accurate diagnosis (Shivani, Goldsmith & Anthenelli, 2002). The majority of alcoholics who came into the Haight Ashbury Detox Clinic for treatment were initially diagnosed as suffering from depression, but after treatment and abstinence began (often taking a month or more), the percentage of depressed clients dropped dramatically (from approximately 70% to 30%).

At the other end of the spectrum, a hasty diagnosis of alcohol dependence can attribute all of the erratic behavior to the effects of the drug and miss the psychiatric diagnosis. The client with co-occurring disorders keeps relapsing because the more serious psychiatric problems have not been addressed. Experience has shown that if indeed there is a true dual diagnosis, both conditions must be treated to achieve an effective recovery. Some research of bipolar patients with alcoholism found it important to discover which illness came first because those who exhibited the bipolar illness first were slower to recover (Strakowski, DelBello, Fleck, et al., 2005).

These problems are especially confusing with psychiatric diagnoses of antisocial personality disorder (ASPD) and borderline personality disorder (BPD). The symptoms of these two illnesses are very common in those who seek treatment.

The symptoms of high impulsivity, no remorse for causing harm to others, and an inability to learn from mistakes are found in ASPD and among drug abusers (Dom, Hulstijn & Sabbe, 2005). BPD is characterized by intense negative emotions such as depression, self-hatred, anger, and hopelessness, and these individuals often use impulsive maladaptive behaviors such as suicidal actions and substance abuse to deal with their feelings.

To diagnosis borderline personality disorder or antisocial personality disorder, the symptoms should exist outside of the drug-seeking/using behavior and should have existed prior to the drug use. There is much debate as to the actual incidence of these diseases, particularly BPD, because its symptoms often shift from moment to moment and can be drug induced. Some treatment personnel refer to the diagnosis of BPD as a "catchall diagnosis" when the real problems aren't clear. Patients who actually have these problems

are difficult to treat and consume a disproportionate amount of the staff's time.

One evaluation of public and private inpatient
alcohol-abuse programs measured the incidence
of ASPD at 15%) for male alcoholics and 5% for
female alcoholics. Conversely, 80% of those with
ASPD develop substance dependence (Schuckit,
2000; Schuckit, Tipp, Bucholz, et al., 1997). In one
older study of alcohol treatment admissions, the
incidence of BPD was 13%) (Nace, Saxon & Shore,
1983). Among admissions for any drug abuse, the
incidence of BPD was 17% (Nace, Saxon, Davis,
et al, 1991).

Alcohol & Pregnancy

Maternal Drinking

"When I was pregnant with my daughter Casey, I was drinking between three
and four liters of wine daily until I was
about eight months and got into the
recovery network. And consequently
she was born with fetal alcohol effects.
She also had a hole in her heart, her
digestive system was all messed up, she
hadprojectile vomiting, and she didn't
gain any weight for about a month."

—24-year-old recovering alcoholic

Alcohol use during pregnancy is the leading
cause of mental retardation in the United States
(May & Gossage, 2001; West & Blake, 2005).

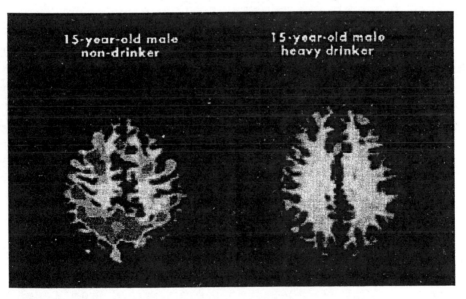

FIGURE 6. The brain images show the differences between the brain of a young male nondrinker
and that of a heavy drinker. The red and pink show brain activity during a memory task. Brain activity in the young heavy drinker is greatly suppressed, leading to problems in later life. According\to
one study; 47% of those who begin drinking alcohol before the age of 14 become alcohol dependent
at some time in their lives compared with 9% of those who wait until age 21.

Courtesy of Susan Tapert, Ph.D., University of California, San Diego

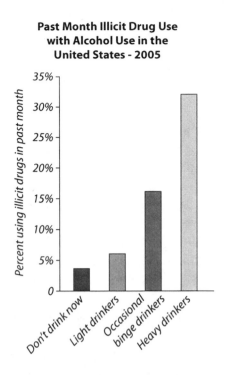

Past Month Illicit Drug Use with Alcohol Use in the United States - 2005

Percent using illicit drugs in past month

Don't drink now / Light drinkers / Occasional binge drinkers / Heavy drinkers

FIGURE 7. This chart shows that excessive drinking is associated with the use of other illicit drugs. Whether it's the association with other people who drink and use drugs, the lowering of inhibitions that makes other drug use acceptable, or the desire for stronger and more-intense experiences, the association is quite clear. In terms of percentages, 83% of the illicit-drug use is marijuana and 17% is cocaine. (SAMHSA, 2006)

Excess drinking during pregnancy also increases the number of miscarriages and infant deaths, causes more problem pregnancies, and gives rise to smaller and weaker newborns (NIAAA, 2000).

A survey of pregnant women in the United States found that:

- 12.4% drank some alcohol during several months of pregnancy;
- 4% used in a binge pattern;
- 0.7% were heavy drinkers;
- 18% smoked cigarettes; and
- 4.3% used illicit drugs at least once (SAMHSA, 2005).

"I had been using for years before I got pregnant; and when I got pregnant, I tried to stop but I just couldn't do it. I wanted the drug more than I wanted the baby."

—27-year-old recovering alcoholic

Dr. Sarajini Budden, an expert on pregnancy and alcohol at Legacy Emmanuel Children's Hospital in Portland, Oregon, did a survey of the mothers of 293 infants born with fetal alcohol syndrome (FAS) or alcohol-related neurodevelopmental disorder (ARND), both caused by heavy drinking. During their pregnancies about 89% of the women were using alcohol with at least two other drugs, and 49% were using just two drugs, usually alcohol and cocaine. Interestingly, all of them were smoking, so nicotine was included as one of the toxins. Most were single moms, most were school dropouts, most had been or were being physically or sexually abused, and often there was a history of alcohol or drug abuse in the family. There is also a suspicion that a number of the mothers had learning problems in school and possibly were alcohol or drug affected themselves.

Through the University of Washing-. ton in Seattle, two groups of children with FAS were studied. By the time the first group was five years old, 38% of the biological mothers had died as a direct result of their alcoholism. By the time the second group was in early adolescence, 69% of the biological mothers died as a direct result of their alcoholism.

Fetal Alcohol Syndrome (FAS), Alcohol-Related Neurodevelopmental Disorder

(ARND) & Alcohol-Related Birth Defects (ARBD)

"He was very inconsolable. He would take 10 cc of feed; he wouldn't sleep. He slept for maybe 15, 20 minutes at a time, 24-hours a day. That's what we went through, and it was like that for a couple of years. He was a very hard baby to parent, but we loved him."
Foster mother of child with FAS

Certain specific toxic effects of alcohol on a developing fetus are known as fetal alcohol syndrome (FAS), a term coined in 1973 although the diagnosis was first written about in France in 1968 (Jones & Smith, 1973). Initially, it was thought that the defects were the result of malnutrition, but the toxicity of alcohol was eventually recognized as the cause. The symptoms can range from obvious gross physical defects to mental deficits to behavioral problems (Sood, Delaney-Black, Covington, et al, 2001). Not all women who drink heavily during pregnancy bear children with FAS.

In 1996 the Institute of Medicine of the National Academy of Sciences reclassified the effects of prenatal alcohol exposure into five categories. Three categories refer to the facial features and two categories are for alcohol-affected infants without the specific facial features. The last two categories are alcohol-related neurodevelop-mental disorder (ARND), marked by CNS abnormalities, and alcohol-related birth defects (ARBD), marked by any number of physical anomalies (Stratton, Howe & Battaglia, 1996). ARND and ARBD used to be referred to as FAE (fetal alcohol effects) or PFAE (possible fetal alcohol effects), but the complexity of the diagnosis made it necessary to expand the definitions. Because of the wide range of symptoms, the term fetal alcohol spectrum disorder (FASD) is used to refer to this whole range of effects caused by prenatal exposure to alcohol.

There is as yet no definitive test for confirming FAS at birth, and only the most severe cases are diagnosable at that time. The minimal standards for a diagnosis of FAS are:

- retarded growth before and after birth, including height, weight, head circumference, brain growth, and brain size;
- facial deformities, including shortened eye openings, thin upper lip, flattened midface, and missing groove (filtrum) in the upper lip;
- occasional problems with the heart and the limbs; and
- central nervous system involvement, such as delayed intellectual development, neurological abnormalities, behavioral problems, visual problems, hearing loss, and balance or gait problems (Sokol & Clarren, 1989).

In tests of 178 individuals with FAS, IQ test scores ranged from 20 to. 120 with a mean of 79; in 295 individuals who were FAE, PFAE, or ARND, IQ scores ranged from 49 to 142 with a mean score of 90 (Streissguth, Barr, Kogn, et al., 1996). (Mental retardation is defined as an IQ of less than 70.)

Alcohol kills cells and changes the wiring of the fetus's brain. Huge gaps during brain development destroy natural connections that can never be regained. For example, SPECT scans in a Finnish study found smaller brain volume in a group of FAS and FAE children as well as abnormalities in serotonin and dopamine functioning (Riikonen, Nokelainen, Valkoneri, et al., 2005).

Other specific problems associated with FAS as well as ARND in terms of a neurocognitive profile include:

- difficulty with short-term memory,
- problems storing and retrieving information,

- impaired ability to form links and make associations,
- difficulty making good judgments and forming relationships,
- problems controlling temper and aggression,
- oversensitivity to such stimuli as a bright light, loud sound, sharp smell, or certain kinds of textures or tastes.

"Our other son has some of the characteristics like the filtrum, but from every other aspect of it he looks normal But his IQ is low, yet he comes across as being very smart. He has severe behavioral issues."

—Mother of adopted children with
FAS or FAE

These cognitive/behavioral deficits are not unique to alcohol exposure. Many other substances and physiological problems can cause similar conditions in children. For that reason a diagnosis of FASD is often missed in the absence of those unique facial features. Many of the symptoms are not obvious until several years after birth.

"What you're seeing at birth is a disorder of the brain's ability to regulate itself and its emotions; later on, especially in the toddler and preschool years, what you're seeing are problems with sleep and behavior; they're sitting and playing and they're pretty happy and then suddenly out of the blue they become aggressive. They throw temper tantrums, and you really don't know what's going on. But that's the up-and-down emotional instability that these children demonstrate."

—Sarajini Budden, M.D., FAS
specialist, Legacy Emmanuel
Children's Hospital, Portland, OR

Recently, researchers have found that early diagnosis of FASD in newborns plus a supportive environment can give the children a chance at a better, functional life (Streissguth, Bookstein, Barr, et al., 2004).

Worldwide studies estimate that FAS births occur in anywhere from 0.33 to 2.9 cases per 1,000 live births. The incidence can vary greatly (e.g., the rate in one survey in South Africa where alcoholism is rampant was 40 cases per 1,000). The worldwide incidence of ARBD and ARND (which are difficult to diagnose) is probably five to 10 times greater than the incidence of FAS and FAE (Hans, 1998; May, 1996; Pagliaro & Pagliaro, 2003).

In the United States, FAS rates of 0.2 to 1.5 per 1,000 are the accepted figures. African Americans have about 6 FAS births per 1,000; Asians, Hispanics, and Whites have 1 to 2; and American Indians have about 30, although rates from 10 to 120 per 1,000 have been reported in various specific American Indian and Canadian Indian communities (May, Brooke, Gossage, et al., 2000). In the United States, the incidence of ARND and ARBD is three times the incidence of FAS (CDC, 2004).

Critical Period. Because the brain is among the first organs to develop and the last to finish, it appears to be vulnerable throughout pregnancy, although weeks 3 through 8, at the onset of embryogenesis (formation of the embryo), are crucial. For example, the corpus callosum, a crucial structure that connects the cerebral hemispheres, is extremely vulnerable to alcohol use during the sixth to eighth gestational weeks; damage to the basal ganglia affects fine motor coordination and cognitive ability (Rosenberg, 1996). Generally:

- during the first trimester, alcohol interferes with the migration and the organization of brain cells;
- in the second trimester, especially the tenth to twentieth weeks, facial features are greatly affected;
- during the third trimester, the hippocampus is strongly affected, which leads to difficulties encoding visual and auditory information (Coles, 1994; Goodlett & Johnson, 1999; Miller, 1995; Streissguth, 1997).

Critical Dose. Animal models suggest that peak blood alcohol concentration rather than the total amount of alcohol drunk determines the critical level above which adverse effects are seen. A pattern of rapid drinking and the resulting high BAC seems to be the most dangerous style of drinking.

How many drinks are safe during pregnancy? One study concludes that seven standard drinks per week by pregnant mothers are a threshold level below which most neurobehav-ioral effects are not seen. This might lead some healthcare professionals to feel that they need not recommend total abstinence. Seven drinks per week are an average, however, and if a pregnant woman consumes a large number of those drinks in one sitting, the fetus may be much more at risk.

> "I think the message really is that if you know you're pregnant, don't drink because you don't know whether an ounce is going to cause a problem or whether 12 ounces is goinq to cause a problem because it may have a different effect on people."
> —Sarajini Bidden, M.D., FAS specialist, Legacy Emmanuel Children's Hospital, Portland, OR

A recent study in rats showed that when the developing brain is creating neurons and neuronal connections at a furious pace, even one high-dose use episode of drinking will also kill brain cells at a furious pace. The experiment showed that normally 1.5% ofbrain cells die during a certain period in a rat's growth; but in rats exposed to alcohol during that critical period, 5% to 30% of neurons died. When extrapolating these results to humans, the blood alcohol concentration would be 0.20, about twice the legal allowable limit for drivers, and the crucial period would be six months into the pregnancy until the baby is born. During the brain growth spurt, a single prolonged contact with alcohol lasting four hours or more is enough to kill vast numbers of brain cells (Ikonomidou, Bittigau, Ishimaru, et al, 2000).

The U.S. Surgeon General advises that women should not drink at all while pregnant because there is no way to determine which babies might be at risk from even very low levels of alcohol exposure (Hans, 1998; Maier & West, 2001; NIAAA, 1997).

> "I think tike anybody who has a child with FAS or FAE, we have a tendency to take a closer look at people who are not acting quite right. The behaviors are a little bit different, and you start to wonder if there isn't some alcohol in their past."
> —Foster father of 13-year-old with FAS

Paternal Drinking

> "For children whose fathers have chanced to beget them in drunkenness are wont to be fond of wine, and to be given to excessive drinking."

—Plutarch, Moralia: The Education of
Children, A.D. 110

As noted in Chapter 2, genetic transmission of alcoholism by fathers is strongly suspected. There is now evidence that some of the detrimental effects of alcohol on the fetus may also be transmitted by paternal alcohol consumption. Researchers are unable to say definitively whether paternal exposure to alcohol results in FAS or in some other damage. In laboratory tests alcoholic-sired rats of nonalcohol-using mothers produced male offspring with disturbed hormonal functions and spatial learning impairments. Adolescent male rats subjected to high alcohol intake produced both male and female offspring suffering from abnormal development, including decreased body weight (Bielawski, Zaher, Svinarich, et al, 2002).

Observations of male children of alcoholic fathers indicate no gross physical deficits but do show an association with intellectual and functional deficits in these offspring. In addition to the deficits in verbal, thinking, and planning skills, sons of male alcoholics exhibit further deficiencies in visual/spatial skills, motor skills, memory, and learning (NIAAA, 2000).

Some explanations of the causes of these abnormalities suggest that alcohol may mutate genes in sperm, kill off certain kinds of sperm, or biochemically and nutritionally alter semen and influence sperm (Little & Sing, 1986).

Aggression & Violence

In a situation involving violence, there are usually three people involved: the victim, the perpetrator, and one or more bystanders. The victim can be the recipient of physical or sexual assault (by a spouse or parent). The perpetrator can be of any age; the common denominator being anger often with alcohol thrown into the mix. Most often the bystanders are children who witness violence in their homes or neighborhoods.

"I've always just been an angry child, growing up with a lot of anger that's been stuffed. And then its like on the fifth drink I'm a party girl, but on the seventh drink I'd kick in your car door, you know. I'd just totally change to that Dr. Jekyll and Mr. Hyde syndrome. There's no end to my anger when I drink. Mine comes from a lot of past abuse as a kid and it comes from just not fitting in."

—18-year-old female recovering
alcoholic

Most research suggests that a tendency to violence already resides in some people and is due to a combination of factors (heredity, environment, and alcohol or other drugs) working together to biochemically and emotionally put them at risk (Hines & Saudino, 2005; Koenen, 2005; Stoff & Cairns, 2005).

"He was a pretty mean guy when he wasn't drunk when I think about it, so it is really hard for me to tell. But I know that when people are addicted and are alcoholics, they can be dry drunks, which makes them just as mean when they're not using as when they are."

—38-year-old victim of domestic
violence

Among many neurochemical effects, alcohol has been shown to increase aggression by interfering with GABA (the main inhibitory neurotransmitter) in ways that provoke intoxicated people with pre-existing aggressive tendencies. In addition, alcohol decreases the action and the levels of serotonin thus lowering impulse control (Javors, Tiouririne & Prihoda, 2000; Miczek, Fish, Almeida, et al., 2004). Lowered impulse control can cause drinkers to act out their aggressive impulses but also makes them less able to stop drinking once they have started (Gustafson, 1994).

> "On a typical Friday night, at least 50% of our calls will be some kind of alcohol and drug violent behavior situation whether it be a shooting, a stabbing, or a beating. A lot of those involve significant others, a spouse, or cohabitants."
>
> —Emergency medical technician, San Francisco Fire department

Even the expectation that alcohol will make one braver can lead people to be more aggressive—even if they are drinking a nonalcoholic beverage that they believe contains alcohol (Bushman, 1997; Higley, 2001). Drinking can impair information processing, leading a drinker to misjudge social cues, thereby overreacting to a neutral, "Hello, how are you?" from the opposite sex. Misjudging intentions can also cause a person to perceive a threat where none exists, leading to a violent overreaction (Miczek, Fish, de Almeida, et al., 2004).

Based on victim reports, 15% of robberies, 26% of aggravated assaults, and 50% of all homicides involved alcohol use. About 30% of the victims of violent crime reported that the offender had been drinking alcohol at the time of the offense. Not only had the offenders been drinking but their blood alcohol concentrations were two or three times the drunk-driving threshold: levels of 0.18 for probationers, 0.20 for local jail inmates, and an incredible 0.28 for state prisoners at the time of their offenses. In domestic-violence situations, the association is particularly important—alcohol is involved at least three-fourths of the time (Bureau of Justice Statistics, 1998 & 2006; NIAAA, 2000; Roizen, 1997).

In a study in Memphis, Tennessee, that examined police calls for domestic violence in that city, 92% of the perpetrators had used alcohol and 67% had used cocaine on the day of the assault. Almost half of the perpetrators had been loaded on alcohol and/or cocaine often during the past 30 days. Other studies (Figure 5-7) showed similar results.

> "The use of alcohol would really bring out the hit man in me. I mean, I could talk to my partner or whoever fairly good if I was sober, but after I started drinking the deep emotions really would come out."
>
> —28-year-old male in an anger management class

Alcohol encourages the release of pent-up anger, hatred, and desires discouraged by society, especially in people prone to violence. Alcohol can also undermine moral judgment and reasoning; so when someone drinks, the common sense that would keep that person out of trouble is often suppressed (Collins & Messerschmidt, 1993).

> "Seems like alcohol is always referred to as this 'liquid courage,' you know? And I guess it depends where you're at: courage to do what? Courage to ask a girl on a date that you hadn't had the courage to do before, or courage to dance like a fool on the floor, or is it courage to beat your wife or beat your girlfriend 'cause you didn't have the guts to do it before?"
>
> —College peer counselor

There are three major kinds of interpersonal violence, and one can escalate into another: emotional violence, physical violence, and sexual violence. The most common form of violence as well as the most underreported is emotional violence, which includes verbal abuse often caused by alcohol's freeing effect on the tongue.

"If you talk about someone being emotionally violated, who goes to jail for that? You don't have amy bruises that you can see, but there are scars there."

—36-year-old ex-wife of an alcoholic

Any type of violence can cause permanent biochemical changes in the victim that can make them more susceptible to drug abuse and other emotional problems. Magnetic resonance imaging (MRI) studies in 1997 at Yale and Harvard Universities showed that severely abused children had permanent changes to the brain. These changes often led to more behavioral problems, including hyperactivity, impulsive behavior, increased aggression, exaggerated fears and nightmares, trouble keeping a job, and difficulty with relationships. The studies showed that the changes could also be caused by severe emotional abuse.

"It doesn't matter if alcohol was in-volved in the situation. He raped me. There's more attention paid to the fact that there was alcohol involved than the fact that a woman was assaulted and that her life changed and that all of these things happened as a result of that. Alcohol's involved in almost every social situation, but it doesn't mean that we recognize it or validate it."

—22-year-old female college senior (rape victim)

Depending on the study, 34% to 74% of sexual-assault perpetrators had been drinking as had 30% to 79% of the victims. In most cases the perpetrator and the victim are drinking simul-taneously; rarely is the victim . drinking alone (Abbey, Zawacki, Buck, et al, 2001).

Driving Under The Influence

"An officer can pull up to a traffic light, and the person is staring straight ahead and their face is up against the wind-shield of the car. Those are all indicators that the person might be under the influence of intoxicants. The people whom we arrest try to stall as much as they can. They'll ask for a lawyer, they'll ask all kinds of questions, they'll try to let enough time go by. But it's been our experience that it doesn't help. The alcohol's gonna be in their system."

—Lt. Rich Walsh, Ashland, OR, Police Department

Approximately 40% of motor vehicle fatalities (16,885) in 2005 involved alcohol use. About 90% of those involved had a BAC of 0.08 or higher (le-gally drunk). Another 275,000 persons were in-jured in crashes where alcohol was present. Over the past 10 years, however, there has actually been an 18% drop in the rate of fatalities. In addition, of the 3 million traffic-related accidents, 1 million were alcohol related (Hingson & Winter, 2003; National Highway Traffic Safety Administration

[NHTSA], 2005 & 2006). According to the National Highway Traffic Safety Administration (NHTSA):

- more than 1 in 4 drivers gets behind the wheel within two hours of drinking;
- on any weekday night between 10 p.m. and 1 a.m., 1 in 13 drivers is legally drunk; on weekend mornings between 1 and 6 a.m., 1 in 7 drivers is drunk (Miller, Lestina & Spicer, 1996);
- of those convicted of DUI, 61% drank beer only, 2% drank wine only, 18% drank liquor only, and 20% drank more than one type of alcoholic beverage; and
- alcohol-related crashes cost an estimated $148 billion in the United States every year (NHTSA, 2005, NIAAA, 2000).

Because alcohol is a depressant, susceptibility to traffic accidents and fatalities is usually directly related to the blood alcohol level: coordination is decreased, and judgment is impaired. Some skills are impaired at even a 0.02 BAC, such as the ability to divide attention between two or more visual inputs. At a 0.05 BAC, eye movement, glare resistance, visual perception, and reaction time are affected (Moskowitz, Burns, Fiorentino, et al, 2000; Moskowitz & Fiorentino, 2000). Impairment for other forms of transportation also begins at relatively low BAC levels. Flight simulators show impaired pilot performance at 0.04 BAC and for up to 14 hours after reaching BACs between 0.10 and 0.12 (Yesavage & Leirer, 1986).

"A number of years ago, I did a test in which I brought a number of individuals down to the police department; I had them drink various amounts of alcohol and then drive a short obstacle course. Some were social drinkers and some didn't drink at all except on very rare occasions. What! found was this: One of the social drinkers felt he did the driving test fairly well and that he felt absolutely fine to drive. I told him I would have arrested him for driving under the influence. When I put him on the Breathalyzer machine, his was the highest blood alcohol of everybody there. This overconfidence in drinkers is fairly common. The people who didn't drink very often and actually had much less to drink than this individual were saying when they took the driving test, 'There's no way in the world that I'd drive.' Their Breathalyzer results were way under the limit."

—Traffic Safety Officer, Ashland, OR, Police department

The laws in the United States do not make exceptions. When the BAC is over the legal limit of 0.08, the officer does not have to prove that the person is impaired; the driver is guilty per se. Usually, though, an officer will first observe the driver for telltale signs; the officer will then pull the driver over and test coordination and physical abilities for physical or mental impairment before requiring a breath or blood test. One of the most effective tests given on the spot is the eye nystagmus test.

"For some reason alcohol affects the eyeballs, and the eyeball will start jerking if it tries to follow a moving finger or object. It's amazing: you can watch people's eyes just twitching away when they're under the influence. They can't follow the finger to the side; they're turning their whole head back and forth."

—Lt. Rich Walsh, Ashland, OR, Police
Department

Among those arrested for DUI, two-thirds have never been arrested before, so laws and programs have to be aimed at all segments of the population. In fact, a majority of drivers in fatal alcohol-related crashes did not have a DUI conviction on their record, and many did not have a history of problem drinking (Baker, Braver, Chen, et al., 2002; NHTSA, 2006). More important, only one driver is arrested for every 300 to 1,000 drunk-driving trips, so effective enforcement can be a daunting task (Voas, Wells, Lestina, et al., 1997).

Quite a few prevention strategies have reduced the number of alcohol-related traffic fatalities and injuries over the years:

- lowering the BAC limit from 0.10 to 0.08;
- imposing administrative license revocation in which a police officer or other official can immediately confiscate the license of a driver whose BAC exceeds the legal limit;
- increasing the minimum legal drinking age to 21 years;
- having zero-tolerance laws for drivers under 21 (i.e., prohibiting driving with any alcohol or a minimum of alcohol in the system [0.01 or 0.02 BAC for drivers under 21]); these laws have reduced alcohol-related crashes involving youth by 17% to 50%;
- impounding or towing vehicles of drunk drivers;
- requiring mandatory treatment for. DUI arrestees; and
- training alcohol servers and mandating sanctions and liability; legally servers have to stop serving drinkers who seem intoxicated.

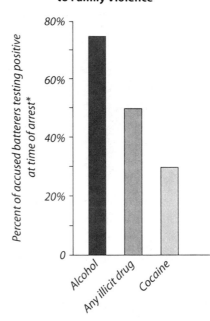

*Figures do not total 100% since many abusers take more than one substance.

FIGURE 8. Three out offour of those arrested for family violence tested positive for alcohol. Half had used some illicit drug, and more than one in four tested positive for cocaine. The National Research Council

There is no single prevention strategy that is most effective. The best results seem to occur with communitywide efforts when a combination of the above suggestions, along with media campaigns, police training, high school and college prevention programs, and better control of liquor sales, are implemented.

Injuries & Suicide

"I was medicating myself, covering it up. I would take a sports bottle of wine with me to work in the morning, and I was operating heavy machinery. I would go home for lunch, refill it, and come back and drive a forklift and operate this thing with spinning blades—and it's just insanity."

—40-year-old female recovering alcoholic

Medical examiner reports indicate that alcohol dramatically increases the risk of injury:

- Emergency room studies confirm that 15% to 25% of emergency patients tested positive for alcohol or reported alcohol use, with relatively high rates among those involved in fights, assaults, and falls.
- Alcoholics are 16 times more likely to die in falls and 10 times more likely to become burn or fire victims.
- The U.S. Coast Guard reported that 31% of boating fatalities had a BAC of 0.10 or more.
- In the workplace up to 40% of industrial fatalities and 47% of injuries involved alcohol. (Bernstein & Mahoney, 1989; National Clearinghouse on Alcohol and Drug Information [NCADI], 2006; SAMHSA, 2005)

"Putting a guy in the ground did nothing for our feeling indestructible, you know, kids that we were. That age of, 'God, we're young and strong and there's nothing we can't do. There are no consequences to this behavior.' And even seeing it, going to the funeral, watching the hearse drive by, it was like, 'Duh, didn't make the connection.'"

—40-year-old recovering alcoholic, concerning a friend who died while driving drunk

Among adult alcoholics, suicide rates are twice as high as for the general population and even greater than the non-mentally ill population; rates also increase with age. One reason for the increase in suicide with age is that the longer the alcoholism, the greater the social, health, and interpersonal problems. The alcoholic suicide victim is typically White, middle-aged, male, and unmarried with a long history of drinking. Additional risk factors for suicide include depression, loss of job, living alone, poor social support, and other illnesses.

"I just didn't want to live. I mean, my family and people that I love so much, I feel like they hated to see me coming, and it's something that I wouldn't wish on anybody to go through. I was drinking on a day-to-day basis, just drinking—and then I wound up at the hospital. I had tried to commit suicide, and they put me in the psych ward."

—38-year-old female recovering alcoholic

Epidemiology

Patterns Of Alcohol Consumption

It is difficult to get accurate, comparable, and consistent alcohol use data in other countries, but as Table 5-5 (earlier in this chapter) points out, most European countries have higher per-capita alcohol consumption rates than the United States while most Asian countries have lower per-capita consumption. These differences result from a combination of physiological, cultural, social, religious, and legal factors.

Culture is one of the main determinants of how a person drinks (Health-EU, 2006). Different drinking patterns are found in the so-called wet and dry drinking cultures in Europe and North

America (although some recent research suggests that the distinctions aren't as clear-cut as they were once thought to be).

Wet drinking cultures (e.g., Austria, Belgium, France, Italy, and Switzerland) sanction daily or almost daily use and integrate social drinking into everyday life. In France children are served watered-down wine at the dinner table (Vaillant, 1995). Wet cultures consume more wine and beer— five times the amount of wine drunk in dry cultures.

Dry drinking cultures (e.g., Denmark, Finland, Norway, and Sweden) restrict the availability of alcohol and tax it more heavily. Dry cultures consume more distilled spirits— almost 1.5 times the amount in wet cultures—and are characterized by binge-style drinking, particularly by males on weekends.

Canada, England, Germany, Ireland, the United States, and Wales exhibit combinations of both wet and dry cultures. In such mixed drinking cultures, patterns such as binge drinking in social situations are common. A relatively higher incidence of violence against women is found in mixed drinking cultures than in dry or wet cultures, probably because binge drinking often occurs in social situations.

Chinese families generally don't drink much, often because of cultural pressures. In Japan and South Korea, however, social pressures to drink are very strong. In Japan most of the men and half of the women drink, yet their alcoholism rate is half of that in the United States.

In Russia vodka is traditionally drunk in large quantities between meals. Vodka is the preferred drink because 500 years previously Czar Ivan the Terrible forcibly replaced the sale of beer and mead with state-controlled vodka, served in state-run taverns. Alcoholism became so rampant in Russia over the centuries that in 1985 Premier Mikhail Gorbachev severely restricted the availability of alcohol almost to the point of prohibition. The number of illegal stills and the consumption of anything with alcohol in it, such as shoe polish and insecticides, soared. In one year, despite prohibition, 11.000 Russians died of alcohol and alcohol-related poisonings. When many of the restrictions were lifted, the number of alcohol-poisoning deaths is reported to have soared to 40,000. When the restrictions had been in place, Russian male life expectancy started to increase. Once the restrictions were lifted, male life expectancy dropped six years. Drinking on the job is one of the major consequences of the easy availability of alcohol and a culture that has few recovery programs (Badkhen, 2003; Bobak, 1999; Courtwright, 2001; Davis, 1994; Segal, 1990).

In England recently about half the country's 60,000 pubs curbed the promotion of happy hours and removed the 11 p.m. closing hour, which had encouraged binge drinking and expelled thousands of drunks onto the streets at one time. These

TABLE 7. Bac Vs. Chances Of Being Killed In A Single-Vehicle Crash

Blood Alcohol Concentration	Chances of Being Killed
0.02-0.04	1.4 times normal
0.05-0.09	11.0 times normal
0.10-0.14	48.0 times normal
0.15 and above	380.0 times normal

Source: Zador, 1991

TABLE 8. Permissible Bac Limits In Other Countries

Country	Permissible BAC
United States	0.08
Austria, Canada, Germany, Switzerland, United Kingdom	0.08
Australia	0.05-0.08
Belgium, Finland, France, Israel, Netherlands	0.05
Japan	0.03
Poland, Sweden	0.02

are strong changes for a country with a tradition of warm beer and darts at the local pub. About 70% of Britons drink regularly, with two-thirds of the alcohol consumption in beer. In a recent campaign to stem alcoholism, Britons were urged to reduce their average daily consumption to just three drinks a day.

In the United States, much drinking is done in social settings away from lunch and dinner tables. In a land of many different cultures and lifestyles, there is a wide variety of culturally influenced drinking customs. The 18-to-25 age group is the most likely to binge drink (SAMHSA, 2006).

Population Subgroups

Men

In all age groups, men drink more per drinking episode than women do, regardless of the culture. Much of this difference has to do with the cultural acceptability of male drinking and the disapproval of female drinking. The other reason for the difference reflects men's ability to more efficiently metabolize higher amounts of alcohol. As expected, men also have more adverse social and legal consequences and develop problems with alcohol abuse or alcohol dependence at a higher rate than women.

Women

Women's alcohol problems become greater in their thirties, not in their twenties as for men (Blume & Zilberman, 2005). Alcohol-dependent women as a group drink about one-third less alcohol than alcohol-dependent men (Center for Science in the Public Interest, 2006).

The magnitude of the genetic influence in women from one or two alcoholic parents hasn't been as widely examined as in men, but a survey

of research seems to indicate a similar genetic susceptibility between men and women (Prescott, 2002). In fact, the rate of alcoholism in relatives of females diagnosed with alcoholism is somewhat higher than in relatives of male alcoholics.

Several studies demonstrate that even low levels of drinking in women with a certain genetic susceptibility can result in major health consequences such as an increase in breast cancer (Thun, Peto, Lopez, et al, 1997; Zhang, Lee, Manson, et al, 2007). Proportionally more women than men die from cirrhosis of the liver, circulatory disorders, suicide, and accidents. As mentioned, female alcoholics have a 50% to 100% higher death rate than male alcoholics. But just as health problems develop after sustained heavy drinking, some health disorders, especially depression, may precede heavy drinking and even contribute to it. Also, because women get higher BACs than men from the same amount of alcohol drunk, negative health consequences develop faster for women than for men (Maher, 1997; NIAAA, 1997; Register, Cline & Shively, 2002).

Because society more readily accepts the alcoholic male but disdains the alcoholic female, women are less likely to seek treatment for alcoholism but are quicker to utilize mental health services when, in fact, their primary problem is alcohol or other drugs. Women are also more likely to enter treatment when their physical or mental health is suffering, whereas men are more likely to seek treatment when they have problems with their employment or with the law (Gomberg, 1991; Kinney, 2005; Ross, 1989).

Adolescents

Adolescence is often a time when one feels invulnerable or at the very least does not give full credence to the cautions of others. Drinking alcohol and smoking tobacco are the two most obvious activities. All research seems to indicate that the younger one starts smoking or drinking, the more likely he or she will have a problem with tobacco or alcohol later in life. Almost one-third of all teenagers report having their first drink before they were 13 years old, most often due to peer encouragement.

> "I was a city kid, and it was pretty muck a standard rite of passage when you're 12, 13, 14 to, you know, one way or another get your hands on a six-pack for a Saturday night—and that's how drinking started for all of us in my neighborhood."

> —22-year-old recovering alcoholic

In a major survey of students, Monitoring the Future, the percentage of teenagers who had been drunk in the past month:

eighth grade	6.2%
tenth grade	18.8%
twelfth grade	30.0%

Interestingly, the percentages that reported daily use were only 0.5%, 1.3%, and 3.1%, respectively, emphasizing the binge nature of teenage drinking (Johnston, O'Malley, Bachman, et al, 2006C).

Adolescent binge drinkers were also 17 times more likely to smoke than non-binge drinkers, a combination that can aggravate one's health with gastrointestinal, respiratory, or other problems.

The three most popular locations for adolescent drinking were in someone's home, outdoors, and in a moving car or truck. The latter two choices often lead to driving under the influence (Windle, 2003).

Because adolescence is a time of intense emotional growth, the disin-hibiting effects of alcohol can encourage unsafe sexual practices, which lead to higher rates of unplanned pregnancies, sexual aggression, and sexually transmitted diseases.

Adolescents' heavy involvement in alcohol (and other drugs) tends to limit emotional growth; so, when they stop using, they often have remained emotionally the same age as when they started. Recovery is therefore not just a matter of stopping use but also learning what they failed to grasp during their use.

College Students & Learning

> "We drank quite a bit in my dorm and, generally, when somebody came into my dorm room on a weekend night, you had to take a bong—a beer bong. And we'd have the funnel that held like two and a half beers, and it was just the rule. We kinda pressured people to keep up, like you had to stay with the crowd."

> —College student in his junior year

It used to be that only college students, away from the control of their parents, began heavy drinking. But in the 1990s and 2000s, the age of first use and heavy use dropped to where many students had "done it all" by the time they finished their senior year in high school. Studies have shown that the majority of students (as high as 86%) kept the same pattern of drinking from high school to College (Reifman & Watson, 2003). In college many of them refined those habits or cut back. The problem is that because so much development takes place during high school and college years, drinking usually has negative effects on learning and maturation.

> "Often it's the style of drinking, not experimentation, that gets college students in trouble. Many think the name of the game is to get drunk. They drink

too fast, they drink without eating, they play drinking games or contests, or they binge drink. But because they drink heavily only once or twice a week, they think that there is no problem. But there usually is a problem: lower grades, disciplinary action, or behavior they regret, which usually means sexual behavior."

—Shauna Quinn, drug and alcohol counselor, California State University, Chico

Forty-four percent of college students admit to binge drinking at least once every two weeks (Wechsler, Lee, Kuo, et al, 2002). Binge drinking (many students, particularly males, object to the term) is defined as having five or more drinks at one sitting for males, four for females. About half of the students in one study who admitted to binge drinking also admitted that their grades fell into the C-to-F range. Many binge drinkers missed classes on a regular basis (O'Malley & Johnston, 2002). In a national study, there was a direct correlation between the number of drinks consumed per week and the grade-point average (Table 5-11).

Notice that women's grades start to deteriorate at slightly less than half the drinking level it takes for men's grades to go down. The National Household Survey on Drug Abuse (Figure 5-10) indicates that the higher the level of educational attainment, the more likely was the current use (not necessarily abuse) of alcohol. This seems a contradiction with the statistics about grade performance; however, the rate of heavy alcohol use in the 18-to-34 age group among those who had not completed high school was twice that of those who had completed college. In general, college students learn to moderate their drinking before they graduate.

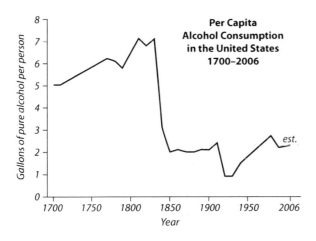

FIGURE 9. In the United States, the per-capita consumption of pure alcohol at present is 2.2 gallons, but, as this chart shows, the rate has varied wildly with the rise and fall of prohibition movements, health concerns, and availability of a good water supply.

Adapted from David F. Musto's "Alcohol in American History," Scientific American, April 1996 (SAMHSA, 2006)

"Secondhand drinking is a large problem on a college campus, and it is a problem on our campus. We have a lot of students complain about their roommate or their boyfriend or girlfriend you know, being drunk, violence occurring, vandalism occurring, being unable to study, having to stay up all night with that person who may have had too much to drink and they need to stay with them to make sure they make it through the night and they don't die from alcohol poisoning."

—Shauna Quinn, drug and alcohol counselor, California State University, Chico

"I guess studying on the weekends was a lot more difficult because a lot of people tend to party and drink a lot more, People banging on the walls and coming into your room, trying to get you to come out and party with them. On a Friday or Saturday night,you had to take your studies elsewhere."

—College senior, Southern Oregon University

In general:

- male students binge somewhat more than female students (48.6% to 40.9%);
- white students (50.2%) are more likely to binge than Hispanic (34.4%), Asian/Pacific Islander (26.2%), or Black (21.7%) students; and
- fraternity members (75.4%) drink more than dormitory residents (45.3%), off-campus residents (54.5%o), or married

residents (26.5%) (Wechsler, Lee, Kuo, et al., 2002).

Unfortunately, the tendency to binge drink in college leads to about 1,700 deaths per year, 696,000 physical assaults, 599,000 injuries, and 97,000 sexual assaults (Hingson, Heeren, Winter, et al., 2005).

Older Americans

"I visited my granddad in the retirement center/nursing home when he was 93 years old. He showed me the medicine cabinet. It was a small closet that, when opened by a nurse, revealed dozens of bottles of alcohol—whiskey, rum, scotch, vodka, and a variety of wines—each one with the name of one of the elderly residents, depending on the health of the patient, they could have one or two

TABLE 9. Alcohol Abuse Or Dependence Within The Past Month

	Males	Females
Any alcohol use	58.19%	45.9%
Binge drinkers	30.5%	15.2% (5 or more drinks on the same occasion at least once in the past 30 days)
Heavy drinkers	10.3%	3.1% (5 or more drinks per day at least 5 or more days in the past 30 days)

Source: SAMSHA, 2006

TABLE 10. Women & Alcohol Problems

More Likely to Have Drinking Problems	Less Likely to Have Drinking Problems
Younger women	Older women (60+)
Loss of role (mother, job)	Multiple roles (married, stable, work outside the home)
Never married	Married
Divorced, separated	Widowed
Unmarried and living with a partner	Children in the home
White women	Black women
Using other drugs	Hispanic women
Experiencing sexual dysfunction	Nondrinking spouse
Victim of childhood sexual abuse	

Source: National Institute on Drug Abuse, 1994

drinks a day for their health. He was still healthy at 96 when a fall killed him."

—42-year-old grandson

People who are 65 years or older constitute the fastest-growing segment of the U.S. population. From 6% to 21% of elderly hospital patients, 20% of elderly psychiatric patients, and 14% of elderly emergency room patients exhibit symptoms of alcoholism (American Medical Association, 1996). One study indicates that approximately 2.5 million older adults have alcohol-related problems (NIAAA, 2004).

Research indicates that patterns of drinking persist into old age and that the amount and the frequency of drinking are a result of general trends in society rather than the aging process. Hip fractures, one of the most debilitating injuries that occurs to the elderly, increase with alcohol consumption mainly due to decreases in bone density caused by the deleterious effects of alcohol (Adams, Yuan, Barboriak, et al., 1993; Blow, 2003). In nursing homes as many as 49% of the patients have drinking problems, although some nursing homes are used to hospitalize problem drinkers, so the rate may seem higher than the general population (Joseph, 1997). Another problem is that, the average American over 65 years old takes two to seven prescription medications daily, so alcohol/prescription drug interactions among older people are quite common (Korrapati & Vestal, 1995). Pharmacologic research has found more than 150 prescription and over-the-counter medications that interact negatively with alcohol (NIAAA, 2003).

About one-third of elderly alcohol abusers are of the late-onset variety (Rigler, 2000). Some older people may increase their drinking because of isolation, retirement, more leisure time, financial pressures, depression over health, loss of friends or a spouse, lack of a day-to-day structure, or simply the access to and availability of alcohol in the home or at friends' homes. The elderly alcohol abuser is less likely to be in contact with a workplace, the criminal justice system, or drug-abuse treatment providers. Thus it may be more difficult to identify elderly abusers and get them help. This is also because of a more tolerant attitude toward drinking by the elderly. The common reaction is So what, if they are heavy drinkers? At their age, they deserve it They ve contributed to society and what harm could it do now anyway?

"Give strong drink unto him that is ready to perish, and wine unto those that be of heavy hearts."
—Proverbs 37:6

Diagnosis of drug or alcohol problems in the elderly is often difficult because of the coexistence of other physical or mental problems that become much more prevalent due to the aging process. Dementia, depression, hypertension, arrhythmia, psychosis, and panic disorder are just some of the conditions whose symptoms are mimicked by either the use of or the withdrawal from alcohol and other drugs (Gambert, 2005). It is often up to the physicians seeing these patients for medical conditions to recognize alcohol problems and do brief interventions to get them help.

Even with all the reasons and the pressures to drink, however, people 65 and older have the lowest prevalence of problem drinking and alcoholism. There are several reasons for the lower rates:

- People who become alcohol abusers or alcoholics usually do so before the age of 65, suggesting a high degree of self-correction or spontaneous remission with age.
- Cutting down on drinking or giving up drinking may be related to the relatively high cost of alcohol for those on a fixed income.

- The body is less able to handle alcohol because liver function declines with age. The general aging process also decreases tolerance and slows metabolism, so the older drinker often has to limit intake.
- Side effects are increased if someone is ill or is taking medications thus encouraging temperance.

"For certainly, old age has a great sense of calm and freedom; when the passions relax their hold, then, as Sophocles says we are freed from the grasp not of one mad master only, but of many."

—Plato, *The Republic*, 30 B.C.E
(translated by Benjamin Jowett)

TABLE 11. Average Number Of Drinks Per Week, By Grade Average

Grade Average	Drinks Per Week		
	Males	Females	Overall
A	5.4	2.3	3.3
B	7.4	3.4	5.0
C	9.2	4.1	6.6
DorF	14.6	5.2	10.1

Source: College Core Study of 56 four-year and 22 two-year colleges by Southern Illinois University, Carbondale, 1993

College Binge Drinking in the 1990s

A Continuing Problem Results of the Harvard School of Public Health 1999 College Alcohol Study

By Henry Wechsler, PhD; Jae Eun Lee, DrPH; Meichun Kuo, ScD; Hang Lee, PhD

Abstract: *In 1999, the Harvard School of Public Health College Alcohol Study resurveyed colleges that participated in the 1993 and 1997 surveys. Responses to mail questionnaires from more than 14000 students at 119 nationally representative 4-year colleges in 39 states were compared with responses received in 1997 and 1993. Two of 5 students (44%) were binge drinkers in 1999, the same rate as in 1993. However, both abstention and frequent binge-drinking rates increased significantly. In 1999, 19% were abstainers, and 23% were frequent binge drinkers. As before, binge drinkers, and particularly frequent binge drinkers, were more likely than other students to experience alcohol-related problems. At colleges with high binge-drinking rates, students who did not binge drink continued to be at higher risk of encountering the secondhand effects of others' heavy drinking. The continuing high level of binge drinking is discussed in the context of the heightened attention and increased actions at colleges. Although it may take more time for interventions to take effect, the actions college health providers have undertaken thus far may not be a sufficient response.*

Key Words: *alcohol-related problems, binge drinking, college students, secondhand effects of binge drinking*

In 1993, the Harvard School of Public Health College Alcohol Study (CAS) surveyed a random sample of students at 140 colleges in 39 states and the District of Columbia. The survey constituted the first attempt to study drinking patterns in a nationally representative sample of college students.

The findings, first published in December 1994,[1] received widespread national attention.

The study's authors described a style of drinking that they designated as "binge" drinking, defined as the consumption of five or more drinks in a row for men and four or more for women,

Henry Weschsler, Jae Eun Lee, Meichun Kuo, & Hang Lee, "College Binge Drinking in the 1990s: A Continuing Problem—Results of the Harvard School of Public Health 1999 College Alcohol Study," *American Journal of College Health*, vol. 48, issue 5, pp. 199-21. Copyright © 2000. Reprinted with permission.

at least once in the 2 weeks preceding the survey. The tern hinge drinking was used by Wechsler and colleagues several years before in a study of Massachusetts college students' alcohol use.[2] The term is now used in the media as a catchword to designate college drinking that leads to serious problems. Following the publication of the initial CAS results, there was greater media attention to alcohol-related tragedies among college students, including deaths in a variety of circumstances: acute alcohol poisonings, falls, drownings, automobile collisions, fires, and hypothermia resulting from exposure. Such drastic consequences underscore the multitude of other, less severe, outcomes of binge drinking.

Heightened public interest in binge drinking prompted changes in the way colleges addressed the problem. Until the mid-1990s, student drinking issues were largely the responsibility of alcohol educators and deans of students. Since then, in association with extensive media coverage and the release of several national studies of drinking behavior, college presidents are often involved. Many of them are frequently included in statewide and regional coalitions that address the problem jointly.

Other indications that college alcohol issues have been placed on the national agenda are such developments as passage of a resolution by the US House of Representatives and the Senate to address binge drinking; a National Institute on Alcoholism and Alcohol Abuse special task force on college drinking, as well as a special grant program to focus on this issue; a Centers for Disease Control and Prevention (CDC) health risk survey for college students; and frequent features on binge drinking in major television network news magazine programs. The Robert Wood Johnson Foundation has established an initiative, the Matter of Degree program, which provides funding to universities to develop comprehensive environmental-change approaches by establishing college/community coalitions to address the problem of student drinking.

In 1997, the CAS survey of students was repeated at the original colleges with new samples. That survey found little change in the intervening 4 years in the overall rates of binge drinking. For the 116 colleges in that analysis, a minor drop occurred in the proportion of binge drinkers, from 44.1% in 1993 to 42.7% in 1997. However, the study uncovered an increase in the prevalence of both frequent binge drinking and abstention. A polarization effect was observed, resulting in two sizable groups of students on campus: those who did not drink at all (19%) and those who binge drank three or more times in a 2-week period (21%). Students in the latter group of frequent binge drinkers were found to consume a median of 14.5 drinks per week, and this group accounted for 68% of all the alcohol consumed by college students.[3]

Despite all of the attention focused on binge drinking by colleges and the media and the initial actions to reduce alcohol-related problems, little change in student drinking levels occurred on the national level between 1993 and 1997. The CAS was repeated in 1999 to examine overall levels of binge drinking and to determine whether the trend toward increased polarization of drinking behavior on campus had continued.

Method

Sample of Colleges

In 1999, we resurveyed 128 schools from the original list of 140 colleges that were surveyed in 1993 and the 130 colleges surveyed in 1997. The 128 schools were located in 39 states and the District of Columbia. The original 1993 sample was selected from a list of accredited 4-year colleges provided by the American Council on

Education. The sample was selected using probability sampling proportionate to the size of undergraduate enrollment at each institution. In 1999, we obtained student samples using the same procedures we had used in the first two surveys. Details of the sample and research design of the 1993 and 1997 surveys are described elsewhere.[1,4]

In 1999, as in the previous surveys, we asked administrators at each college to provide a random sample of 225 undergraduates drawn from the total enrollment of full-time students. The attrition of 10 colleges in 1997 and 2 colleges in 1999 was primarily the result of the college administrators' inability to provide a random sample of students and their mailing addresses to us within the time requirements for the study.

In conducting the data analyses, we excluded schools that failed to meet the minimal criteria for response rate. To be part of the 3-year comparison sample described in this report, a school had to have a response rate of at least 50% in two of the three surveys and a rate of at least 40% in the third. For all 3 survey years, 119 schools met these criteria, and we dropped 9 from the analyses. When we compared the binge-drinking rates of the 119 retained in 1999 with the corresponding rates of all 128 participating in 1999, we found that they were identical. Dropping the low-response schools did not change the results of the survey. Similar comparisons for the 1997 and 1993 rates of these schools with those of the total samples in those years also revealed no differences.

The sample of 119 colleges presents a national cross-section of 4-year colleges. Two thirds of the colleges sampled are public institutions, and one third are private. In terms of student enrollments, two fifths of the schools (44%) are large (more than 10000 students), one fifth (23%) are medium sized (5001 to 10000 students), and nearly one third (34%) are small (5000 students or fewer). About two thirds are located in an urban or suburban setting and one third are in small-town or rural settings. Fifteen percent are affiliated with a religious denomination, and 5% enroll women only.

Questionnaire

The 1999 survey repeated standard questions used in 1993 and 1997 about alcohol, tobacco, and other drug use, as well as lifestyle, demographic, and other background characteristics. These questions were adapted from previous large-scale, national studies.[2,5,6] The questionnaire instructed participants to define a drink in equivalent amounts of alcohol: a 12-oz (360 mL) bottle or can of beer, a 4-oz (120 mL) glass of wine, a 12-oz (360 mL) bottle or can of wine cooler, or a shot of liquor (1.25 oz or 37 mL), either straight or in a mixed drink. Questions also inquired about students' experiences with prevention programs and school alcohol and tobacco policies.

The Measure of Binge Drinking

Heavy episodic or binge drinking was defined as the consumption of at least five drinks in a row for men or four drinks in a row for women during the 2 weeks before the completion of the questionnaire. In the past decade, large-scale epidemiologic studies of youth alcohol use have employed five drinks in a row as a measure of heavy drinking, and this has become a standard measure in both secondary school populations [the University of Michigan's National Institute of Drug Abuse (NIDA)-sponsored Monitoring the Future study[5]] and college populations (Core Institute Survey,[7] National College Health Risk Behavior Survey[8]). In an analysis of the 1993 CAS data,[9] a gender-specific definition ("five/four") of binge drinking provided a measure of equivalent alcohol-related problems for college men and women.

The CAS gender-specific measure of binge drinking was constructed from responses to four questions: (a) gender; (b) recency of last drink; (c) drinking five or more drinks during the past 2 weeks; and (d) drinking four or more drinks during the past 2 weeks. Missing data for any of these questions resulted in the exclusion of that student's responses from the analysis of binge drinking. We excluded 2.6% of the responses in 1993, 1.4% in 1997, and 2.3% in 1999.

We defined *frequent binge drinker*s as those students who had binged three or more times in the past 2 weeks (or more than once a week, on average), *occasional binge drinkers* were those students who had binged one or two times in the same period. *Nonbinge drinkers* were those students who had consumed alcohol in the past year but had not binged in the previous 2 weeks, and *abstainers* were those students who had consumed no alcohol in the past year.

Students who had consumed alcohol in the past 30 days were asked to report on the number of occasions they had a drink of alcohol in the past month. The response categories were 1 to 2 occasions, 3 to 5 occasions, 6 to 9 occasions, 10 to 19 occasions, 20 to 39 occasions, and 40 or more occasions. In response to a question asking whether getting drunk was a reason for drinking, students who responded very important, important, or somewhat important, as opposed to not important, were considered to have the drinking style of "drinking to get drunk." High school binge drinking was defined as the amount of alcohol usually consumed during the last year of high school, using the same five/four measure.

Students who drank alcohol in the past year were asked a series of questions about their experiences with alcohol-related problems during the current school year, including 12 health and behavioral consequences of one's own drinking. All students were asked 8 questions about the consequences of other students' drinking

(secondhand effects). We examined these secondhand effects among students who were not binge drinkers (nonbinge drinkers and abstainers) and lived on campus (ie, were residents of on-campus dormitories or fraternity/sorority houses). In this article, data on alcohol-related sexual assaults and unwanted sexual advances, problems that most frequently affect women, are presented for women only. We divided colleges into high-binge institutions (more than 50% of students are binge drinkers); middle-binge level (36%-50%), and low-binge (35% or lower) on the basis of the aggregated binge-drinking behavior of their students.

Mailing and Response Rate

In all three surveys, questionnaires were mailed directly to students at the end of February. Three separate mailings were sent within a 3-week period: first a questionnaire, then a remmder postcard, followed by a second questionnaire. Mailings were timed to avoid the period immediately preceding and following spring break so that students would be responding to questions concerning their behavior during a time when they were on campus. The students' responses were voluntary and anonymous. The study therefore received exempt status from the institutional review committees. To encourage students to respond, we offered an award of one $1,000 prize to a student whose name was drawn from among students responding within 1 week; a $500 award and 10 $100 awards were offered to students whose names were drawn from a pool of all who responded.

Response rates varied among the colleges that participated in the 1993, 1997, and 1999 surveys. Average response rates were 60% in 1999 (range = 49%-83%), 60% in 1997 (range = 40%-88%), and 70% in 1993 (range = 41%-100%).

We used two procedures to examine potential bias introduced by nonresponders. The response rates at individual colleges were not associated with their binge-drinking rates. The Pearson correlation coefficient between a college's binge rate and its response rate was -.029 (p = .753) in 1999, .006 (p = .949) in 1997, and -.014 (p = .879) in 1993. In addition, we adjusted for response rates in the multiple logistic regression models in all of the analyses.

Data Analysis

We used chi-square analysis to compare student characteristics and outcomes of interest between the 3 survey years. Prevalence of outcomes over the 3 survey years was indicated by percentages and their percentage changes, and tested for significance, using the chi-square test. We employed logistic regression to assess the odds of an alcohol-related problem or behavior for binge drinkers compared with nonbinge drinkers. In this article, we report adjusted odds ratios (ORs) and 95% confidence intervals for student and college characteristics, based on the logistic regression model. In addition, we employed the generalized estimating equations (GEE)[10,11] approach to fitting the logistic regression models. Because it uses the clustered outcomes appropriate to our sampling scheme, the GEE provides more robust standard errors of the OR estimates. The GEE procedure resulted in little or no difference in the estimated ORs, compared with the ordinary logistic regression models, and provided slightly greater standard errors of the estimate. When appropriate, we used the GEE-based standard errors to perform the significance tests. We also used this method in the time-trend analysis of frequent binge drinking and abstaining over the three surveys, adjusting for class year, sex, and race.

Four percent of the participants were sampled in both the 1997 and 1999 surveys. However, we found no statistical evidence of reduced variation in the sample resulting from these duplicated respondents, and therefore they remained in the analysis.

To facilitate comparisons between the 1993, 1997, and 1999 data, we used data from only those respondents at the 119 schools that met the inclusion criteria for relatively high response rates in all survey years. Thus, the 1999 findings are slightly different (usually 1% or less) from those previously reported in articles reporting data for the 140 colleges in 1993[1] and the 116 colleges[3] in 1997.

Results

Composition of the Student Samples

In 1999, 3 of 5 (61%) respondents were women. This was higher than the national rates (55%) of undergraduate women at 4-year institutions.[12] Perhaps this was attributable, at least in part, to the inclusion of 6 women's colleges. Four of 5 (78%) of the respondents were White, and 15% were more than 23 years of age. The background characteristics of the students at the 119 colleges were similar to those found in 1993 and 1997. However, because each of the three survey samples consisted of more than 14000 students, even small differences were statistically significant (Table 1).

In 1999, the proportion of women in the CAS was higher than in 1993 and 1997, and the proportion of White and older students in 1999 was lower than in 1993 and 1997. Because both of these demographic characteristics were associated with drinking outcome, we controlled the multi-variate comparisons of drinking and other behaviors in the three survey samples for those characteristics.

Student Drinking Behavior

Data on drinking patterns of students in the three surveys are presented in Table 2. In 1999, as in previous years, approximately 2 of 5 students' self-reported drinking behaviors met our criteria for

TABLE 1
Repeated Measures Binge-Drinking Rate
Among 119 Schools (N= 476)

Variable	Coeff	SE	p
Intercept (rate in 1993)	0.4388	0.0232	<.0001
Year (0, 4, 6, 8)	0.0033	0.0028	.2483
Response rate			
High (> 70%)	Reference		—
Middle (50–70%)	−0.0239	0.0318	.4516
Low (< 50%)	2.6254	2.3185	.2575
Year × Low Response			
Rate interaction	−0.0274	0.0239	.2515

Note. Year was coded as 0 (1993), 4 (1997), 6 (1999), and 8 (2001).

TABLE 2
College Student Patterns of Alcohol Use: 1993, 1997, 1999, and 2001

Drinking pattern	% prevalence in each survey				Change over time		Test for linear time trend p
	1993[a]	1997[b]	1999[c]	2001[d]	2001 vs 1993 OR	95% CI	
Past year drinking							
Total	83.6	80.3	79.8	80.7	0.82	0.76, 0.89***	<.0001
Female	82.9	79.7	80.5	81.3	0.90	0.81, 0.99*	.0039
Male	84.2	81.0	79.0	79.9	0.75	0.66, 0.84***	<.0001
Binge drinkers							
Total	43.9	43.2	44.5	44.4	1.02	0.96, 1.09	.4354
Female	39.0	38.4	39.4	40.9	1.08	1.00, 1.17	.1078
Male	49.2	48.5	50.2	48.6	0.97	0.89, 1.07	.9970
Abstainers							
Total	16.4	19.6	19.8	19.3	1.22	1.13, 1.32***	<.0001
Female	17.0	20.3	19.2	18.7	1.12	1.02, 1.24*	.0042
Male	15.7	18.9	20.5	20.1	1.35	1.19, 1.52***	<.0001
Non–binge drinkers							
Total	39.7	37.2	35.7	36.3	0.86	0.81, 0.92***	<.0001
Female	44.0	41.4	41.4	40.4	0.87	0.80, 0.93***	<.0001
Male	35.1	32.6	29.4	31.3	0.85	0.77, 0.93***	<.0001
Occasional binge drinkers							
Total	24.3	22.2	21.9	21.6	0.86	0.80, 0.92***	<.0001
Female	21.9	19.4	19.2	20.0	0.89	0.81, 0.97**	.0005
Male	26.8	25.3	24.9	23.4	0.84	0.75, 0.93***	.0004
Frequent binge drinkers							
Total	19.7	21.0	22.6	22.8	1.21	1.13, 1.30***	<.0001
Female	17.1	18.9	20.3	20.9	1.28	1.17, 1.40***	<.0001
Male	22.4	23.2	25.3	25.2	1.16	1.05, 1.29***	.0006

Note. OR = odds ratio; CI = confidence interval.
[a]n = 15,282. [b]n = 14,428. [c]n = 13,954. [d]n = 10,904.
*p < .05; **p < .01; ***p < .001.

binge drinking. The proportion of binge drinkers, therefore, did not change among most student subgroups between 1993 and 1999, with two notable exceptions. Binge drinking decreased among dormitory residents and increased among students living off campus (Table 3).

Even though the overall rate of binge drinking did not change between 1993 and 1999, other changes were evident. In 1999, drinking on college campuses continued a trend toward becoming more strongly polarized: almost 1 in 5 students (19%) was an abstainer, and almost 1 in 4 (23%) was a frequent binge drinker. The numbers of students in these two groups increased over the 3 survey years. To examine the 1993 to 1999 trends among abstainers and frequent binge drinkers, adjusting for year in class, race, and sex, we used the GEE. The result showed a significant

TABLE 3
Patterns of College Student Binge Drinking Among Subpopulations, 1993, 1997, 1999, and 2001

| Characteristic | % prevalence in each survey | | | | Change over time | | Test for linear time trend *p* |
| | 1993[a] | 1997[b] | 1999[c] | 2001[d] | 2001 vs 1993 | | |
					OR	95% CI	
Gender							
Female	39.0	38.4	39.4	40.9	1.08	1.00,1.17	.1078
Male	49.2	48.5	50.2	48.6	0.97	0.89,1.07	.9970
Ethnicity							
Non-Hispanic	44.3	43.7	44.8	45.2	1.04	0.97,1.12	.2620
Hispanic	39.7	37.7	41.0	34.4	0.80	0.65,0.97*	.2166
White	49.5	48.2	50.1	50.2	1.03	0.96,1.11	.3406
Black/African American	16.7	18.5	17.5	21.7	1.38	0.97,1.68	.1455
Asian/Pacific Islander	23.1	24.4	23.3	26.2	1.18	0.88,1.57	.4384
Native American Indian/ Other	39.3	37.9	42.6	33.6	0.78	0.65,0.94**	.1812
Age (y)							
<21	45.5	44.6	44.9	43.6	0.93	0.85,1.01	.1172
21–23	48.1	47.5	50.3	50.2	1.09	0.98,1.20	.0558
≥24	28.5	28.8	29.1	30.9	1.12	0.92,1.37	.3325
Year in school							
Freshman	42.9	42.8	42.0	42.4	0.98	0.85,1.12	.6591
Sophomore	45.4	44.6	44.9	42.8	0.90	0.80,1.01	.1281
Junior	44.4	44.8	46.3	45.9	1.06	0.94,1.20	.2375
Senior	42.8	41.7	45.6	44.9	1.09	0.97,1.21	.0645
Residence							
Non-substance-free residence hall	46.7	45.8	44.5	45.3	0.94	0.85,1.05	.1478
Substance-free residence hall	34.7	32.5	32.1	35.3	1.03	0.80,1.33	.9912
Fraternity/sorority	83.4	82.6	80.3	75.4	0.61	0.42,0.89*	.0237
Off campus, alone, or with a roommate	54.1	53.5	56.2	54.5	1.02	0.89,1.15	.4451
Off campus, with a spouse	18.5	20.8	22.9	26.5	1.60	1.24,2.05***	.0002
Off campus, with parents	29.7	28.3	29.8	30.1	1.02	0.88,1.18	.8096
Fraternity/sorority member	67.4	67.4	65.2	64.3	0.87	0.74,1.03	.1030

Note. OR = odds ratio; CI = confidence interval.
[a] *n* = 15,282. [b] *n* = 14,428. [c] *n* = 13,954. [d] *n* = 10,904.
**p* < .05; * *p* < .01; ** *p* < .001.

increase in abstainers during the 4-year period from 1993 to 1997 (OR = 1.21, *p* < .0001) and no change (OR = 0.97, *p* = .51) during the 2-year period from 1997 to 1999. Overall, we observed a significant increase in the number of abstainers from 1993 to 1999 (OR = 1.18, *p* < .0001). The number of frequent binge drinkers significantly increased during the 4-year period, 1993 to 1997 (OR = 1.11, *p* < .0126), and continued to increase significantly during the 2-year period, 1997 to 1999 (OR = 1.01, *p* = .024). Overall, we noted a significant increase in frequent binge drinkers from 1993 to 1999 (OR = 1.20, *p* < .0001).

When we took student characteristics into account, the rise in abstention and frequent binge drinking was significant between 1993 and 1999 in most student subgroups. The growth in abstention between 1993 and 1997 was significant in both men (*p* < .001) and women (*p* < .001). However, an increase in the numbers of women who abstained occurred in 1997, whereas the increase in men's abstaining was significant in both 1997 and 1999 (*p* < .001, see Table 4). A significant rise in abstention was reported among Hispanic (*p* < .001), African American (*p* < .05), Asian (*p* < .05), freshmen students (*p* < .05), and in residents

TABLE 4
Drinking Styles of Students Who Consumed Alcohol, 1993, 1997, 1999, and 2001

| | % prevalence in each survey | | | | Change over time | | |
| | | | | | 2001 vs 1993 | | Test for linear |
Drinking style	1993[a]	1997[b]	1999[c]	2001[d]	OR	95% CI	time trend p
Drank on 10 or more occasions in the past 30 days							
Total	18.1	21.1	23.1	22.6	1.33	1.21, 1.46***	< .0001
Women	12.3	15.1	16.4	16.8	1.44	1.27, 1.64***	< .0001
Men	23.9	27.2	30.1	29.2	1.31	1.14, 1.50***	< .0001
Was drunk ≥ 3 times in the past 30 days							
Total	23.4	29.0	30.2	29.4	1.36	1.25, 1.48***	< .0001
Women	18.9	24.4	25.0	24.6	1.40	1.26, 1.55***	< .0001
Men	28.0	33.6	35.8	34.9	1.38	1.22, 1.57***	< .0001
Drinks to get drunk†							
Total	39.9	53.5	47.7	48.2	1.40	1.31, 1.51***	< .0001
Women	35.6	48.4	42.4	42.4	1.33	1.23, 1.45***	< .0001
Men	44.4	59.1	53.8	55.2	1.54	1.39, 1.71***	< .0001

Note. Only students who drank alcohol in the last year are included. OR = odds ratio; CI = confidence interval.
†Report that drinking "to get drunk" is an important reason for drinking.
[a]$n = 12,708.$ [b]$n = 11,506.$ [c]$n = 10,825.$ [d]$n = 8,783.$
*** $p < .001.$

of dormitories ($p < .001$) and fraternity/sorority houses ($p < .01$). In the meantime, a significant rise in frequent binge drinking occurred among students who were binge drinkers in high school.

The data in Table 5 show changes in the prevalence of binge drinking in terms of college characteristics. In comparing colleges in various categories according to characteristics of the institution, we found that the prevalence of binge drinking at most types of colleges did not change between 1993 and 1999. Where significant changes emerged, as in the case of competitive standings of institutions, there was no clear pattern or direction of change. The abstainer and frequent binge-drinker rates at most types of colleges increased between 1993 and 1997 and did not change between 1997 and 1999. The rise in both abstention and frequent binge drinking between 1993 and 1999 occurred in most college subgroups (Table 6).

From 1993 to 1999, an increase in binge-drinking rates was observed at 53% of the 119 participating

colleges but was statistically significant at only 7 schools (6%). A decrease in binge-drinking rates was observed at almost an equal number of participating colleges (47%) and was statistically significant for only 8 schools (7%). Thus, the results indicating no change among students at all colleges are reinforced when individual colleges are examined.

The polarization in college drinking appeared when we examined data from individual colleges from 1993 to 1999. An increase in abstention was observed at 3 out of 4 colleges (77%), and was statistically significant for 19 (16%) schools. This was in contrast to decreases in abstainers at only 23% of the colleges; none of the decreases reached statistical significance. An increase in frequent binge drinkers was observed at 83 (70%) out of 119 colleges and was statistically significant for 11% of schools. On the other hand, we observed a decrease in frequent binge drinkers at only 30% of colleges. It was statistically significant for only 3 (3%) schools.

TABLE 5
Changes in Binge-Drinking Rates Among Women at All-Women's and Coeducational Colleges, 1993, 1997, 1999, 2001

Variable	1993	1997	1999	2001	OR	95% CI†
% of students in						
all-women's schools	2.8	4.5	4.5	4.7		
Binge						
All-women's	24.5	27.4	29.8	32.1	1.36	0.99, 1.86
Coed (only women)	39.3	38.7	39.7	41.2	1.08	0.99, 1.17
Abstainers						
All-women's	25.9	25.9	20.9	20.7	0.76	0.63, 0.93**
Coed (only women)	16.8	20.3	19.1	18.6	1.13	1.01, 1.26*
Frequent binge						
All-women's	5.3	8.9	12.9	11.9	2.19	1.60, 2.99***
Coed (only women)	17.4	19.3	20.5	21.2	1.27	1.15, 1.40***

Note. OR = odds ratio; CI = confidence interval.
†Controlled for age, race, and response rate.
*$p < .05$; * *$p < .01$; * *$p < .001$.

Drinking Style

The data in Table 7 indicate changes in drinking style among students who drank alcohol in the past year. The intensity of their drinking increased significantly between 1993 and 1999. In 1999, a greater percentage of both male and female students drank on 10 or more occasions; usually binged when they drank; were drunk three or more times in the past month; and drank to get drunk. Although we found a general increase in drinking intensities from survey to survey, the strongest increase had occurred by 1997.

Prevalence of Alcohol-related Problems

In 1999, the prevalence of each of 12-alcohol-related educational, interpersonal, health, and safety problems among college men and women who drank any alcohol in the past year was significantly higher than in 1993. These increases had occurred by 1997, and additional increases did not appear between 1997 and 1999. In fact, some problems decreased significantly between 1997 and 1999 but were still significantly higher than in 1993.

Risk of Alcohol-related Problems

In the 1999 study, as in the previous studies, occasional binge drinkers and frequent binge drinkers were more likely to experience alcohol-related problems than those who drank alcohol but did not binge (Table 8). Occasional binge drinkers were 5 times as likely as nonbinge drinkers to report they had experienced 5 or more of 12 different alcohol-related problems, whereas frequent binge drinkers were 21 times as likely to do so. This result is consistent with previous years. Frequent binge drinkers, in contrast to nonbinge drinkers, were 4 to 15 times more likely to experience a particular problem as a result of their drinking.

Secondhand Binge Effects

We examined the secondhand binge effects experienced by nonbinge drinkers and abstainers who lived in dormitories or fraternity or sorority residences. In 1999, as in 1993 and 1997, the most frequent problems were (a) being interrupted while studying or being awakened at night (58%), (b) having to take care of a drunken fellow student (50%), and (c) being insulted or humiliated

TABLE 6
Alcohol-Related Problems Among Students Who Drank Alcohol, 1993, 1997, 1999, and 2001

| Alcohol-related problem | Prevalence in % | | | | Change over time | | |
| | 1993[a] | 1997[b] | 1999[c] | 2001[d] | 2001 vs 1993 | | Test for linear time trend p |
					OR	95% CI	
Miss a class	26.9	31.1	29.9	29.5	1.14	1.06, 1,23***	< .0001
Get behind in school work	20.5	24.1	24.1	21.6	1.07	0.99, 1.16	.0004
Do something you regret	32.1	37.0	36.1	35.0	1.13	1.06, 1.21***	< .0001
Forget where you were or what you did	24.7	27.4	27.1	26.8	1.12	1.03, 1.21**	.0005
Argue with friends	19.6	24.0	22.5	22.9	1.22	1.13, 1.31***	< .0001
Engage in unplanned sexual activities	19.2	23.3	21.6	21.3	1.14	1.06, 1.24***	.0002
Not use protection when you had sex	9.8	11.2	10.3	10.4	1.07	0.97, 1.19	.1840
Damage property	9.3	11.7	10.8	10.7	1.16	1.04, 1.30**	.0031
Get into trouble with the campus or local police	4.6	6.4	5.8	6.5	1.43	1.25, 1.65***	< .0001
Get hurt or injured	9.3	12.0	12.4	12.8	1.42	1.29, 1.57***	< .0001
Require medical treatment for an overdose	0.5	0.6	0.6	0.8	1.76	1.07, 2.91*	.0334
Drove after drinking	26.6	29.5	28.8	29.0	1.12	1.04, 1.21**	.0010
Have ≥ 5 different alcohol-related problems	16.6	20.8	19.9	20.3	1.28	1.27, 1.39***	< .0001

Note. Analysis limited to only those who drank alcohol in the past year. % is the prevalence of those who had the problem one or more times since the beginning of the school year. OR = odds ratio; CI = confidence interval.
[a]n = 12,708. [b]n = 11,506. [c]n = 10,825. [d]n = 8,783.
*p < .05; **p < .01; ***p < .001.

(29%). About 3 out of 4 students (77%) experienced at least one secondhand effect.

We found no clear pattern of change in the rates of secondhand effects in the 3 survey years. Some problems, such as experiencing an unwanted sexual advance and having to take care of a drunken student, increased significantly. Other problem experiences, such as being pushed, hit, or assaulted, or being the victim of sexual assault or date rape, decreased significantly.

Secondhand Binge Effects at High-binge, Medium-binge, and Low-binge Campuses

In 1999. as in the previous study, students who did not binge drink and who lived in a dormitory or fraternity or sorority house on high-binge campuses were twice as likely as nonbinge drinkers and abstainers on low-binge campuses to report experiencing any of the secondhand effects listed in the study. In addition, they were three times as likely to report at least one such effect (Table 9).

Comment

A Cautionary Note About Student Surveys

The CAS is based on self-reported responses to a mail survey and is subject to sources of error associated with this approach. First, respondents may intentionally or unintentionally distort their answers. However, a number of studies support the validity of self-reports of alcohol use.[13,15]

| Secondhand effect | % prevalence in each survey | | | | Change over time | | Test for linear time trend p |
| | 1993[a] | 1997[b] | 1999[c] | 2001[d] | 2001 vs 1993 | | |
					OR	95% CI	
Been insulted or humiliated	29.5	28.9	29.5	29.2	0.99	0.86, 1.14	.9423
Had a serious argument and quarrel	16.8	19.0	19.2	19.0	1.16	0.97, 1.39	.0700
Been pushed, hit, or assaulted	10.4	9.8	10.0	8.7	0.82	0.65, 1.04	.1793
Had your property damaged	12.7	13.8	13.1	15.2	1.23	1.00, 1.52	.1161
Had to take care of drunken student	45.3	49.6	50.0	47.6	1.10	0.96, 1.26	.0330
Had your studying/sleeping interrupted	59.9	61.9	58.2	60.0	1.00	0.87, 1.16	.5890
Experienced an unwanted sexual advance	16.5	18.7	18.9	19.5	1.23	1.04, 1.46*	.0169
Been a victim of sexual assault or date rape†	1.9	2.7	1.1	1.0	0.51	0.28, 0.93*	.0407
≥ 2 secondhand effects	53.1	55.5	55.4	55.2	1.09	0.94, 1.26	.1636

Note. Included only abstainers and non–binge drinkers in dorms or fraternity/sorority house. OR = odds ratio; CI = confidence interval.
†Women only.
[a]n = 12,708. [b]n = 11,506. [c]n = 10,825. [d]n = 8,783.
*$p < .05$.

The same pattern of responses among different student subgroups is present in all 3 years of the study, as well in other major studies of college alcohol use.[5,7,16]

Second, another possible source of bias may be introduced through sample attrition or nonresponse. Although we received responses from 60% of the students in the random samples in 1999 and 1997, these rates were lower than the 1993 rate (70%). However, the binge-drinking rates in the CAS in all 3 survey years were almost identical to rates obtained by other researchers who used different sampling methods.[5,7,8] Furthermore, the statistical controls we used to examine potential bias revealed no association between student nonresponse and binge-drinking rates in any of the 3 survey years.

The CAS did not have an equivalent time period in investigating change over the 6-year period. It is possible that changes during the 2-year period from 1997 to 1999 may be more difficult to detect than changes over the years from 1993 to 1997. We urge readers to use caution in interpreting our finding that the rates changed more between 1993 and 1997 than between 1997 and 1999.

Finally, the data presented in this article describe all colleges in the sample or college sub-groupings. Within these national norms, individual colleges may vary extensively. For example, although the national binge-drinking rate is 44%, the rate ranged from less than 1% at the lowest binge school to 76% at the highest.

Findings and Conclusion

Surveys of representative samples of college students at 119 colleges in 39 states in 1993, 1997, and 1999 have yielded remarkably similar rates of binge drinking over the past 6 years. Two of 5 college students were classified as binge drinkers in each of the three surveys. Although no change occurred in the overall binge-drinking rate, the nature of drinking among students who drink has become more extreme, with a significant increase in heavier drinking throughout the entire 6 years. We noted increases in the number of frequent binge drinkers between 1993 and 1999, as well as in the proportion of students who were drunk three or more times, who drank on 10 or more occasions, who usually binged when they drank,

TABLE 8
Attendance and Heavy Drinking at Select On-Campus and Off-Campus Venues

Venue	% prevalence in each survey				Change over time		
					2001 vs 1993		Test for linear time trend p
	1993[a]	1997[b]	1999[c]	2001[d]	OR	95% CI	
Dorm event or party							
% attending	29.1	32.2	30.3	29.2	1.01	0.91, 1.11	.5836
% consuming ≥ 5 drinks	4.4	9.6	7.3	6.2	1.43	1.16, 1.76***	.0002
Fraternity/sorority party							
% attending	39.5	33.4	32.6	32.4	0.73	0.67, 0.80***	< .0001
% consuming ≥ 5 drinks	14.7	15.4	13.9	12.5	0.82	0.74, 0.91***	.0012
Off-campus party							
% attending	66.7	69.4	72.5	72.0	1.28	1.17, 1.41***	< .0001
% consuming ≥ 5 drinks	23.9	29.1	29.9	30.3	1.38	1.26, 1.51***	< .0001
Off-campus bar							
% attending	73.3	68.9	70.8	70.5	0.87	0.80, 0.95**	.0012
% consuming ≥ 5 drinks	22.6	23.2	23.9	32.5	1.65	1.49, 1.83***	< .0001

Note. Percentage is based on the total students in the survey who drank alcohol in the past 30 days. OR = odds ratio; CI = confidence interval.
[a]n = 10,671. [b]n = 9,447. [c]n = 8,875. [d]n = 7,364.
**p < .01; ** *p < .001.

and who drank to get drunk. Among drinkers, the proportion of frequent binge drinkers increased from 23.4% in 1993 to 28.1% in 1999. During the same 6 years, the rates of abstaining from alcohol increased from 15.4% to 19.2%.

Most of the increase in abstention had occurred by 1997. These patterns of change have resulted in greater polarization in drinking behaviors on campuses. Although 2 out of 3 students who live in fraternity or sorority houses are binge drinkers, 1 in 3 (33.2%) students who lives in a campus residence hall or dormitory lives in an alcohol-free residence. An additional 12.6% of the respondents who did not currently live in such housing indicated that they would like to live in alcohol-free quarters.

From 1993 to 1999, the proportion of binge drinkers remained very similar for almost all subgroups of students and in all types of colleges. The same types of students who had the highest rates of binge drinking in 1993 and 1997 continued to have those high rates in 1999. Among the students most likely to binge drink were fraternity or sorority house residents and members of Greek organizations and students who were White, male, and were binge drinkers in high school. The students least likely to binge drink continued to be African American or Asian, aged 24 years or older, married, and who were not binge drinkers in high school.

The only exception to the lack of change in binge drinking during the 6-year period related to place of residence. Binge-drinking rates decreased among students living in dormitories and increased among students living off campus. This finding may be important in understanding current efforts at prevention of high-risk drinking.

In recent years, some debate has occurred about the five/four measure of binge drinking (five drinks for men, four for women).[17] Does it overstate the problem or label normative behavior as deviant? Findings from this study continue to

TABLE 9
Exposure to Educational Materials

| Educational material | % prevalence in each survey | | | | Change over time | | Test for linear time trend p |
| | 1993[a] | 1997[b] | 1999[c] | 2001[d] | 2001 vs 1993 | | |
					OR	95% CI	
Direct educational programs							
Lectures, meetings, or workshops	14.7	16.9	18.8	17.9	1.27	1.14, 1.41***	< .0001
Special college course	6.4	7.8	9.0	8.7	1.39	1.20, 1.60***	< .0001
Indirect educational programs							
Mailings or handouts	34.2	34.3	35.5	33.0	0.95	0.85, 1.06	.8663
Posters or signs	67.6	65.5	67.4	63.6	0.84	0.75, 0.94**	.0253
Announcement or articles	57.2	55.0	57.9	53.6	0.86	0.77, 0.97*	.1281

Note. OR = odds ratio; CI = confidence interval.
[a]*n* = 15,282. [b]*n* = 14,428. [c]*n* = 13,954. [d]*n* = 10,904.
*p < .05; **p < .01; ***p < .001.

show that students who drink at these levels, particularly those who do so more than once a week, experience a far higher rate of problems than other students. For example, frequent binge drinkers are likely to miss classes (OR = 16.9), to vandalize property (OR = 9.7), and to drive after drinking (OR = 7.6). Indeed, the frequent binge drinkers are also more likely to experience 5 or more different alcohol-related problems (OR = 21.1).

Students on campuses that have many binge drinkers experienced higher rates of secondhand problems, compared with students on campuses with lower rates of binge drinking. Students who did not binge drink and lived on high-binge campuses were twice as likely to report being assaulted, awakened, or kept from studying by drinking students than were nonbinge drinkers and abstainers at low-binge campuses. A student who did not binge drink on a high-binge campus was 3 times more likely than his or her counterpart on a low-binge campus to report at least one secondhand effect. These findings indicate that students who drink at the binge level create problems for themselves and for other students at their colleges. Indeed, we have previously reported that

frequent binge drinkers consumed two thirds of all the alcohol college students drink. They also accounted for more than three fifths of the most serious alcohol-related problems on campus.

Some Future Thoughts: Going Beyond the Data

In a companion article in this issue, we report on a survey of college administrators views and actions in dealing with binge drinking.[18] Their responses indicate that they have a great deal of concern about student drinking and that most colleges are taking actions to address the problem. Why, then, do rates of binge drinking continue to be this high? Why do we find an increase in the most extreme forms of drinking? Perhaps not enough time has passed since the initial studies attracted attention to the serious problem of college alcohol abuse for change to occur.

Another explanation may be related to the types of actions college officials are taking. Almost all colleges employ educational approaches to effect change. Certainly that is an appropriate strategy for academic institutions. Yet, we know that most students have received information about drinking and that those groups with the highest binge-drinking rates (athletes and fraternity members) have received the most information (Nelson TF, Wechsler H, unpublished data, 1999).[19] Although these educational programs are reaching the right target audiences, they have not resulted in decreased binge drinking and we cannot expect this strategy to accomplish this difficult task by itself.

The apparent inadequacy of even targeted educational efforts to change problem drinking among high-risk groups is not surprising. Public health is increasingly recognizing that education and information alone are not enough to change behavior. In our opinion, we need more support from additional, complementary initiatives. Prevention efforts must work on the alcohol supply, and they must increase the involvement of role models, those who shape opinions, and policy makers beyond the college campus, including community members and students' families.

The finding that binge drinking decreased among students living on campus but increased among those living off campus may reflect the current focus of prevention efforts. Without involving the community and the way alcohol is marketed, efforts to decrease binge drinking may simply displace it.

A comprehensive approach to student binge drinking should consider such factors as

- Alcohol marketing, outlet density, price, special promotions, and the volume in which alcohol is sold.
- Drinking history of students before they come to college. Working with high schools to decrease binge drinking should result in reducing the problem in colleges.
- Assuring alcohol-free social and recreational activities for students on weekends so that they have more to do than just "party."

- Increasing educational demands in terms of Friday classes and exams to reduce the length of the weekend and provide full-time education for full-time tuition.
- Enacting control policies and enforcing them, recognizing that the heaviest binge drinkers will not change unless forced to do so. These students do not think they have a drinking problem. They consider themselves moderate drinkers, and they are not ready to change. They may require an offer they cannot refuse. "Three strikes and you're out" (a punishment appropriate to the level of the violation) and parental notification may be strategies needed for these students. Although social marketing may be effective for some students (eg, those who are less committed to the binge-drinking lifestyle), it may not succeed with others.

Finally, there are no magic solutions. Just as no single technique applies to all students, no single approach applies to all colleges. Colleges differ in the roles that factors, such as fraternities, intercollegiate athletics, and drinking traditions, play on campus, as well as in the academic demands they make on student performance and the options that students have for recreation and social life. Alcohol control laws and their enforcement differ in the state and local communities in which colleges are located. All of these factors must be taken into consideration in planning a comprehensive response to student binge drinking.

Acknowledgment

This study was supported by the Robert Wood Johnson Foundation. We gratefully acknowledge the assistance of the Center for Survey Research of the University of Massachusetts, Boston; Dr Anthony M. Roman, for conducting the mail survey; Jeff Hansen and Mark Seibring, for the preparation of the data; and Toben Nelson and Dr Elissa Weitzman, for the preparation of the manuscript.

Note

For further information, please address communications to Henry Wechsler, PhD, Department of Health and Social Behavior, Harvard School of Public Health, 677 Huntington Avenue, Boston, MA 02115 (e-mail: hwechsle@hsph.harvard.edu).

References

Wechsler H, Davenport A, Dowdall G, Moevkens B, Castillo S. Health and behavioral consequences of binge drinking in college: A national survey of students at 140 campuses. JAMA. 1994;272(21):1672-1677.

Wechsler H, Isaac N. "Binge" drinkers at Massachusetts colleges: Prevalence, drinking style, time treads, and associated problems. JAMA. 1992;267:2929-2931.

Wechsler H, Molnar B, Davenport A, Baer J. College alcohol use: A Ml or empty glass? J Am Coll Health. 1999;47 (6):247-252.

Wechsler H, Davenport A, Dowdall G, Grossman S, Zanakos S. Binge drinking, tobacco, and illicit drug use and involvement in college athletics: A survey of students at 140 American colleges. J Am Coll Health. 1997;45(5): 195-200.

Johnston LD, O'Malley PM, Bachman JG. National Survey Results on Drug Use From the Monitoring the Future Study, 1975-1995. Vol II, College Students and Young Adults. US Dept of Health and Human Services; NIH Publication number 98-4140;* 1997.

Wechsler H, Dowdall GW, Maenner G, Gledhill-Hoyt J, Lee H. Changes in binge drinking and related problems among American college students between 1993 and 1997. JAm Coll Health 1998;47:57-68.

Presley CA, Meilman PW, Cashin JR, Lyerla R. Alcohol and Drugs on American College Campuses: Use, Consequences, and Perceptions of the Campus Environment Vol IV: 1992-94. Carbondale, IL: Southern Illinois University; 1996.

Douglas KA, Collins JL, Warren C, et al. Results from the 1995 National College Health Risk Behavior Survey. JAm Coll Health. 1997;46(2):55-66.

Wechsler H, Dowdall G, Davenport A, Rimm E. A gender-specific measure of binge drinking among college students. Am J Public Health. 1995;85:982-985.

Liang KY, Zeger SL. Longitudinal data analysis using generalized linear models. Biometrik. 1992;73:12-22.

Zeger SL, Liang KY, Albeit PS. Models for longitudinal data: A generalized estimating equation approach. Biometrics. 1988;44:1049-1060.

US Dept of Education. Digest of Education Statistics. Washington, DC: National Center of Educational Statistics; 1998.

Frier MC, Bell RM, Ellickson PL. Do Teens Tell the Truth? The Validity of Self-Report Tobacco Use by Adolescents. Santa Monica, CA: RAND; 1991. RAND publication N-3291-CHF.

Cooper AM, Sobell MB, Sobell LC, Maisto SA. Validity of alcoholics[5] self-reports: Duration data. IntJAddict. 1981;16: 401-406.

Midanik L. Validity of self-report alcohol use: A literature review and assessment. Brit J Addict. 1988;83:1019-1030.

Centers for Disease Control and Prevention. Youth Risk Behavior Surveillance: National College Health Risk Behavior Survey, United States. MMWR. 1997;46(SS-6):l-54.

Wechsler H, Austin SB. Binge drinking: The five/four mea-sure. J Stud Alcohol. 1998;59(1): 122-124.

Wechsler H, Kelly K, Weitzman E. What colleges are doing about student binge drinking: A survey of college administrators. JAm Coll Health. 2000;48:219-226.

Wechsler H, Nelson T, Weitzman E. From knowledge to action: How Harvard's college alcohol study can help your campus design a campaign against student alcohol abuse. Change. In press.

Barron's Profiles of American Colleges. Hauppauge, NY: Barron's Educational Series; 1996.

Henry Wechsler, Jae Eun Lee, and Meichun Kuo are all with the Department of Health and Social Behavior at the Harvard School of Public Health in Boston, and Hang Lee is with the Center for Vaccine Research and Department of Pediatrics at the University of California Los Angeles School of Medicine in Torrance.

A Brief History of Opiates, Opioid Peptides, and Opioid Receptors

By Michael J. Brownstein

> "Presently she cast a drug into the wine of which they drank to lull all pain and anger and bring forgetfulness of every sorrow."
>
> —*The Odyssey*, Homer
> (Ninth century B.C.)

It is hard to decide when and where the opium poppy was first cultivated. It may have been grown for its seeds before people discovered how to prepare meko- nion from the leaves and fruits of the plant or opium (from "opos," the Greek word for juice) from the liquid that appears on the unripe seed capsule when it is notched.

The use of written records to decipher the early history of opium use and abuse is hard because descriptions of drugs by ancient authors are often ambiguous. The preparation described by Homer—given by Helen, the daughter of Zeus, to Telemachus and his friends to help them forget their grief over Odysseus' absence—was attributed to Homer's imagination by Theophrastus (300 B.C.) who was himself aware of the method used to produce opium. Other writers (e.g., Diskourides,

A.D. 60) have argued that the drug alluded to by Homer contained henbane, the active ingredient of which is scopolamine. Most modern pharmacologists including Schmiedeberg (1) and Lewin (2) feel that Helen administered opium to the men. Indeed, Kritikos and Papadaki (3) have suggested that Telemachus may not have experienced any of the toxic effects of opium because he and his contemporaries used it habitually.

Despite difficulties in interpreting ancient writings and archeological data, a picture of opium use in antiquity does emerge from them. There is general agreement that the Sumerians, who inhabited what is today Iraq, cultivated poppies and isolated opium from their seed capsules at the end of the third millenium B.C. They called opium "gil," the wordforjoy, and the poppy "hulgil," plant of joy. It appears that opium spread from Sumeria to the remainder of the old world.

At first opium may have been employed as a euphoriant in religious rituals, taken by mouth or inhaled from heated vessels (4). Knowledge of its use may initially have been confined to priests representing gods who healed the sick and gods

Michael J. Brownstein, "A Brief History of Opiates, Opioid Peptides, and Opioid Receptors," *Proceedings of the National Academy of Sciences of the United States of America*, vol. 90, no. 12, pp. 5391-5393. Copyright © 1993 by the National Academy of Sciences. Reprinted with permission.

of death as well. It was given along with hemlock to put people quickly and painlessly to death, and it came to be used medicinally. The Ebers Papyrus (ca. 1500 B.C.), for example, includes the following description of a "'remedy to prevent excessive crying of children" (see ref. 2, p. 35): "Spenn, the grains of the Spenn (poppy)-plant, with excretions of flies found on the wall, strained to a pulp, passed through a sieve and administered on four successive days. The crying will stop at once." This remedy and others containing opium (such as spongia somnifera, sponges soaked in opium used to relieve pain during surgery) were dangerous because they varied in potency and rate of absor- bance. Consequently, many physicians were wary of using them.

Most authors[1] agree that, as early as the eighth century A.D., Arab traders brought opium to India (6) and China (7) and that between the tenth and thirteenth centuries opium made its way from Asia Minor to all parts of Europe. With the drug came addiction. Starting in the sixteenth century, manuscripts can be found describing drug abuse and tolerance in Turkey, Egypt, Germany, and England. Nowhere was the problem of addiction greater than in China where the practice of smoking opium began in the mid- seventeenth century after tobacco smoking was banned. Efforts to suppress the sale and use of opium failed because the British, later joined by the French, forced the Chinese to permit opium trade and consumption.

In 1806, Serturner (8, 9) isolated the active ingredient in opium and named it morphine after the god of dreams, Morpheus. (Codeine was isolated from opium a few years later.) Pure morphine, a weak base or alkaloid, the structure of which is shown in Fig. 1, could be made in large amounts. After the invention of the hy- podermic syringe and hollow needle in the 1850s, morphine began to be used for minor surgical procedures, for postoperative and chronic pain, and as an adjunct to general anesthetics. In fact, it was Claude Bernard who first investigated the use of morphine for premedicating experimental animals. He found that it reduced the amount of chloroform needed to produce anesthesia.

Unfortunately, morphine had just as much potential for abuse as opium and was not terribly safe to use either. Consequently, a great deal of energy was spent trying to develop a safer, more efficacious, nonaddicting opiate. In 1898, heroin was synthesized and pronounced to be more potent than morphine and free from abuse liability. This was the first of several such claims for novel opiates. To date, none has proven valid.

In 1939, the search for a synthetic substitute for atropine culminated seren- dipitously in the discovery of meperidine (10), the first opiate with a structure altogether different from that of morphine. This was followed in 1946 by the synthesis of methadone (11), another structurally unrelated compound with pharmacological properties similar to those of morphine. The abstinence syndrome seen when methadone consumption ceases is different from that of the natural alkaloid. Its onset is slower, it lasts longer, and it is less intense. Furthermore, it is orally active. Therefore, it is given to human addicts by clinicians as a substitute for morphine. Stable

---

[1] The Arabian system of medicine, including the use of opium, was introduced into India by Muslims in the ninth century A.D. The Greeks, however, were using Indian drugs by the third century B.C., and conversely, opium seems to have been employed in Indian folk remedies in the same period. As for China, opium was mentioned in the medical book K'ai-pao-pen-tsao in A.D. 973. The recent discovery of silk in the hair of a tenth century B.C. Egyptian mummy (5) indicates that there may have been regular traffic on the "Silk Road" in ancient times. One might infer from the above that opium was known, if not widely used, on both the Indian subcontinent and in Asia well before the eighth century A.D.

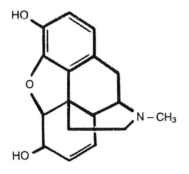

FIGURE 1. Morphine (pKb = 6.13). Heroin, diacetylmorphine, is more lipid soluble than morphine and enters the brain more readily. Heroin is converted to 6-monoacetylmorphine and morphine, which are responsible for its actions on central peripheral targets.

methadone addicts can lead reasonably normal lives, and the drug can gradually be withdrawn when they no longer desire to use it.

In 1942, Weijlard and Erikson (12) produced nalorphine (TV-allylnormorphine), the first opiate antagonist (13). This compound could reverse the respiratory depression produced by morphine and precipitate the abstinence syndrome in addicts. In spite of the fact that nalorphine counters the actions of morphine, it is effective as an analgesic agent. This is because it is a mixed agonist-antagonist. Its utility as a pain killer is limited since it often produces anxiety and dysphoria, but its discovery led to the development of additional compounds, such as naloxone, that are relatively pure opiate antagonists.

By the mid-1960s, it was becoming clear that the actions of opiate agonists, antagonists, and mixed agonist-antagonists could best be explained by actions on multiple opiate receptors. Goldstein et al. (14) suggested that radiolabeled drugs might be used to demonstrate the existence of these receptors and to characterize them. Their efforts to do this failed, however, because they could not obtain radioligands with high specific activities. In 1973, Pert and Snyder (15), Simon et al. (16),

and Terenius (17) succeeded almost simultaneously in showing that there are stereospecific opiate binding sites in the central nervous system and, soon afterwards, these receptors were found to have a nonuniform distribution there (38, 39). People reasoned that the opiate receptors might be the targets of neurotransmitters—endogenous opiates. This argument was strengthened when Akil et al. (18) found that footshock stress induced analgesia, which was partially reversed by naloxone. They inferred that stress must cause the release of opiatelike compounds.

In 1975, Kosterlitz and Waterfield (19) observed that brain extracts contain a factor that inhibits acetylcholine release from nerves innervating the guinea pig ileum. This inhibition was blocked by naloxone. The factors responsible for these effects proved to be pentapeptides (20): Tyr-Gly-Gly-Phe-Met (Met-en- kephalin) and Tyr-Gly-Gly-Phe-Leu (Leu-enkephalin). It soon became obvious that the Met-enkephalin sequence was present on the N terminus of another molecule, β-endorphin (21), a fragment of 0-lipotropin that had been isolated several years earlier from pituitary extracts. Like the enkephalins, β-endorphin proved to have a high affinity for brain opioid receptors.

Another group of peptides structurally related to the enkephalins were identified in 1981 (22). The first of these was named dynorphin. Finally, a fourth family of opioid peptides was shown to be present in the skin of the frog *Phyllomedusa bicolor* (23). These peptides, now known collectively as deltorphins, are quite unusual; they contain d-amino acids. The first such species characterized had the sequence Tyr-d-Met-Phe-His-Leu-Met- Asp-NH$_2$.

Not unexpectedly, each of the opioid peptides is made as part of a larger precursor protein. In mammals there are three such precursors—proenkephalin (24), prodynorphin (25), and proopiomelanocortin (26). Proenkephalin gives rise to four Met-enkephalins, one Leu-enkephalin, one Met-enkephalin-Arg^6- Phe^7, and one Met-enkephalin-Arg^6- Gly^7-Leu^8. Additional larger fragments of proenkephalin have been isolated from tissues. These may be incompletely processed or, possibly, opioid ligands in their own right.

Prodynorphin also gives rise to several biologically active peptides all of which contain the Leu-enkephalin sequence. These include dynorphin A, dynorphin B, α-neoendorphin, and β-neoendorphin. Proopiomelanocortin is the precursor for corticotropin and a-melanotropin along with β-endorphin. In total the three precursors described above give rise to more than 20 candidate opioid ligands. In addition, there is evidence that proteolysis of milk proteins generates opioid peptides (casorphins) in vitro (27) and that morphine-like compounds may occur naturally in mammals (28). That there were many potential ligands gave credence to the suggestion, mentioned earlier, that there might be more than one opioid receptor.

The first conclusive evidence for this was provided by Martin et al. (29). They performed a detailed analysis of the neu- rophysiological and behavioral properties of several opiate compounds and looked for "cross tolerance" among the opiates as well (i.e., the ability of a drug to prevent withdrawal symptoms after removal of a second drug from an animal tolerant to it). The results of these experiments suggested the existence of three types of receptors named after the drugs used in the studies: μ (morphine), κ (ke- tocyclazocine), and a (SKF 10,047 or AT-allylnormetazocine). The a receptor is now generally thought not to be an opioid receptor.

After they discovered the enkephalins, Kosterlitz and his colleagues (30) wanted to know which receptor(s) they act on. They found that morphine was more effective than the enkephalins in inhibiting electrically induced contractions of the guinea pig ileum. Surprisingly, the peptides were more active than morphine in inhibiting contraction of the mouse vas defferens. Furthermore, the action of enkephalins on the vas deferens was comparatively insensitive to naloxone. Based on these observations, Kosterlitz and his colleagues (30) proposed that a fourth type of opioid receptor, the 8 receptor, must be present in the vas deferens.

Unlike the enkephalins, the dynorphin- related peptides appear to bind principally to κ receptors, β-endorphin interacts with both fi and 8 sites as does Met-enkephalin-Arg^6-Gly^7-Leu^8. Interestingly, the deltorphins, as their name implies, are highly selective δ receptor agonists. In fact, iodinated and tritiated deltorphins are considered prototypic δ ligands.

Additional prototypic ligands have been developed for each of the opioid receptors (Table 1). These ligands and others like them are bound with high affinity and specificity, and they have been used for receptor binding as well as anatomical, physiological, and pharmacological studies. The results of these studies have suggested that there are subtypes of μ, κ, and δ receptors (see ref. 31). All of these receptors have high affinity for compounds with one common structural feature: a protonated amine juxtaposed to an aromatic ring (see Fig. 1).

The opioid receptors are all acknowledged to be guanine nucleotide binding (G)-protein-coupled. Both μ and δ receptors mediate the inhibition of adenylate cyclase (32) and the activation of inwardly rectifying potassium channels (33). κ and δ receptors have also been shown to inhibit the opening of voltage- dependent calcium channels (34).

Attempts to purify opioid receptors to homogeneity were thwarted by their paucity in most tissues and their lability after detergent solubilization (35). Until this year, the structure of opioid receptors remained a mystery. Now two groups

TABLE 1. Opioid receptor ligands

Receptor	Agonist	Antagonist	Agonist effect(s)
μ	Morphiceptin DAGO Normorphine Sufentanyl	Naloxone	Analgesia Respiratory depression Miosis Reduced gastrointestinal motility Nausea Vomiting Euphoria
δ	Deltorphin DPDPE DADLE	ICI 154,126 ICI 174,864	Supraspinal analgesia
κ	U 50,488 Trifluadom	MR2266	Analgesia (spinal level) Miosis (weak) Respiratory depression (weak) Dysphoria

DAGO, Tyr-d-Ala-Gly-MePhe-Gly-ol; DPDPE, [d-Pen^2,d-Pen^5]enkephalin; Pen, penicillamine; DADLE, [d-Ala^2,d-Leu^5]enkephalin; deltorphin II, Tyr-d-Ala-Phe-Glu-Val-Val-Gly- NH2; morphiceptin, /3-caso-morphin-(l-4)-amide or Tyr-Pro-Phe-Pro-NH2.

of investigators have published descriptions of the expression cloning of cDNAs encoding the 8 receptor on the neuroblas- toma-glioma (NG108-15) cells (36, 37). This receptor proved to be a member of the rhodopsin receptor superfamily. As expected, it is coupled to the inhibitory G protein Gi and inhibits activation of adenylate cyclase. It binds [d-Pen^2,d- Pen^5]enkephalin (DPDPE), [d-Ala^2,d- Leu^5]enkephalin (DADLE), and other 5-specific ligands with high affinity. It has considerably lower affinity for U 50,488 and dynorphin, and very low affinity for morphiceptin and Tyr-d-Ala-Gly-Me- Phe-Gly-ol (DAGO). It is stereospecific and has a marked preference for (-)- naloxone and levorphanol vs. (+)- naloxone and levorphanol. Thus, unlike receptor candidates cloned earlier, it behaves just as one might have expected it to.

The description of a 8 receptor marked the beginning of the race for additional members of the opioid receptor family, and a k- 1 receptor with high affinity for U 50,488 has been cloned

(40). Surely a new chapter in the annals of opiate research is about to be written.

1. Schmiedeberg, O. (1918) Schr. Wiss. Ge- sellsch. (Strassburg) 36, 1-29.
2. Lewin, L. (1931) Phantastica (Dutton, New York).
3. Kritikos, P. G. & Papadaki, S. P. (1967) Bull. Narc. 19 (3), 17-38.
4. Kritikos, P. G. & Papadaki, S. P. (1967) Bull. Narc. 19 (4), 5-10.
5. Lubec, G., Holaubek, J., Feldl, C., Lubec, B. & Strouhal, E. (1993) Nature (London) 362, 25.
6. Dwarakanath, S. C. (1965)Bull. Narc. 17 (1), 15-19.
7. Fort, J. (1965) Bull. Narc. 17 (3), 1-11.
8. Serturner, F. W. A. (1806) J. Pharm. f. Arzte. Apoth. Chem. 14, 47-93.
9. Serturner, F. W. A. (1817) Gilbert's Ann. d. Physik. 25, 56-89.
10. Eisleb, O. & Schaumann, O. (1939) Dtsch. Med. Wochenschr. 65, 967-968.

11. Scott, C. C. & Chen, K. K. (1946) J. Pharmacol. Exp. Ther. 87, 63-71.

12. Weijlard, J. & Erikson, A. E. (1942) J. Am. Chem. Soc. 64, 869-870.

13. Unna, K. (1943) J. Pharmacol. Exp. Ther. 79, 27-31.

14. Goldstein, A., Lowney, L. I. & Pal, B. K. (1971) Proc. Natl. Acad. Sci. USA 68, 1742-1747.

15. Pert, C. B. & Snyder, S. H. (1973) Science 179, 1011-1014.

16. Simon, E. J., Hiller, J. M. & Edelman, I. (1973) Proc. Natl. Acad. Sci. USA 70, 1947-1949.

17. Terenius, L. (1973) Acta Pharmacol. Toxicol. 33, 377-384.

18. Akil, H., Madden, J., Patrick, R. L. & Barchas, J. D. (1976) in Opiates and Endogenous Opioid Peptides, ed. Koster- litz, H. (Elsevier, New York), pp. 63-70.

19. Kosterlitz, H. W. & Waterfield, A. A. (1975) Annu. Rev. Pharmacol. Toxicol. 15, 29-47.

20. Hughes, J., Smith, T. W., Kosterlitz, H. W., Fothergill, L. A., Morgan, B. A. & Morris, H. R. (1975) Nature (London) 258, 577-579.

21. Bradbury, A. F., Smyth, D. G., Snell, C. R., BirdsaU, N. J. M. & Hulme, E. C. (1976) Nature (London) 260, 793795.

22. Goldstein, A. G., Fischli, W., Lowney, L. I., Hunkapiller, M. & Hood, L. (1981) Proc. Natl. Acad. Sci. USA 78, 72197223.

23. Erspamer, V., Melchiorri, P., Falconeri- Erspamer, G., Negri, L., Corsi, R., Severing C., Barra, D., Simmaco, M. & Kriel, G. (1989) Proc. Natl. Acad. Sci. USA 86, 5188-5192.

24. Noda, M., Furutani, Y., Takahashi, H., Toyosato, M., Hirose, T., Inayama, S., Nakanishi, S. & Numa, S. (1982) Nature (London) 295, 202-206.

25. Kakidani, H., Furutani, Y., Takahashi, H., Noda, M., Morimoto, Y., Hirose, T., Asai, M., Inayama, S., Nakanishi, S. & Numa, S. (1982) Nature (London) 298, 245-249.

26. Nakanishi, S., Inoue, A., Kita, T., Na- kamura, M., Chang, A. C. Y., Cohen, S. N. & Numa, S. (1979) Nature (London) 278, 423-427.

27. Henschen, A., Lottspeich, F., Brantl, V. & Teschmacher, H. (1979) Hoppe-Sey- ler's Z. Physiol. Chem. 360, 1211-1216.

28. Donnerer, J., Cardinale, G., Coffey, J., Lisek, C. A., Jardine, I. & Spector, S. (1987) J. Pharmacol. Exp. Ther. 242, 583-587.

29. Martin, W. R., Eades, C. G., Thompson, J. A., Huppler, R. E. & Gilbert, P. E. (1976) J. Pharmacol. Exp. Ther. 197, 517-532.

30. Lord, J. A. H., Waterfield, A. A., Hughes, J. & Kosterlitz, H. W. (1977) Nature (London) 267, 495-499.

31. Adler, B., Goodman, R. R. & Pasternak, G. W. (1990) in Handbook of Chemical Neuroanatomy, eds. Bjorklund, A., Hokfelt, T. & Kuhar, M. J. (Elsevier, New York), Vol. 9, Part 2, pp. 359-393.

32. Burns, D. L., Hewlett, E. L., Moss, J. & Vaughan, M. (1983) J. Biol. Chem. 258, 1435-1438.

33. North, R. A., Williams, J. T., Sur- prenant, A. & Christie, M. J. (1987) Proc. Natl. Acad. Sci. USA 84, 54875491.

34. Tsunoo, A., Yoshii, M. & Narahashi, T. (1986) Proc. Natl. Acad. Sci. USA 83, 9832-9836.

35. Loh, H. H. & Smith, A. P. (1990) Annu. Rev. Pharmacol. Toxicol. 30, 123-147.

36. Evans, C. J., Keith, D. E., Jr., Morrison, H., Magendzo, K. & Edwards, R. H. (1992) Science 258, 1952-1955.

37. Kieffer, B. L., Belfort, K., Gaveriaux- Ruff, C. & Hirth, C. G. (1992) Proc. Natl. Acad. Sci. USA 89, 12048-12052.

38. Hiller, J. M., Pearson, J. & Simon, E. J. (1973) Res. Commun. Chem. Pathol. Pharmacol. 6, 1052-1062.

39. Kuhar, M. J., Pert, C. B. & Snyder, S. H. (1973) Nature (London) 245, 447451.

40. Yasuda, K., Raynor, K. Kong, H., Breder, C. D., Takeda, J., Reisine, T. & Bell, G. I. (1993) Proc. Natl. Acad. Sci. USA 90, in press.

Stimulants

By Glen Hanson, Peter J. Venturelli, and Annette E. Fleckenstein

Did You Know?

- The first therapeutic use of amphetamines was in inhalers to treat nasal congestion.
- Methylphenidate (Ritalin) is a type of amphetamine used to treat hyperactive (attention deficit hyperactivity disorder) children.
- Illegal methamphetamine can be easily made from drugs found in common over-the-counter (OTC) decongestants and some herbal products.
- Smoking "freebased" or "crack" cocaine is more dangerous and more addicting than other forms of administration.
- Using high doses of amphetamines or cocaine can cause behavior that resembles schizophrenia.
- Caffeine is the most frequently used stimulant in the world.
- Herbal stimulants promoted as "natural highs" contain CNS stimulants that can cause high blood pressure, seizures, and strokes.
- Ephedrine found in natural herbal products has caused fatal cardiovascular problems in unsuspecting athletes and was recently removed from the list of FDA-approved OTC products.

Learning Objectives

On completing this chapter you will be able to:

- Explain how amphetamines work.
- Identify the FDA-approved uses for amphetamines.
- Recognize the major side effects of amphetamines on brain and cardiovascular functions.
- Identify the terms speed, ice, run, high, and tweaking as they relate to amphetamine use.
- Explain what "designer" amphetamines are and how Ecstasy compares to methamphetamine.
- Explain what "club drugs" are.

- Trace the changes in attitude toward cocaine abuse that occurred in the 1980s and explain why they occurred.
- Compare the effects of cocaine with those of amphetamines.
- Identify the different stages of cocaine withdrawal.
- Discuss the different approaches to treating cocaine dependence.
- Identify and compare the major sources of the caffeinelike xanthine drugs.
- List the principal physiological effects of caffeine.
- Compare caffeine dependence and withdrawal to that associated with the major stimulants.
- Understand the potential dangers of using herbal stimulants such as ephedra.
- Identify the role of the FDA in regulating herbal stimulants.

Introduction

Stimulants are substances that cause the user to feel pleasant effects such as a sense of increased energy and a state of euphoria, or "high." This effect is likely due to the ability of these drugs to release dopamine (Deslandes et al. 2002). The user may also feel restless and talkative and have trouble sleeping. High doses administered over the long term can produce personality changes or even induce violent, dangerous, psychotic behavior. Methamphetamine addicts make notoriously bad decisions that hurt them and their loved ones. The following is a quote from a former methamphetamine user: "For 5 months I hung out with a crew who cooked meth. My job was to write bad checks to get ingredients to make it. This was my life. My house was a mess and I couldn't take care of anyone including myself. I weighed 100 pounds and stayed up for weeks at a time because I never ran out of gas. ... I also picked my eye for no reason, until it would get so swollen and red it would stay shut for days. I had my first son when I was 26 and later gave up my second son for adoption because I was such a mess. . . . My mother called social services and made sure that I was not allowed to take care of my children" (Snider 2007).

Many users self-medicate psychological conditions (for example, depression) with stimulants. Because the initial effects of stimulants are so pleasant, these drugs are repeatedly abused, leading to dependence.

In this chapter, you will learn about two principal classifications of stimulant drugs. Major stimulants, including amphetamines and cocaine, are addressed first, given their prominent role in current drug abuse problems in the United States. The chapter concludes with a review of minor stimulants — in particular, caffeine. The stimulant properties of over-the-counter (OTC) sympathomimetics and "herbal highs" are also discussed. (Because nicotine has unique stimulant properties, it is covered separately in Chapter 11 on tobacco.)

Major Stimulants

All major stimulants increase alertness, excitation, and euphoria; thus, these drugs are referred to as uppers. The major stimulants are classified as either Schedule I ("designer" amphetamines) or Schedule II (amphetamine and cocaine) controlled substances because of their abuse potential. Although these drugs have properties in common, they also have unique features that distinguish them from one another. The similarities and differences of the major stimulants are discussed in the following sections.

Amphetamines

More than 12 million Americans have abused methamphetamine and 1.5 million of these users are addicted to this potent stimulant (Partnership 2007). Amphetamines are potent synthetic central nervous system (CNS) stimulants capable of causing dependence due to their euphorigenic properties and ability to eliminate fatigue. Despite their addicting effects, amphetamines can be legally prescribed by physicians. Consequently, amphetamine abuse occurs in people who acquire their drugs by both legitimate and illicit means (McCaffrey 1999).

The History of Amphetamines

The first amphetamine was synthesized by the German pharmacologist L. Edeleano in 1887, but it was not until 1910 that this and several related compounds were tested in laboratory animals. Another 17 years passed before Gordon Alles, a researcher looking for a more potent substitute for ephedrine (used as a decongestant at the time), self-administered amphetamine and gave a firsthand account of its effects. Alles found that when inhaled or taken orally, amphetamine dramatically reduced fatigue, increased alertness, and caused a sense of confident euphoria (Grinspoon and Bakalar 1978).

Because of Alles's impressive findings, the Benzedrine (amphetamine) inhaler became available in 1932 as a nonprescription medication in drugstores across America. The Benzedrine inhaler, marketed for nasal congestion, was widely abused for its stimulant action but continued to be available OTC until 1949. Because of a loophole in a law that was passed later, not until 1971 were all potent amphetamine-like compounds in nasal inhalers withdrawn from the market (Grinspoon and Bakalar 1978; McCaffrey 1999).

Owing to the lack of restrictions during this early period, amphetamines were sold to treat a variety of ailments, including obesity, alcoholism, bed-wetting, depression, schizophrenia, morphine and codeine addiction, heart block,

head injuries, seasickness, persistent hiccups, and caffeine mania. Today, most of these uses are no longer approved as legitimate therapeutics but would be considered forms of drug abuse.

World War II provided a setting in which both the legal and "black market" use of amphetamines flourished (Grinspoon and Bakalar 1978). Because of their stimulating effects, amphetamines were widely used by the Germans, Japanese, and British in World War II to counteract fatigue. By the end of World War II, large quantities of amphetamines were readily available without prescription in seven types of nasal inhalers.

In spite of warnings about these drugs' addicting properties and serious side effects, the U.S. armed forces issued amphetamines on a regular basis during the Korean War and, in fact, may still make it available to pilots in the Air Force to relieve fatigue. Amphetamine use became widespread among truck drivers making long hauls; it is believed that among the earliest distribution systems for illicit amphetamines were truck stops along major U.S. highways. High achievers under continuous pressure in the fields of entertainment, business, and industry often relied on amphetamines to counteract fatigue. Homemakers used them to control weight and to combat boredom from unfulfilled lives. At the height of the U.S. epidemic in 1967, some 31 million prescriptions were written for **anorexiants** (diet pills) alone.

Today, a variety of related drugs and mixtures exist, including amphetamine substances such as dextroamphetamine (Dexedrine), methamphetamine (Desoxyn), and amphetamine itself. Generally, if doses are adjusted, the psychological effects of these various drugs are similar, so they will be discussed as a group. Other drugs with some of the same pharmacological properties are phenme-trazine (Preludin) and methylphenidate (Ritalin). Common slang terms for amphetamines include *speed, crystal, meth, bennies, dexies, uppers, pep pills, diet pills, jolly beans, copilots, hearts, footballs, white crosses, crank, and ice.*

How Amphetamines Work

Amphetamines are synthetic chemicals that are similar to natural neurotransmitters such as norepinephrine (noradrenaline), dopamine, and the stress hormone epinephrine (adrenaline). The amphetamines exert their pharmacological effect by increasing the release and blocking the metabolism of these catecholamine substances as well as serotonin (see Chapter 4), both in the brain and in nerves associated with the sympathetic nervous system. Because amphetamines cause release of norepinephrine from sympathetic nerves, they are classified as sympathomimetic drugs. The amphetamines generally cause an arousal or activating response (also called the fight-or-flight response) that is similar to the normal reaction to emergency situations, stress, or crises.

Amphetamines also cause alertness so that the individual becomes aroused, hypersensitive to stimuli, and feels "turned on." These effects occur even without external sensory input. This activation may be a very pleasant experience in itself, but a continual high level of activation may convert to anxiety, severe apprehension, or panic.

Amphetamines have potent effects on dopamine in the reward (pleasure) center of the brain (see Chapter 4). This action probably causes the "flash" or sudden feeling of intense pleasure that occurs when amphetamine is taken intravenously. Some users describe the sensation as a "whole-body orgasm," and many associate intravenous metham-phetamine use with sexual feelings. The actual effect of these drugs on sexual behavior is quite variable and dependent on dose (McCaffrey 1999).

What Amphetamines Can Do

A curious condition commonly reported with heavy amphetamine use is behavioral stereotypy, or getting hung up. This term refers to a simple activity that is done repeatedly. An individual who is "hung up" will get caught in a repetitious thought or act for hours. For example, he or she may take objects apart, like radios or clocks, and carefully categorize all the parts, or sit in a tub and bathe all day, persistently sing a note, repeat a phrase of music, or repeatedly clean the same object. This phenomenon seems to be peculiar to potent stimulants such as the amphetamines and cocaine. Similar patterns of repetitive behavior also occur in psychotic conditions, which suggests that the intense use of stimulants such as amphetamines or cocaine alters the brain in a manner like that causing psychotic mental disorders (American Psychiatric Association [APA] 2000) and can lead to violent behavior.

Key Terms

anorexiants
    drugs that suppress appetite for food
behavioral stereotypy
    meaningless repetition of a single activity

Chronic use of high doses of amphetamines causes dramatic decreases in the brain content of the neurotransmitters dopamine and serotonin that persist for months, even after drug use is stopped (Gehrke et al. 2003). These decreases have been shown to reflect damage to the CNS neurons that release these transmitters. It is not clear why this neuronal destruction occurs, although there is evidence that the amphetamines can stimulate production of very reactive molecules, called free radicals, which in turn damage brain cells (Riddle et al. 2006).

Until 1970, amphetamines were prescribed for a large number of conditions, including depression, fatigue, and long-term weight reduction. In 1970, the Food and Drug Administration (FDA), acting on the recommendation of the National Academy of Sciences, restricted the legal use of amphetamines to three medical conditions: (1) narcolepsy, (2) attention deficit hyperactivity disorder (ADHD), and (3) short-term weight reduction programs (APA2000).

Narcolepsy Amphetamine treatment of narcolepsy is not widespread because this condition is a relatively rare disorder. The term narcolepsy comes from the Greek words for numbness and seizure. A person who has narcolepsy falls asleep as frequently as 50 times a day if he or she stays in one position for very long. Taking low doses of amphetamines helps keep narcoleptic people alert.

Attention Deficit Hyperactivity Disorder This common behavioral problem in children and adolescents involves an abnormally high level of physical activity, an inability to focus attention, and frequent disruptive behavior. Four to six percent of children and adults have ADHD (Polanczyk and Rohole 2007) The drug commonly used to treat children with ADHD is the. amphetamine-related methylphenidate or Ritalin (discussed later in this chapter).

Weight Reduction The most common use of amphetamines is for the treatment of obesity. Amphetamines.and chemically similar compounds are used as anorexiants to help obese or severely overweight people control appetite.

Amphetamines are thought to act by affecting the appetite center in the hypothalamus of the brain, which causes the user to decrease food intake. The FDA has approved short-term use of amphetamines for weight loss programs but has warned of their potential for abuse. Many experts believe that the euphoric effect of amphetamines is the primary motivation for their continued use in weight reduction programs. It is possible that many obese people have a need for gratification that can be satisfied by the euphoric feeling this drug produces (Wang et al. 2004). If the drug is taken away, these individuals return to food to satisfy their need and sometimes experience "rebound," causing them to gain back more weight than they lost. Some persons who become addicted to amphetamine-like substances begin illicit use of these drugs by trying to prevent weight gain or to lose weight on their own without the guidance of a physician (APA 2000).

Side Effects of Therapeutic Doses

The two principal side effects of therapeutic doses of amphetamines are (1) abuse, which has already been discussed at length, and (2) cardiovascular toxicities. Many of these effects derive from the amphetamine-induced release of epinephrine from the adrenal glands and norepinephrine from the nerves associated with the sympathetic nervous system. The effects include increased heart rate, elevated blood pressure, and damage to vessels, especially small veins and arteries (Drug War Facts 2004; Swan 1996). In users with a history of heart attack, coronary arrhythmia, or hypertension, amphetamine toxicity can be severe or even fatal.

Current Misuse

Because amphetamine drugs can be readily and inexpensively synthesized in makeshift

---

Key Terms

narcolepsy
   a condition causing spontaneous and uncontrolled sleeping episodes

---

laboratories for illicit sale, can be administered by several routes, and cause a more sustained effect, these drugs are more popular than cocaine in many parts of the United States (Johnston 2007). Surveys suggest that there was a decline in the abuse of amphetamines in the late 1980s and early 1990s in parallel with a similar trend in cocaine abuse (Johnston 1996). However, in 1993, the declines were replaced by a rise in the number of persons abusing amphetamines. By 2001, approximately 5.6% of high school seniors used amphetamines at least each month. Currently, approximately 5.7% of high school seniors in the United States are regularly using amphetamines (Johnston 2007). In general, 4-5% of the population has abused methamphetamine. Of those who become addicted, many end up in the criminal justice system, accounting for about 30% of the court cases in the United States (Leinwand ,2007).

Because of the potential for serious side effects, U.S. medical associations have asked all physicians to be more careful about prescribing amphetamines. Presently, use is recommended only for narcolepsy and some cases of hyperactivity in children (Drug Facts and Comparisons 2005; Hoffman and Lefkowitz 1995). In spite of FDA approval, most medical associations do not recommend the use of amphetamines for weight loss. Probably less than 1% of all prescriptions now written are for amphetamines, compared with 8% in 1970.

Amphetamine abusers commonly administer a dose of 10 to 30 milligrams. Besides the positive effects of this dose — the "high" — it can cause hyperactive, nervous, or jittery feelings that encourage the use of a depressant such as a benzodiazepine, barbiturate, or alcohol to relieve the discomfort of being "wired" (Hoffman and Lefkowitz 1995).

A potent and commonly abused form of amphetamine is speed, an illegal methamphetamine available as a white, odorless, bitter-tasting crystalline powder for injection. Methamphetamine is a highly addictive stimulant that is often cheaper and much longer lasting than cocaine (American Council for Drug Education 2007). The profit for the speed manufacturer is substantial enough to make illicit production financially attractive. Because the cost ranges from $10 to $20 a dose, it is sometimes known as the "poor man's cocaine" (Leinwand 2007). Methamphetamine is relatively easy and inexpensive to make. The illicit manufacturers are usually individuals without expertise in chemistry. Such people, referred to as "cookers," produce methamphetamine batches by using cookbook-style recipes (often obtained in jail or over the Internet). The most popular recipe uses common OTC ingredients — ephedrine, pseu-doephedrine, and phenylpropanolamine — as precursor chemicals for the methamphetamine. To discourage the illicit manufacture of this potent stimulant, the Comprehensive Methamphetamine Control Act was passed in October 1996. This law increases penalties for trafficking in methamphetamine and in the precursor chemicals used to create this drug and gives the government authority to regulate and seize these substances (Comprehensive Methamphetamine Control Act 2008).

Due to the ease of production and the ready availability of chemicals used to prepare methamphetamine, this drug has become particularly problematic in the United States and has been declared the number 1 drug problem in the majority of counties across the country (Rutledge 2006). Traditional methamphetamine users have been white, male, blue-collar workers over 26 years of age, although currently there also is a disturbingly high rate of use in adolescents (3-5% annual use; Johnston 2007) and use by young women is on the rise in some regions of the United States. There has been higher abuse of this drug in the western United States, illustrated by the fact that methamphetamine dependence dominates the treatment systems in this region (National Institute on Drug Abuse [NIDA] 2007d). In contrast, methamphetamine abuse is much less common on the East Coast. In general, production and trafficking are rampant throughout the West and Midwest areas, with the highest levels occurring in California, Arizona, and Utah. However, the methamphetamine problem is moving across the country, with Iowa, Missouri, and Tennessee being particularly affected, and there are increasing reports of its use in the South and some Northeast areas (Leinwand 2007; NIDA 2007d).

Today, so-called meth or speed labs are frequently raided by law enforcement agencies across the country as local drug entrepreneurs try to grab a share of the profits. In 2003, law enforcement agencies shut down more than 17,000 illegal methamphetamine labs, most of which were in the western United States. This number decreased to 7,347 in 2006 (Leinwand 2007). The laboratory operators are usually well armed, and the facilities are frequently booby-trapped with explosives. Not surprisingly, these operations pose a serious threat to their neighbors (U.S. Department of Justice 2003a) and to residents, especially children, in the structure that contains the lab (U.S. Department of Justice 2002; see "Here and Now" Innocent Victims of Meth). Law enforcement personnel and firefighters are also at risk when dealing with methamphetamine labs owing to ignitable, corrosive, reactive, and toxic chemicals that might explode, start a fire, emit toxic fumes, or cause serious injury at the site. The toxic chemicals can create fumes that contaminate neighboring buildings, the water supply, or soil. These labs are especially dangerous when they are set up in poorly ventilated rooms (Kennedy 1999; see "Here and Now," Chemical Toxins Associated with Meth Labs).

Although still a problem, the incidences of "mom and pop" neighborhood methamphetamine labs are decreasing dramatically across the nation. This is the result of federal and state laws that limit access to large quantities of precursor drugs found in OTC decongestants. The new statutes require these decongestant products be kept behind the pharmacy counter, and the quantity sold to a customer must be minimal in order to limit access (Leinwand 2007; see "Holding the Line," Cold Restrictions). While decreasing the number of meth labs in the United States, this strategy unfortunately has had minimal effect on actual supplies of this drug for illegal sales. Methamphetamine is being smuggled across U.S. borders from Mexico (Berkes 2007) and is being manufactured by criminal organizations from chemicals diverted by the ton from Asian pharmaceutical companies (Haus 2006; Randolph 2007). It is estimated that currently 90% of meth is imported, keeping supplies abundant and cost low (Leinwood 2007).

Patterns of High-Dose Use Amphetamines can be taken orally, intravenously, or by smoking. The intensity and duration of effects vary according to the mode of administration. The "speed

---

Key Term

speed
   an injectable methamphetamine used by drug addicts
precursor chemicals
   chemicals used to produce a drug

Key Terms

ice
   a smokable form of methamphetamine
rush
   initial pleasure after amphetamine use that includes racing heartbeat and elevated blood pressure

Innocent Victims of Meth

In almost one quarter of meth labs seized, children ares found who have been exposed to the toxins used to "cook" the drug as well as the emotional and physical abuse of parents more preoccupied with satisfying their addiction than caring for their children. Burners have been left on next to a baby's crib. Bottles filled with potent acids are stored in the refrigerator, Children have been starved and 3-year-olds left to care for themselvesi and also care for a baby brother or sister while their mom or dad binges on meth for days or even weeks and then crash into a sleeping stupor. Explosive ingredients are abundant with vaporized drugs, contaminating the food, drinking water, clothing, and even the air. Officials must decide what to do with children abused and injured both physically and emotionally by parents who ignore their children's basic needs because they are so preoccupied with obtaining their next meth fix. Reports are that meth addiction has caused foster-care programs across the country to be swamped with young victims.

Source: Tseng, N. "Children Fall by Wayside in Meih-Addicted Homes " Orlando Sentinel (11 September 2005) B1.

freak" uses chronic, high doses of amphetamines intravenously and is often infected with HIV (see Chapter 16) (NIDA, Research Report 2000). Another approach to administering amphetamines is smoking ice, which can cause effects as potent, but perhaps more prolonged and erratic, than intravenous doses. The initial effect (after 5 to 30 minutes) of these potent stimulants is called the rush and includes a racing heartbeat and elevated blood pressure, metabolism, and pulse. During this phase, the user has powerful impressions of pleasure and enthusiasm. The next stage is the high (4 to 16 hours after drug use) when the person feels aggressively smarter, energetic, talkative, and powerful and may initiate and complete highly ambitious tasks. The amphetamine addict tries to maintain the high for as long as possible with continual drug use leading to extended mental and physical hyperactivity; this is referred to as a run or binge and can persist from 3 to 15 days. Persistent use of these drugs, such as methamphetamine, to maintain the high for long periods of time is called tweaking. The tweaker often has neither slept nor eaten much for 3 to 15 days and

can be extremely irritable and paranoid and have an elevated body temperature, a condition known as hyperpyrexia. This is a potentially dangerous stage for medical personnel or law enforcement officers because if the tweaker becomes agitated, he or she can respond violently to the efforts of others to help. To relieve some of the side effects of the extensive use of methamphetamine, tweakers often use a depressant such as alcohol, barbiturates, benzodiazepines, or opioid narcotics. The consequences of such a drug combination are to intensify negative feelings and worsen the dangers of the drug. Tweakers are frequently involved in domestic violence and frequently injure their children and partners (Transitions 2007). Withdrawal follows for 30 to 90 days, including feelings of depression and lethargy. During this phase, craving can be intense and the abuser may even become suicidal. Because a dose of methamphetamine often relieves these symptoms, many addicts in treatment return to abusing this stimulant (Prevline 1999).

After the first day or so of a run, unpleasant symptoms become prominent as the dosage is increased. Symptoms commonly reported at this stage are teeth grinding, disorganized patterns of thought and behavior, stereotypy,

irritability, self-consciousness, suspiciousness, and fear. Hallucinations and delusions that are similar to a paranoid psychosis and indistinguishable from schizophrenia can occur (APA 2000). The person is likely to show aggressive and antisocial behavior for no apparent reason, although recent brain imaging studies have revealed that addictions to the amphetamines can cause long-term damage to the brain's inhibitory control centers (Kuehn 2007). Severe chest pains, abdominal discomfort that mimics appendicitis, and fainting from overdosage are sometimes reported. "Cocaine bugs" represent one bizarre effect of high doses of potent stimulants such as amphetamines: The user experiences strange feelings, like insects crawling under the skin. The range of physical and mental symptoms experienced from low to high doses is summarized in "Signs and Symptoms" Summary of the Effects of Amphetamines on the Body and Mind.

Key Terms

high

4 to 16 hours after drug use; includes feelings of energy and power

run

intense use of a stimulant, consisting of multiple administrations over a period of days

binge

similar to a run, but usually of shorter duration

tweaking

repeated administration of methamphetamine to maintain the high

hyperpyrexia

elevated body temperature

Cold Restrictions

As of September 30, 2006, it became somewhat more difficult for a person with a cold, and a lot more difficult for persons desiring to make methamphetamine from decongestant ingredients, to obtain adequate OTC cold medicine for their needs. This is due to a federal law to stop the manufacture of methamphetamine in illegal meth labs found in homes, garages, or basements. To achieve this objective, the new restrictions require customers to show a picture ID to purchase cold medicine such as NyQuil Cold & Flu, Actifed Cold & Allergy, and Claritin-D. These and similar decongestant products that contain drugs that can be converted into methamphetamine must be kept behind the store counters. Customers must sign a logbook identifying what they purchased and where they live. The logbook remains on file for 2 years. This law restricts purchase to 3-6 grams of product/day and 9 grams/month.

Toward the end of the run, the adverse symptoms dominate. When the drug is discontinued because the supply is exhausted or the symptoms become too unpleasant, an extreme crash can occur, followed by prolonged sleep, sometimes lasting several days. On awakening, the person is lethargic, hungry, and often severely depressed. The amphetamine user may overcome these unpleasant effects by smoking ice or injecting speed, thereby initiating a new cycle (APA 2000).

Continued use of massive doses of amphetamine often leads to considerable weight loss, sores in the skin, poor oral hygiene and deterioration of the teeth (Rauscher 2006), nonhealing ulcers, liver disease, hypertensive disorders, cerebral hemorrhage (stroke), heart attack, kidney damage, and seizures (Hall and Hando 1993; Kinkead and Romboy 2004). For some of these effects, it is impossible to tell whether they are caused by the drug, poor eating habits, or other factors associated with the lifestyle of people who inject methamphetamine.

Speed freaks are generally unpopular with the rest of the drug-taking community, especially "acid-heads" (addicts who use lysergic acid diethylamide [LSD]), because of the aggressive, unpredictable behavior associated with use of potent stimulants. In general, drug abusers who take high doses of these agents, such as amphetamines or cocaine, are more likely to be involved in violent crimes than those who abuse other drugs (Drug Enforcement Agency [DEA] 2007). Heavy users are generally unable to hold steady jobs because of their drug habits and often have a parasitic relationship with the rest of the illicit drug-using community.

Although claims have been made that amphetamines do not cause physical dependence, it is almost certain that depression (sometimes suicidal), lethargy, muscle pains, abnormal sleep patterns, and, in severe cases, suicide attempts occur after high chronic doses as part of withdrawal (Cantwell and McBride 1998; NIDA Diagnosis 2000). During withdrawal from amphetamine use, the dependent user often turns to other drugs for relief (Cantwell and McBride 1998). Rebound from the amphetamines is opposite to that experienced with withdrawal from CNS depressants (see Chapter 6).

Although the effects of amphetamines on the unborn fetus are not fully understood, some animal studies suggest that there is a possibility of long-term problems in the offspring. However, these findings remain to be verified in humans (Slamberova et al. 2007). There is evidence that repeated high-dose use of amphetamines, such as methamphetamine, by adolescents or adults causes long-term and perhaps permanent damage to both dopamine and serotonin systems of the brain (Cohen 2006; Hanson et al. 2004). This brain damage may result in persistent episodes of psychosis (Yui et al. 1999) as well as long-lasting memory, motor impairment, and cognitive deficits. (Hanson et al. 2004; Volkow et al. 2001). Abuse of amphetamines often seriously damages personal relationships with friends, associates, and even family members. Particularly disturbing is the increasing methamphetamine use by young mothers. Moms on meth have claimed that use of this stimulant makes them feel invincible, and like they can run around the world — and then do it again. They claim to lose weight, but they also can lose their instinct to mother their children as they become obsessed with the drug (Holt 2005). Consequently, children are being exposed to dangerous levels of this drug in many forms (see "Here and Now," Small Towns, Big Problems: The Female Methamphetamine Epidemic).

Treatment

Admissions for treatment of methamphetamine addiction have more than doubled since 2000 (Join Together 2006). The dependence disorder caused by the amphetamines is very hard, but not impossible, to treat successfully. Many of the methamphetamine addicts do not self-refer, but are forced into treatment by drug courts and other components of the criminal justice system (Newswise 2007). This has led to a dramatic rise

Signs & Symptoms Summary of the Effects of Amphetamines on the Body and Mind

	BODY	MIND
Low dose	Increased heartbeat.	Decreased fatigue
	Increased blood pressure	Increased confidence
	Decreased appetite	Increased feeling of alertness
	Increased breathing rate	Restlessness, talkativeness
	Inability to sleep	Increased irritability
	Sweating	Fearfulness, apprehension
	Dry mouth	Distrust of people
	Muscle twitching	Behavioral stereotypy
	Convulsions	Hallucinations
	Fever	Psychosis
	Chest pain	
	Irregular heartbeat	
High dose	Death due to overdose	

Small Towns, Big Problems: The Female Methamphetamine Epidemic

Methamphetamine is causing a drug-related epidemic never before experienced in this country. Its abuse and devastating social effects are popping up in communities across the country and greatly taxing public social services in unanticipated ways. For example, 10 years ago social workers in Missoula, Montana, rarely heard of people abusing methamphetamine — let alone had to deal with these addicts. That situation has now changed. Today local and state governments find themselves overrun by the methamphetamine plague.

One of the most striking aspects of this drug's abuse in Montana is its effect on, and appeal to, young adult women. Typically, state figures show that the number of women seeking treatment for drug addiction are considerably lower than the number of men in the same situation; in 20CW, however, roughly equal numbers of men and women sought help for methamphetamine as their primary addiction. Clearly, the destructive influence of methamphetamine abuse is taking an enormous toll on homes and families. In Missoula alone, almost half of the 137 children placed in the care of Family Services were removed from their homes due to use of methamphetamine by their mothers. Likewise, Montana's criminal justice system for women offenders is being overwhelmed. In 2004, the Montana State Prison for Women was filled for the first time, principally due to the methamphetamine epidemic in this population.

Women who are addicted to methamphetamine often do not do well in conventional drug treatment Because of the potent addicting properties of this drug, they typically struggle with the requirements of probation or parole and often end up back in prison. While it is not clear why this stimulant is so seducing to young women, it is apparent that "this drug is a massive black hole. It's swallowing these people alive. It takes a miracle to put these families back together again."

Source: "Escalation in Methamphetamine Use Also Leads to Escalation In Social 5ervice," Health & Medicine Week (14 February 2005).

in admissions to treatment for methamphetamine dependence in many parts of the country (Health and Medicine Week 2006). Presently, the most effective treatments for amphetamine addiction are behavioral interventions to help modify thinking patterns, improve cognitive skills, change expectations, and increase coping with life's stressors. Amphetamine support groups also appear to be successful as adjuncts to behavioral therapies. There currently are no well-established pharmacological treatments for amphetamine dependency. Approaches used for cocaine have been tried with some success. Antidepressant medication may help relieve the depression that occurs during early stages of withdrawal (Los Angeles Times 2005; NIDA, Research Report 2000).

Amphetamine Combinations

As previously mentioned, amphetamines are frequently used in conjunction with a variety of other drugs such as barbiturates, benzodiazepines, alcohol, and heroin (Nuckols and Kane 2003).

Amphetamines intensify, prolong, or otherwise alter the effects of LSD, and the two types of drugs are sometimes combined. The majority of speed users have also had experience with a variety of psychedelics or other drugs. In addition, people dependent on opiate narcotics frequently use amphetamines or cocaine. These combinations are called speedbaSls (Wikipedia 2007b).

"Designer" Amphetamines

Underground chemists can synthesize drugs that mimic the psychoactive effects of amphetamines. Although the production of such drugs diminished in the early 1990s, their use by American teens surged in the late 1990s and early 2000s, but decreased in 2003 and 2004 and remained low in 2006 (Johnston 2007). These substances have become known as "designer drugs" (Christophersen 2000).

Designer amphetamines sometimes differ from the parent compound by only a single element. These "synthetic spinoffs" pose a significant abuse problem because often several different designer amphetamines can be made from the parent compound and still retain the abuse potential of the original substance.

For many years, the production and distribution of designer amphetamines were not illegal, even though they were synthesized from controlled substances. In the mid-1980s, however, the DEA actively pursued policies to curb their production and sale. Consequently, many designer amphetamines were outlawed under the Substance Analogue Enforcement Act (1986), which makes illegal any substance that is similar in structure or psychological effect to any substance already scheduled, if it is manufactured, possessed, or sold with the intention that it be consumed by human beings (Beck 1990).

The principal types of designer amphetamines are:

- Derivatives from amphetamine and methamphetamine that retain the CNS stimulatory effects, such as methcathinone ("cat").
- Derivatives from amphetamine and methamphetamine that have prominent hallucinogenic effects in addition to their CNS stimulatory action, such as MDMA (Ecstasy).

Because the basic amphetamine molecule can be easily synthesized and readily modified, new amphetamine-like drugs occasionally appear on the streets. Although these designer amphetamines are thought of as new drugs when they first appear, in fact most were originally synthesized from the 1940s to the 1960s by pharmaceutical companies trying to find new decongestant and anorexiant drugs to compete with the other amphetamines. Some of these compounds were found to be too toxic to be marketed but have been rediscovered by "street chemists" and are sold to unsuspecting victims trying to experience a new sensation. Table 10.1 lists some of these designer amphetamines.

Some designer drugs of abuse that are chemically related to amphetamine include DOM (STP), methcathinone (called cat or bathtub speed), MDA, and MDMA (or methylenedioxymethamphetamine, called Ecstasy, X, E, XTC, or Adam). All of these drugs are currently classified as Schedule I agents.

MDMA (Ecstasy) Among the designer amphetamines, MDMA continues to be the most popular. It gained widespread popularity in the United States throughout the 1980s, and its use peaked in 1987 despite its classification as a Schedule I drug in 1985 by the DEA. At the height of its use, 39% of the undergraduates at Stanford University reported having used MDMA at least once (Randall 1992a). In the late 1980s and early 1990s, use of MDMA declined in this country, but about this time it was "reformulated": This

TABLE 1. "Designer" Amphetamines

Amphetamine Derivative	Properties
Methcathinone ("cat")	Properties like those of methamphetamine and cocaine
Methylenedioxymethamphetamine (MDMA, "Ecstasy")	Stimulant and hallucinogen
Methylenedioxyamphetamine (MDA)	More powerful stimulant and less powerful hallucinogen than MDMA
H-Methylaminorex	CNS stimulant like amphetamine
A/,A/-Dimethylamphetamine	One-fifth potency of amphetamine
H-Thiomethyl-2,5-dimethoxyamphetamine	Hallucinogen
Para-methoxymethamphetamine	Weak stimulant

reformulation was not in a pharmacological sense but in a cultural context.

The "rave" scene in England provided a new showcase for MDMA or Ecstasy (Randall 1992a). Partygoers attired in "Cat in the Hat" hats and psychedelic jumpsuits paid $20 to dance all night to heavy electronically generated sound mixed with computer-generated video and laser light shows. An Ecstasy tablet could be purchased for the sensory enhancement caused by the drug (Randall 1992b). At one time, it was estimated that as many as 31% of English youth from 16 to 25 years old had used Ecstasy (Grob et al. 1996). The British rave counterculture and its generous use of Ecstasy were exported to the United States in the early 1990s. High-tech music and video trappings were encouraged by low-tech laboratories that illegally manufactured the drug and shipped it into this country. Ecstasy rapidly became the drug of choice for many young people in the United States (Cloud 2000) looking for a novel "chemical" experience. The availability of Ecstasy tablets dramatically escalated in the United States, as demonstrated by the report that the DEA seized approximately 400,000 of these tablets in 1997, which increased to more than 9 million tablets seized in 2000 (Aarons 2000). Most of these illegal drugs originate in European countries such as the Netherlands and are smuggled into the United States (U.S. Department of Justice 2003b). The association of Ecstasy with raves has continued. Because of its frequent association with raves, clubs, and bars, MDMA has been referred to as a dub drag (Leshner 2000). At its peak in 2000, Ecstasy was being used by 11% of all U.S. high school seniors. During the next few years, however, the popularity of this drug declined; in 2006, only 6% of high school seniors reported use (Johnston 2007).

Some have compared the rave culture of the past decade and its use of MDMA to the acid-test parties of the 1960s and the partygoers' use of LSD and amphetamines (Cloud 2000; Randall 1992a). This drug is said by some not to cause dependence, but intense use appears to be able to cause addiction. Incidents of medical emergencies caused by MDMA reported by hospitals from 1999 to 2001 almost doubled, suggesting that during this period more intense use of this drug caused severe dependence (U.S. Department of Justice 2003b). However, part of the explanation

---

Key Terms

speedballs
combinations of amphetamine or cocaine with an opioid narcotic, often heroin

---

for the recent dramatic reduction in MDMA use by young populations appears to be a perceived increase in the "risk" of this drug (Johnston 2007).

MDMA was first inadvertently discovered in 1912 by chemists at E. Merck in Darmstadt, Germany (Grob et al. 1996). No pharmaceutical company has ever manufactured MDMA for public marketing, and the FDA has never approved it for therapy. MDMA was first found by the DEA on the streets in 1972 in a drug sample bought in Chicago (Beck 1990). The DEA earnestly began gathering data on MDMA abuse a decade later, which led to its classification as a Schedule I substance in 1985 despite the very vocal opposition by a number of psychiatrists who had been giving MDMA to patients since the late 1970s to facilitate communication, acceptance, and fear reduction (Beck 1990). Some health professionals believe that MDMA should be made available to clinicians for the treatment of some psychiatric disorders such as fear and anxiety (Benedetti 2002; Cloud 2000). In fact, with FDA approval, small trial studies are being conducted to test the safety of this drug (Drug Monkey 2007). MDMA and related designer amphetamines are somewhat unique from other amphetamines in that, besides causing excitation, they have prominent hallucinogenic effects (Tancer and johanson 2007; see Chapter 12). These drugs have been characterized as combining the properties of amphetamine and LSD (Schifano et al. 1998). The psychedelic effects of MDMA are likely caused by release of the neurotransmitter serotonin (Tancer and Johanson 2007). After using hallucinogenic amphetamines, the mind is often flooded with irrelevant and incoherent thoughts and exaggerated sensory experiences and is more receptive to suggestion.

MDMA is often viewed as a "smooth amphetamine" and does not appear to cause the severe depression, "crash," or violent behavior (U.S. Department of Justice 2003b) often associated with frequent high doses of the more traditional

Key Terms

club drug
   drug used by young adults at dance parties such as raves

amphetamines. MDMA was originally thought to be nonaddictive; however, some reports suggest that addiction does occur when high doses of this drug are used (Jansen 1999). Many users tend to be predominantly positive when describing their initial MDMA experiences (Cloud 2000). They claim the drug causes them to dramatically drop their defense mechanisms or fear responses while they feel an increased empathy for others (Benedetti 2002). Combined with its stimulant effects, this action often increases intimate communication and association with others (Cloud 2000; Goldstein 1995). However, heavy users often experience adverse effects, such as loss of appetite, grinding of teeth, muscle aches and stiffness, sweating, rapid heartbeat, hostility, anxiety, and altered sleep patterns (Gamma et al. 2000; Good-child and Johnson 2005; Morland 2000; Parrott et al. 2000). In addition, fatigue can be experienced for hours or even days after use. In high doses, MDMA can cause panic attacks and severe anxiety (NIDA 2007c). There is evidence that these high doses can seriously damage serotonin neurons in the brain and cause long-term memory deficits and psychological disturbances in some people (Lyles and Cadet 2003; Parrott 2001).

Along with the increases in MDMA-related emergencies, there has been an increase in MDMA-related deaths. Although the 76 MDMA-linked deaths in the United States during 2001 are tragic, compared to other drugs of abuse such as cocaine and heroin, this number is relatively small (DEA 2003). The leading causes of deaths associated with MDMA use appear to be complications from either hyperthermia (related to heatstroke), metabolic problems, or underlying heart problems (DEA 2003).

Methylphenidate: A Special Amphetamine

Methylphenidate (Ritalin) is related to the amphetamines but is a relatively mild CNS stimulant that has been used to alleviate depression. Research now casts doubt on its effectiveness for treating depression, but it is effective in treating narcolepsy (a sleep disorder). As explained previously, Ritalin has also been found to help calm children suffering from attention deficit hyperactivity disorder (ADHD) and is currently the drug of choice for this indication. The stimulant potency of Ritalin lies between that of caffeine and amphetamine. Although it is not used much on the street by hardcore drug addicts, there are frequent reports of use by high school and college students because of claims that it helps them to "study better," "party harder," and experience a buzz (Hinkle and Winck-ler 1996; Khan 2003). However, there is no evidence when used properly and taken orally that this drug will cause serious dependence or addiction. Recent statistics from the Monitoring the Future Survey suggest that in 2006, 4.4% of high school seniors used this drug for nonmedical purposes (Johnston 2007). Because of its potential for abuse, some critics claim its medical use in the treatment of childhood ADHD may increase the likelihood that patients will later abuse drugs. However, this has not been found to be the case (Barkley et al. 2003). High doses of Ritalin can cause tremors, seizures, and strokes. Ritalin has been classified as a Schedule II drug, like the other prescribed amphetamines. Its principal mechanism of action is to block the reuptake of dopamine and noradrenaline into their respective neurons; thus, its pharmacological action is more like cocaine than methamphetamine.

Cocaine

In the so-called War on Drugs, cocaine eradication has been considered to be a top priority. The tremendous attention directed at cocaine reflects the fact that from 1978 to 1987 the United States experienced the largest cocaine epidemic in history. Antisocial and criminal activities related to the effects of this potent stimulant have been highly visible and widely publicized.

As recently as the early 1980s, cocaine use was not believed to cause dependency because it did not cause gross withdrawal effects, as do alcohol and narcotics (Goldstein 1994). In fact, a 1982 article in Scientific American stated that cocaine was "no more habit forming than potato chips" (Van Dyck and Byck 1982). This perception has clearly been proven false; cocaine is so highly addictive that it is readily self-administered not only by human beings but also by laboratory animals (personal observation). Surveys suggest that during 2000, 2.7 million chronic and 3.0 million casual cocaine users lived in the United States (Office of National Drug Control Policy [ONDCP] 2003).

There is no better substance than cocaine to illustrate the "love-hate" relationship that people can have with drugs. Many lessons can be learned by understanding the impact of cocaine and the social struggles that have ensued as people and societies have tried to determine their proper relationship with this substance.

The History of Cocaine Use

Cocaine has been used as a stimulant for thousands of years. Its history can be classified into three eras, based on geographic, social, and therapeutic considerations. Learning about these eras can help us understand current attitudes about cocaine.

The First Cocaine Era

The first cocaine era was characterized by an almost harmonious use of this stimulant by South American Indians living in the regions of the Andean Mountains and dates back to about 2500 B.C. in Peru. It is believed that the stimulant properties of cocaine played a major role in the advancement of this isolated civilization, providing its people with the energy and motivation to realize dramatic social and architectural achievements while being able to endure tremendous hardships in barren, inhospitable environments. The Erythroxylon coca shrub (cocaine found in the leaves) was held in religious reverence by these people until the time of the Spanish conquistadors (Golding 1993).

The first written description of coca chewing in the New World was by the explorer Amerigo Vespucci in 1499:

> They were very brutish in appearance and behavior, and their cheeks bulged with the leaves of a certain green herb which they chewed like cattle, so that they could hardly speak. Each had around his neck two dried gourds, one full of that herb in their mouth, the other filled with a white flour-like powdered chalk. . . . [This was lime, which was mixed with the coca to enhance its effects.] When I asked . . . why they carried these leaves in their mouth, which they did not eat, . . . they replied it prevents them from feeling hungry, and gives them great vigor and strength. (Aldrich and Barker 1976, p. 3)

It is ironic that there are no indications that these early South American civilizations had any significant social problems with cocaine, considering the difficulty it has caused contemporary civilizations. There are three possible explanations for their lack of negative experiences with coca:

1. The Andean Indians maintained control of the use of cocaine. For the Incas, coca could only be used by the conquering aristocracy, chiefs, royalty, and other designated honor-ables (Aldrich and Barker 1976).
2. These Indians used the unpurified, and less potent, form of cocaine in the coca plant.
3. Chewing the coca leaf was a slow, sustained form of oral drug administration; therefore, the effect was much less potent, and less likely to cause serious dependence, than snorting, intravenous injection, or smoking techniques most often used today.

The Second Cocaine Era

A second major cocaine era began in the 19th century. During this period, scientific techniques were used to determine the pharmacology of cocaine and identify its dangerous effects. It was also during this era that the threat of cocaine to society — both its members and institutions — was first recognized (DiChiara 1993; Musto 1998). At about this time, scientists in North America and Europe began experimenting with a purified, white, powdered extract made from the coca plant.

In the last half of the 19th century, Corsican chemist Angelo Mariani removed the active ingredients from the coca leaf and identified cocaine. This purified cocaine was added into cough drops and into a special Bordeaux wine called Vin Mariani (Musto 1998). The Pope gave Mariani a medal in appreciation for the fine work he had done developing this concoction. The cocaine extract was publicized as a magical drug that would free the body from fatigue, lift the spirits, and cause a sense of well-being, and the cocaine-laced wine became widely endorsed throughout the civilized world (Fischman and Johanson 1996).

Included in a long list of luminaries who advocated this product for an array of ailments were the Czar and Czarina of Russia; the Prince and Princess of Wales; the Kings of Sweden, Norway, and Cambodia; commanders of the French and English armies; President McKinley of the United States; H. G. Wells; August Bartholdi (sculptor of the Statue of Liberty) ; and some 8000 physicians.

The astounding success of this wine attracted imitators, all making outlandish claims. One of these cocaine tonics was a nonalcoholic beverage named Coca-Cola, which was made from African kola nuts and advertised as the "intellectual beverage and temperance drink"; it contained 4 to 12 milligrams per bottle of the stimulant (DiChiara 1993). By 1906, Coca-Cola no longer contained detectable amounts of cocaine, but caffeine had been substituted in its place.

In 1884, the esteemed Sigmund Freud published his findings on cocaine in a report called "Uber Coca." Freud recommended this "magical drug" for an assortment of medical problems, including depression, hysteria, nervous exhaustion, digestive disorders, hypochondria, "all diseases which involve degeneration of tissue," and drug addiction.

In response to a request by Freud, a young Viennese physician, Karl Koller, studied the ability of cocaine to cause numbing effects. He discovered that it was an effective local anesthetic that could be applied to the surface of the eye and permit painless minor surgery to be conducted. This discoveiy of the first local anesthetic had tremendous worldwide impact. Orders for the new local anesthetic, cocaine, overwhelmed pharmaceutical companies.

Soon after the initial jubilation over the virtues of cocaine came the sober realization that with its benefits came severe disadvantages. As more people used cocaine, particularly in tonics and patent medicines, the CNS side effects and abuse liability became painfully evident. By the turn of the 20th century, cocaine was being processed from the coca plant and purified routinely by drug companies. People began to snort or inject the purified form of this popular powder, which increased both its effects and its dangers. The controversy over cocaine exploded before the American public in newspapers and magazines.

As medical and police reports of cocaine abuse and toxicities escalated, public opinion demanded that cocaine be banned. In 1914, the Harrison Act misleadingly classified both cocaine and coca as narcotic substances (cocaine is a stimulant) and outlawed their uncontrolled use.

Although prohibited in patent and nonprescription medicines, prescribed medicinal use of cocaine continued into the 1920s. Medicinal texts included descriptions of therapeutic uses for cocaine to treat fatigue, vomiting, seasickness, melancholia, and gastritis. However, they also included lengthy warnings about excessive cocaine use, "the most insidious of all drug habits" (Aldrich and Barker 1976).

Little of medical or social significance occurred for the next few decades (Fischman and Johanson 1996). The medicinal use of cocaine was replaced mostly by the amphetamines during World War II because cocaine could not be supplied from South America. (Cocaine is not easily synthesized, so even today the supply of cocaine, both legal and illegal, continues to come from the Andean countries of South America.) During this period, cocaine continued to be employed for its local anesthetic action, was available on the "black market," and was used recreationally by musicians, entertainers, and the wealthy. Because of the limited supply, the cost of cocaine was prohibitive for most would-be consumers. Cocaine abuse problems continued as a minor concern until the 1980s.

The Third Cocaine Era

With the 1980s came the third major era of cocaine use. This era started much like the second in that the public and even the medical community were naive and misinformed about the drug. Cocaine was viewed as a glamorous substance and portrayed by the media as the drug of celebrities. Its use by prominent actors, athletes, musicians, and other members of a fast-paced, elite society was common knowledge. By 1982, more than 20 million Americans had tried cocaine in one form or another, compared with only 5 million in 1974 (Green 1985).

The following is an example of a report from a Los Angeles television station in the early 1980s, which was typical of the misleading information being released to the public:

> Cocaine may actually be no more harmful to your health than smoking cigarettes or drinking alcohol; at least that's according to a 6-year study of cocaine use [described in Scientific American]. It concludes that the drug is relatively safe and, if not taken in large amounts, it is not addictive. (Byck 1987)

With such visibility, an association with prestige and glamour, and what amounted to an indirect endorsement by medical experts, the stage was set for another epidemic of cocaine use. Initially, the high cost of this imported substance limited its use. With increased demand came increased supply, and prices tumbled from an unaffordable $100 per "fix" to an affordable $10. The epidemic began.

By the mid-1980s, cocaine permeated all elements of society. No group of people or part of the country was immune from its effects. Many tragic stories were told of athletes, entertainers, corporate executives, politicians, fathers and mothers, high school students, and even children using and abusing cocaine. It was no longer the drug of the laborer or even the rich and famous. It was everybody's drug and everybody's problem (Golding 1993). As one user recounted:

> I think I was an addict. I immediately fell in love with cocaine. I noticed right away it was a drug that you had power with, and I wanted more and more. (From Venturelli's research files, interview with a 22-year-old male, 1995.)

Cocaine prices in the United States recently have been dropping again to about $135/gram of pure cocaine, a price similar to that of the early 1990s. Officials are concerned these low prices will result in increased abuse (CBS News 2007).

Cocaine Production

Because cocaine is derived from the coca plant, which is imported from the Andean countries, the United States' problems with this drug have had a profound effect on several South American countries. With the dramatic rise in U.S. cocaine demand in the early 1980s, coca production in South America increased in tandem. The coca crop is by far the most profitable agricultural venture in some of these countries. In addition, it is easily cultivated and maintained (the coca plant is a perennial and remains productive for decades) and can be harvested several times a year (on average, two to four). The coca harvest has brought many jobs and some prosperity to these struggling economies.

It has been claimed that the U.S. coca eradication program has seriously damaged the fragile economies of poor Latin American countries, such as Bolivia and Peru, causing anti-American sentiment especially in poor rural communities that depend on money from their coca crops

(Caesar 2002). In addition, the spraying of herbicides from U.S.-piloted aircraft to destroy coca harvests is suspected of posing health hazards to the native populations (DeYoung 2003). Because of these problems, there is evidence that the attempts by the U.S. government to control cocaine abuse by eliminating coca crops have not been as successful as hoped (Hall 2003). In fact, some of these countries have initiated a program, to develop products that "legally" contain extract from the coca plant, an effort not likely to be endorsed by the United States (see "Here and Now" Entrepreneurs Promote Addition of Coca to Toothpaste, Shampoo, and Liquor).

Trafficking of illegal cocaine is very profitable and often very dangerous (see "Here and Now," Bloody "Drug War" Fought in Streets of Mexico). Because of the highly addictive nature of cocaine and the profits associated with the illegal purchasing and selling of this drug, criminal groups frequently engage in violent struggles for control of the cocaine market (Weiner 2003).

Cocaine Processing

Cocaine is one of several active ingredients from the leaves of Erythroxylon coca (its primary source). The leaves are harvested two or four times per year and used to produce coca paste, which contains as much as 80% cocaine. The paste is processed in clandestine laboratories to form a pure, white hydrochloride salt powder (Hat-sukami and Fischman 1996). Often, purified cocaine is adulterated (or "cut") with substances such as powdered sugar, talc, arsenic, lidocaine, strychnine, and methamphetamine before it is sold on the streets. Adverse responses to street cocaine are sometimes caused by the additives, not the cocaine itself. The resultant purity of the cut material ranges from 10% to 85%.

Cocaine is often sold in the form of little pellets, called rocks, or as flakes or powder. If it is in pellet form, it must be crushed before use. Such exotic names as Peruvian rock and Bolivian flake are bandied about to convince the buyer that the "stash" is high grade. Other street names used for cocaine have included Mow, snow, flake, C, coke, toot, white lady, girl, cadillac, nose candy, gold dust, and stardust.

Current Attitudes and Patterns of Abuse

Given contemporary medical advances, we have greater understanding of the effects of cocaine and its toxicities and the dependence it produces. The reasons for abusing cocaine are better understood as well. For example, it has been suggested that some chronic cocaine users are self-medicating psychiatric disorders, such as depression, attention deficit disorders, or anxiety (Gunnarsdottir et al. 2000). Such knowledge helps in identifying and administering effective treatment. The hope is that society will never again be fooled into thinking that cocaine abuse is glamorous or an acceptable form of entertainment.

Attempts are being made to use this understanding (either recently acquired or merely re-learned) to educate people about the true nature of cocaine. Such education was likely responsible for trends of declining cocaine use observed from 1987 to 1991 (see Figure 10.1). Decreases occurred in virtually every age group evaluated during this period. Surveys during this time revealed that, in general, cocaine use became less acceptable; these changes in attitude almost certainly contributed to the dramatic reduction in use. From 1992 to 1999 cocaine use rose, but since then it has leveled off (Johnston 2007).

Cocaine Administration

Cocaine can be administered orally, inhaled into the nasal passages, injected intravenously, or smoked. The form of administration is important in determining the intensity of cocaine's effects, its abuse liability, and the likelihood of toxicity (Nathan et al. 1998).

Oral administration of cocaine produces the least potent effects; most of the drug is destroyed in the gut or liver before it reaches the brain. The result is a slower onset of action with a milder, more sustained stimulation. This form is least likely to cause health problems and dependence (Grinspoon 1993). South American Indians still take cocaine orally to increase their strength and for relief from fatigue. Administration usually involves prolonged chewing of the coca leaf, resulting in the consumption of about 20 to 400 milligrams of the drug (DiChiara 1993). Oral use of cocaine is not common in the United States.

"Snorting" involves inhaling cocaine hydrochloride powder into the nostrils, where deposits form on the lining of the nasal chambers and approximately 100 milligrams of the drug passes through the mucosal tissues into the bloodstream (DiChiara 1993). Substantial CNS stimulation occurs in several minutes, persists for 30 to 40 minutes, and then subsides. The effects occur more rapidly and are shorter-lasting and more intense than those achieved with oral administration, because more of the drug enters the brain more quickly. Because concentrations of cocaine in the body are higher after snorting than after oral ingestion, the side effects are more severe. One of the most common consequences of snorting cocaine is rebound depression, or "crash," which is of little consequence after oral consumption. As a general rule, the intensity of the depression correlates with the intensity of the euphoria (Goldstein 1995).

According to studies performed by the National Institute on Drug Abuse, 10% to 15% of those who try intranasal (snorting) cocaine go on to heavier forms of dosing, such as intravenous administration. Intravenous administration of cocaine is a relatively recent phenomenon because the hypodermic needle was not widely available until the late 1800s. This form of administration has contributed to many of the cocaine problems that appeared at the turn of the 20th century. Intravenous administration allows large amounts of cocaine to be introduced very rapidly into the body and causes severe side effects and dependence. Within seconds after injection, cocaine users experience an incredible state of euphoria. The "high" is intense but short-lived; within 15 to 20 minutes, the user experiences dysphoria and is heading for a "crash." To prevent these unpleasant rebound effects, cocaine is readministered every 10 to 30 minutes. Readministration continues as long as there is drug available (NIDA 1998).

This binge activity resembles that seen in the methamphetamine "run," except it is usually shorter in duration. When the cocaine supply is exhausted, the binge is over (Zickler 2001). Several days of abstinence may separate these episodes; the average cocaine addict binges once to several times a week, with each binge lasting 4 to 24 hours. Cocaine addicts claim that all thoughts turn toward cocaine during binges; everything else loses significance. This pattern of intense use is how some people blow all of their money on cocaine.

Freebasing is a method of reducing impurities in cocaine and preparing the drug for smoking. It produces a type of cocaine that is more powerful than normal cocaine hydrochloride. One way to "freebase" is to treat the cocaine hydrochloride with a liquid base such as sodium carbonate or ammonium hydroxide. The cocaine dissolves, along with many of the impurities commonly found in it (such as amphetamines, lidocaine, sugars, and others). A solvent, such as petroleum or ethyl ether, is added to the liquid to extract the cocaine. The solvent containing the cocaine floats to the top and is drawn off with an eyedropper; it is placed in an evaporation dish to dry, and crystal-ized cocaine residue is then crushed into a fine powder, which can be smoked in a special glass pipe (APA 2000).

The effects of smoked cocaine are as intense or more than those achieved through intravenous administration (Fischman and Johanson 1996). The onset is very rapid, the euphoria is dramatic, the depression is severe, the side effects are dangerous, and the chances of dependence are high (NIDA 2007b). The reason for these intense reactions to inhaling cocaine into the lungs is that the drug passes rapidly through the lining of the lungs and into the many blood vessels present; it is then carried almost directly to the brain.

Freebasing became popular in the United States in the 1980s due to the fear of diseases such as AIDS and hepatitis, which are transmitted by sharing contaminated hypodermic needles. But free-basing involves other dangers. Because the volatile solvents required for freebasing are very explosive, careless people have been seriously burned or killed during processing (Seigel 1985). Street synonyms used for freebased cocaine include baseball, bumping, white tornado, world series, and snowtoke.

"Crack"

Between 1985 and 1986, a special type of free-based cocaine known as crack or "rock" appeared on the streets (Hatsukami and Fischman 1996). By 1988, approximately 5% of high school students had tried crack. As of 1992 this number had fallen to 2.6%, by 1999 it rose to 4.6%, but by 2006 it declined again to 2.1% (Johnston 2007). Crack is inexpensive and can be smoked without the dangerous explosive solvents mentioned earlier in the discussion of freebasing. It is made by taking powdered cocaine hydrochloride and adding

sodium bicarbonate (baking soda) and water. The paste that forms removes impurities as well as the hydrochloride from the cocaine. The substance is then dried into hard pieces called rocks, which may contain as much as 90% pure cocaine. Other slang terms for crack include base, black rock, gravel, Roxanne, and space basing.

Like freebased cocaine, crack is usually smoked in a glass water pipe. When the fumes are absorbed into the lungs, they act rapidly, reaching the brain within 8 to 10 seconds. An intense "rush" or "high" results, and later a powerful state of depression, or "crash," occurs. The high may last only 3 to 5 minutes, and the depression may persist from 10 to 40 minutes or longer in some cases. As soon as crack is smoked, the nervous system is greatly stimulated by the release of dopamine, which seems to be involved in the rush. Cocaine prevents resupply of this neurotransmitter, which may trigger the crash.

Because of the abrupt and intense release of dopamine, smoked crack is viewed as a drug with tremendous potential for addiction (APA 2000) and is considered by users to be more enjoyable than cocaine administered intravenously (Fischman and Johanson 1996). In fact, some people with serious cardiovascular disease continue using crack despite knowing their serious risk for heart attacks and strokes (Fischman and Foltin 1992).

Crack and cocaine marketing and use are often associated with criminal activity (APA 2000) such as robberies and homicides (Swan 1995).

In general, crack use has been more common among African American and Hispanic populations than among white Americans. Of special

---

Key Terms

adulterated
 contaminating substances are mixed in to dilute the drugs

concern is the use of crack among women during pregnancy. Children born under these circumstances have been referred to as crack babies. Even though the effects of crack on fetal development are not fully understood, many clinicians and researchers have predicted that these crack babies will impose an enormous social burden as they grow up. However, other experts have expressed concern that the impact of cocaine on the fetus is grossly overstated and have suggested that behavioral problems seen in these children are more a consequence of social environment than direct pharmacological effects (Vidaeff and Mastrobat-tista 2003). This issue is discussed in greater detail later in this section.

It is not coincidental that the popularity of crack use paralleled the AIDS epidemic in the mid-1980s. Because crack administration does not require injection, theoretically the risk of contracting HIV from contaminated needles is avoided. Even so, incidence of HIV infection in crack users is still very high because many crack smokers also use cocaine intravenously, thereby increasing the chances of their becoming HIV infected (see Chapter 16). Another reason for the high incidence of HIV infection (as well as other sexually transmitted diseases, such as syphilis and gonorrhea) among crack users is the dangerous sexual behavior in which these people engage (Castilla et al. 1999). Not only is crack commonly used as payment for sex, but its users are also much less inclined to be cautious about their sexual activities while under the influence of this drug (Ladd and Petry 2003).

Major Pharmacological Effects of Cocaine

Cocaine can have profound effects on several vital systems in the body (Drug Facts and Comparisons 2005). With the assistance of modern technology, the mechanisms whereby cocaine alters body functions have become better understood today. Such knowledge may eventually lead to better treatment of cocaine dependence.

Bloody "Drug War" Fought in Streets of Mexico

Drug cartels ship hundreds of ions of cocaine to the United States. Because of the billions of dollars that can be made from this illegal market, gangs fight each other for control of the production and merchandising of this substance. This competition frequently turns violent, as appeared to be the case in the small Mexican border city of Nuevo Laredo, where nine people were found tortured and killed in April 2003. These assassinations were thought to be the result of a power struggle within the cartels.

Source: Weiner, L [4,9] Linked to Drug War Found Slain Outside Mexican Border City." The New York Times (3 April 2003): A5.

Most of the pharmacological effects of cocaine use stem from enhanced activity of catecholamine (dopamine, noradrenaline, adrenaline) and serotonin transmitters. It is believed that the principal action of the drug is to block the reuptake and inactivation of these substances following their release from neurons. Such action prolongs the activity of these transmitter substances at their receptors and substantially increases their effects. The summation of cocaine's effects on these four transmitters causes CNS stimulation (Woolverton and Johnston 1992). The increase of noradrenaline activity following cocaine administration increases the effects of the sympathetic nervous system and alters cardiovascular activity.

CNS Effects Because cocaine has stimulant properties, it has antidepressant effects as well. Some users self-administer cocaine to relieve severe depression or the negative symptoms of schizophrenia (Markou and Kenny 2002), but in general its short-term action and abuse liability make cocaine unsatisfactory for the treatment

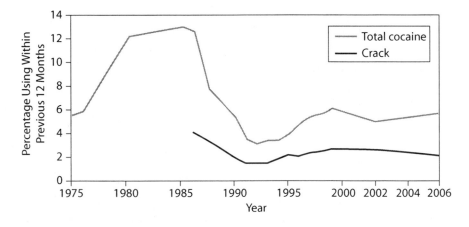

Note: Crack cocaine did riot become widely available until 1986.

Source: Johnston, L. "Monitoring the Future" 2007. Available www.monitoringthefuture.org/pubs/rnonographs/voll_2006.pdf.

FIGURE 1. Trends in cocaine and crack use by high school seniors, 1975-2006. These data represent the percentages of high school seniors surveyed who reported using cocaine during the year.

of depression disorders. The effects of stimulation appear to increase both physical and mental performance while masking fatigue. High doses of cocaine cause euphoria (based on the form of administration) and enhance the sense of strength, energy, and performance. Because of these positive effects, cocaine has intense reinforcing properties, which encourage continual use and dependence (Nathan et al. 1998).

Cocaine addicts can often distinguish between the two phenomena of the rush and the high associated with cocaine administration. Both the rush and the high peak about 3 minutes after use. The rush seems to be associated with elevated heart rate, sweating, and feelings of "speeding" or "being out of control"; the high includes feelings of euphoria, self-confidence, well-being, and sociability. Drug craving also occurs rapidly and is evident as soon as 12 minutes after administration. Interestingly, brain scans of cocaine users have demonstrated that specific brain regions are associated with these drug effects; thus, the rush and craving are linked with different regions of the limbic system in the brain (see Figure 4.6; Stocker 1999).

The feeling of exhilaration and confidence caused by cocaine can easily become transformed into irritable restlessness and confused hyperactivity (APA 2000). In addition, high chronic doses alter personality, frequently causing psychotic behavior that resembles paranoid schizophrenia (APA 2000; Nathan et al. 1998). For example, in an interview with Peter Venturelli, a 17-year-old female explained that a cocaine-abusing friend . . . was so coked up that he' carved the word 'pain' in his arm and poured coke on it. He thought it symbolized something." In addition, cocaine use heightens the risk of suicide, major trauma, and violent crimes (APA 2000). In many ways, the CNS effects of cocaine resemble those of amphetamines, although perhaps with a more rapid onset, a more intense high (due partially to

the manner in which the drugs are administered), and a shorter duration of action (APA 2000).

Besides dependence, other notable CNS toxicities that can be caused by cocaine use include headaches, temporary loss of consciousness, seizures, and death (DrugFacts and Comparisons 2005).

Cardiovascular System Effects Cocaine can initiate pronounced changes in the cardiovascular system by enhancing the sympathetic nervous system, increasing the levels of adrenaline, and causing vasoconstriction (Zickler 2002). The initial effects of cocaine are to increase heart rate and elevate blood pressure. While the heart is being stimulated and working harder, the vasoconstriction effects deprive the cardiac muscle of needed blood (Fischman and Johanson 1996). Such a combination can cause severe heart arrhythmia (an irregular contraction pattern) or heart attack. Other degenerative processes have also been described in the hearts and blood vessels of chronic cocaine users (Kloner and Rezkalla 2003). In addition, the vasoconstrictive action of this sympathomimetic can damage other tissues, leading to stroke, lung damage in those who smoke cocaine, destruction of nasal cartilage in those who snort the drug, and injury to the gastrointestinal tract (Goodger etal. 2005).

Local Anesthetic Effects Cocaine was the first local anesthetic used routinely in modern-day medicine (Musto 1998). There is speculation that in ancient times, Andes Indians of South America used cocaine-filled saliva from chewing coca leaves as a local anesthetic for surgical procedures (Aldrich and Barker 1976). However, this assumption is contested by others (Byck 1987). Even so, cocaine is still a preferred local anesthetic for minor pharyngeal (back part of the mouth and upper throat area) surgery due to its good vasoconstriction (reduces bleeding) and topical, local numbing effects. Although relatively safe when applied topically, significant amounts of cocaine can enter the bloodstream and, in sensitive people, cause CNS stimulation, toxic psychosis, or, on rare occasions, death (Harris and Batki 2000; Medical Letter 1996).

Cocaine Withdrawal

Considerable debate has arisen as to whether cocaine withdrawal actually happens and, if so, what it involves. With the most recent cocaine epidemic and the high incidence of intense, chronic use, it has become apparent that nervous systems do become tolerant to cocaine and that, during abstinence, withdrawal symptoms occur (APA 2000). In fact, because of CNS dependence, the use of cocaine is less likely to be stopped voluntarily than is the use of many other illicit drugs (Sofuoglu et al. 2003). Certainly, if the withdrawal experience is adverse enough, a user will be encouraged to resume the cocaine habit.

The extent of cocaine withdrawal is proportional to the duration and intensity of use. The physical withdrawal symptoms are relatively minor compared with those caused by long-term use of CNS depressants and by themselves are not considered to be life-threatening (MedlinePlus 2007). Short-term withdrawal symptoms include depression (chronic cocaine users are 60 times more likely to commit suicide than nonusers), sleep abnormalities, craving for the drug, agitation, and anhedonia (inability to experience pleasure). Long-term withdrawal effects include a return to normal pleasures, accompanied by mood swings and occasional craving triggered by cues in the surroundings (APA 2000; Mendelson and Mello 1996).

Of particular importance to treatment of chronic cocaine users is that abstinence after bingeing appears to follow three unique stages, each of which must be dealt with in a different manner if relapse is to be prevented. These phases are classified as phase 1, or "crash" (occurs 9

Key Terms

freebasing
    conversion of cocaine into its alkaline form for smoking
crack
    already processed and inexpensive "freebased" cocaine, ready for smoking

---

hours to 4 days after drug use is stopped); phase 2, or withdrawal (1 to 10 weeks); and phase 3, or extinction (indefinite). The basic features of these phases are outlined in Table 10.2 (APA 2000).

Treatment of Cocaine Dependence

Cocaine dependency is classified as a psychiatric disorder by the American Psychiatric Association (APA 2000) and is resulting in a growing number of persons seeking treatment for drug addiction (Piatt et al. 2002). Treatment of this condition has improved as experience working with these patients has increased. Even so, success rates vary for different programs (Nathan et al. 1998). The problem with program assessments is that they often do not take into account patients who drop out. Also, no clear-cut criteria for qualifying success have been established. For example, is success considered to be abstaining from cocaine for 1 year, 2 years, 5 years, or forever?

No one treatment technique has been found to be significantly superior to others or universally effective (Mendelson and Mello 1996; NIDA 2007; Substance Abuse and Mental Health Services Administration [SAMHSA] 1999), nor is there a particularly effective medication to treat cocaine addiction (Piatt et al. 2002). Consequently, substantial disagreement exists as to what is the best strategy for treating cocaine dependency. There is a major ongoing effort by federal agencies and scientists to find effective therapy for cocaine addiction. Most treatments are directed at relieving craving. Major differences in treatment approaches include (1) whether outpatient or inpatient status is deemed appropriate, (2) which drugs and what dosages are used to treat patients during the various stages of abstinence, and (3) what length of time the patient is isolated from cocaine-accessible environments.

It is important to treat each individual patient according to his or her unique needs. Some questions that need to be considered when formulating a therapeutic approach include the following:

Why did the patient begin using cocaine, and why has dependency occurred?

What is the severity of abuse?

How has the cocaine been administered?

What is the psychiatric status of the patient; are there underlying or coexisting mental disorders, such as depression or attention deficit disorder?

What other drugs are being abused along with the cocaine?

What is the patient's motivation for eliminating cocaine dependence?

What sort of support system (family, friends, coworkers, and so on) will sustain the patient in the abstinence effort?

Outpatient Versus Inpatient Approaches The decision as to whether to treat a patient who is dependent on cocaine as an outpatient or an inpatient is based on a number of factors. For example, inpatient techniques allow greater control than outpatient treatment; thus, the environment can be better regulated, the training of the patient can be more closely supervised, and the patient's responses to treatment can be more closely monitored. In

contrast, the advantages of the outpatient approach are that supportive family and friends are better able to encourage the patient, the surroundings are more comfortable and natural, and potential problems that might occur when the patient returns to a normal lifestyle are more likely to be identified. In addition, outpatient treatment is less expensive.

Cocaine-dependent patients should be matched to the most appropriate strategy based on their personalities, psychiatric status, and the conditions of their addiction (Mendelson and Mello 1996). For instance, a cocaine addict who lives in the inner city, comes from a home with other drug-dependent family members, and has little support probably would do better in the tightly controlled inpatient environment. However, a highly motivated cocaine addict who comes from a supportive home and a neighborhood that is relatively free of drug problems would probably do better on an outpatient basis.

Therapeutic Drug Treatment Several drugs have been used to treat cocaine abstinence, some of which are themselves active on dopamine systems, but none has been found to be universally effective (Smith et al. 1999). Table 10.3 lists some drugs that have been used in each of the three principal phases of cocaine abstinence. Besides relieving acute problems of anxiety, agitation, and psychosis, drugs can diminish cocaine craving; this effect is achieved by giving drugs such as bromocriptine or levodopa that stimulate the dopamine transmitter system or the narcotic buprenorphine. As mentioned, the pleasant aspects of cocaine likely relate to its ability to increase the activity of dopamine in the limbic system. When cocaine is no longer available, the dopamine system becomes less active, causing depression and anhedonia, which result in a tremendous craving for cocaine. The intent of these cocaine substitutes is to stimulate dopamine activity and relieve the cravings. Although this approach sometimes works initially, it is temporary. In the third phase

---

Key Term

crack babies
   infants born to women who use crack cocaine during pregnancy

of cocaine abstinence, antidepressants such as desipramine are effective for many cocaine-dependent patients in relieving underlying mood problems and occasional cravings.

The beneficial effects of these drugs are variable and not well studied. There is some debate over their use. Drugs are, at best, only adjuncts in the treatment of cocaine dependence (Carroll et al. 1994). Successful treatment of cocaine abuse requires intensive counseling; strong support from family, friends, and coworkers; and a highly motivated patient. It is important to realize that a complete "cure" from cocaine dependence is not likely; ex-addicts cannot return to cocaine and control its use (Kleber 1992).

Recovery from Cocaine Dependence Although numerous therapeutic approaches exist for treating cocaine addiction, successful recovery is not likely unless the individual will substantially benefit by giving up the drug. Research has shown that treatment is most likely to succeed in patients who are middle-class, employed, and married; for example, 85% of addicted medical professionals recover from cocaine addiction. These people can usually be convinced that they have too much to lose in their personal and professional lives by continuing their cocaine habit. In contrast, a severely dependent crack addict who has no job, family, home, or hope for the future is not likely to be persuaded that abstinence from cocaine would be advantageous, so therapy is rarely successful (Grinspoon 1993). Unfortunately, there currently is no uniformly effective pharmacological treatment available to deal with long-term cocaine addiction, although intensive research to identify such therapeutic agents is under way (SAMHSA 1999).

Polydrug Use by Cocaine Abusers Treatment of most cocaine abusers is complicated by the fact that they are polydrug (multiple drug) users. It is unusual to find a person who abuses only cocaine. For example, many cocaine abusers also use alcohol (Pennings et al. 2002). In general, the more severe the alcoholism, the greater the severity of the cocaine dependence. Alcohol is used to relieve some of the unpleasant cocaine effects, such as anxiety, insomnia, and mood disturbances (Pennings et al. 2002). This drug combination can be dangerous for several reasons:

1. The presence of both cocaine and alcohol (ethanol) in the liver results in the formation of a unique chemical product called cocaethylene, which is created in the reaction of ethanol with a cocaine metabolite. Cocaeth-ylene is often found in high levels in the blood of victims of fatal drug overdoses and appears to enhance the euphoria as well as the cardiovascular toxicity of cocaine (Pennings et al. 2002).

2. Both cocaine and alcohol can damage the liver; thus, their toxic effects on the liver are likely to add together when the drugs are used in combination (Pennings et al. 2002).

3., The likelihood of damaging a fetus is enhanced when both drugs are used together during pregnancy (Pennings et al. 2002).

4. Cardiovascular stress is increased in the presence of both drugs (Pennings et al. 2002).

Like users of amphetamines, cocaine abusers frequently coadminister narcotics, such as heroin; this combination is called a speedball and has been associated with a high risk for HIV infection (NIDA 2007b). Cocaine users sometimes combine their drug with other depressants, such as benzodiazepines, or marijuana to help reduce the severity of the crash after their cocaine binges. Codepen-dence on cocaine and a CNS depressant can complicate treatment but must be considered.

Cocaine and Pregnancy

One of the consequences of widespread cocaine abuse is that since the mid-1980s approximately 1 million babies in the United States have been born to mothers who used cocaine during pregnancy (March of Dimes 2003). Cocaine use during pregnancy is highest in poor, inner-city regions. In the United States, more than $1 billion is spent annually for care of cocaine-using women during their pregnancies. Many of these cocaine babies are abandoned by their mothers and left to the welfare system for care.

It is still not clear exactiy what types of direct effects cocaine has on die developing fetus (Vidaeff and Mastrobattista 2003) . Some early studies have been criticized because (1) the pregnant populations examined were not well defined and properly matched, (2) use of other drugs (such as alcohol) with cocaine during pregnancy was often ignored, and (3) the effects of poor nutrition, poor living conditions, and a traumatic lifestyle were not considered when analyzing the results. Due to these problems, much of the earlier work examining prenatal effects of cocaine is flawed and the conclusions are questionable (Vidaeff and Mastrobattista 2003; Women's Health Week 2006).

It is known that cocaine use during pregnancy can cause vasoconstriction of placental vessels, thereby interfering with oxygen and nutrient exchange between mother and child, or contraction of the uterine muscles, resulting in trauma or premature birth. Current data also suggest that infants exposed to cocaine during pregnancy are more likely to suffer a small head (microencephaly), reduced birthweight, increased irritability, and subtle learning and cognitive deficits (March of Dimes 2003; Singer et al. 2004). Recent findings also suggest that children who had experienced prenatal cocaine exposure have problems with some motor skills, subtie deficits in I.Q., and some minor problems with language development, attention span, and ability to gather and use information (March of Dimes 2003). Clearly, individuals exposed to cocaine during fetal development can function in society, but they frequently require special help. It remains to be seen how these individuals will cope as adults (Schiller and Allen 2005).

Minor stimulants

Minor stimulants enjoy widespread use in the United States because of the mild lift in mood provided by their consumption. The most popular of these routinely consumed agents are methyl-xanthines (commonly called xanthines), such as caffeine, which are consumed in beverages made from plants and herbs. Other minor stimulants are contained in OTC medications, such as cold and hay fever products; these will be mentioned briefly in this chapter but discussed at greater length in Chapter 15. Because of their frequent use, some dependence on these drugs can occur; however, serious dysfunction due to dependence is infrequent. Consequently, abuse of xanthines such as caffeine is not viewed as a major health problem by most health experts (Daly and Fredholm 1998). However, there has been recent concern that many pcople, especially adolescents and young adults, do not appreciate that caffeine is a drug and consume it like a food group resulting in side effects and even trips to the emergency room (Hitti 2006).

Caffeinelike Drugs (Xanthines)

Caffeine is the world's most frequently used stimulant and perhaps its most popular drug (Demos 2001). Beverages and foods containing caffeine are consumed by almost all adults and children living in the United States today (see Table 10.4). In this country, the average daily intake of

TABLE 2. Cocaine Abstinence Phases

	PHASE 1: "CRASH"	PHASE 2: WITHDRAWAL	PHASE 3: EXTINCTION
Time since last binge	24-48 hours	1-10 weeks	Indefinite
Features	Initial Agitation, depression, anorexia, suicidal thoughts Middle Fatigue, no craving, insomnia Late Extreme fatigue, no craving, exhaustion	initial Mood swings, sleep returns, some craving, little anxiety Middle and late Anhedonia, anxiety, intense craving, obsessed with drug seeking	Normal pleasure, mood swings, occasional craving, cues trigger craving

Source: Gawin, F. "Cocaine Addiction: Psychology and Neurophysiology." Science 251 (1991): 1580-1586.

caffeine is approximately 200 mg (the equivalent of approximately 2 cups of coffee), with as many as 30% of Americans consuming 500 mg or more per day (APA 2000). The most common sources of caffeine include coffee beans, tea plants, kola nuts, mate leaves, guarana paste, and yoco bark.

Although the consumption of caffeine-containing drinks can be found throughout history, the active stimulant caffeine was identified by German and French scientists in the early 1820s. Caffeine was described as a substance with alkaloid (basic) properties that was extracted from green coffee beans and referred to as kaffebase by Ferdinand Runge in 1820 (Gilbert 1984). In the course of the next 40 to 60 years, caffeine was identified in several other genera of plants, which were used as sources for common beverages. These included tea leaves (originally the drug was called theiri); guarana paste (originally the drug was called guaranin); Paraguay tea, or mate; and kola nuts. Certainly, the popularity of these beverages over the centuries attests to the fact that

most consumers find the stimulant effects of this drug desirable.

The Chemical Nature of Caffeine

Caffeine belongs to a group of drugs that have similar chemical structures and are known as the xanthines. Besides caffeine, other xanthines are theobromine (means "divine leaf"), discovered in cacao beans (used to make chocolate) in 1842, and theophylline (means "divine food"), isolated from tea leaves in 1888. These three agents have unique pharmacological properties (which are discussed later), with caffeine being the most potent CNS stimulant.

Beverages Containing Caffeine

To understand the unique role that caffeine plays in U.S. society, it is useful to gain perspective on its most common sources: unfermented beverages.

Coffee Coffee is derived from the beans of several species of coffea plants. The Coffea arabica plant grows as a shrub or small tree and reaches 4 to 6 meters in height when growing wild. Coffee beans are primarily cultivated in South America and East Africa and constitute the major cash crop for exportation in several developing countries.

The name coffee was likely derived from the Arabian word kahwa or named after the Ethiopian prince Kaffa. From Ethiopia, the coffee tree was carried to Arabia and cultivated (Kihlman 1977); it became an important element in Arabian civilization and is mentioned in writings dating back to A.D. 900.

Coffee probably reached Europe through Turkey and was likely used initially as a medicine. By the middle of the 17th century, coffeehouses had sprung up in England and France — places to relax, talk, and learn the news. These coffeehouses turned into the famous "penny universities" of the early 18th century where, for a penny a cup, you could listen to some of the great literary and political figures of the day.

Coffee was originally consumed in the Americas by English colonists, although tea was initially preferred. Tea was replaced by coffee following the Revolutionary War. Because tea had become a symbol of English repression, the switch to coffee was more a political statement than a change in taste. The popularity of coffee grew as U.S. boundaries moved west. In fact, daily coffee intake continued to increase until it peaked in 1986, when annual coffee consumption averaged 10 pounds per person. Although concerns about the side effects associated with caffeine use have since caused some decline in coffee consumption, this beverage still plays a major role in the lifestyles of most Americans (McMahon 2001), with approximately 56% of adults in the United States being coffee drinkers in 2006 (Painter 2006).

Tea Tea is made from the Camellia sinensis plant, which is native to China and parts of India, Burma, Thailand, Laos, and Vietnam. Tea contains two xanthines: caffeine and theophylline. As with coffee, the earliest use of tea is not known.

Although apocryphal versions of the origin of tea credit Emperor Shen Nung for its discovery in 2737 B.C., the first reliable account of the use of tea as a medicinal plant appears in an early Chinese manuscript written around A.D. 350. The popular use of tea slowly grew. The Dutch brought the first tea to Europe in 1610, where it was accepted rather slowly; with time, it was adopted by the British as a favorite beverage and became an integral part of their daily activities. In fact, the tea trade constituted one of the major elements of the English economy. Tea revenues made it possible for England to colonize India and helped to bring on the Opium Wars in the 1800s, which benefited British colonialism (see Chapter 9) .

The British were constantly at odds with the Dutch as they attempted to monopolize the tea trade. Even so, the Dutch introduced the first tea into America at New Amsterdam around 1650. Later, the British gained exclusive rights to sell tea to the American colonies. Because of the high taxes levied by the British government on tea

TABLE 3. Medications Used in Treatment of Cocaine Abstinence at Various Phases

PHASE	DRUG	DRUG GROUP (RATIONALE) 1
1. Crash	Benzodiazepines	Depressants (relieve anxiety)
2. Withdrawal	Bromocriptine, levodopa	Dopamine agonists (relieve craving)
3. Extinction	Desipramine, imipramine	Antidepressants (relieve depression and craving)

Source: Mendelson, J., and N. Mello. "Management of Cocaine Abuse and Dependence." New England Journal of Medicine 33H (1996): 965-972.

being shipped to America, tea became a symbol of British rule.

Soft Drinks The second most common source of caffeine is soft drinks. In general, the caffeine content per 12-ounce serving ranges from 30 to 60 milligrams (see Table 10.4). Soft drinks account for most of the caffeine consumed by U.S. children and teenagers; for many people, a can of cola has replaced the usual cup of coffee. Recently, caffeine has been added to juices and even water. These caffeine-containing products have names such as Buzz Water or Water Joe. Americans consumed 574 cans of soft drinks — 70% of which were caffeinated — for every man, woman, and child in 2003 (Kluger 2004).

Social Consequences of Consuming Caffeine-Based Beverages It is impossible to accurately assess the social impact of consuming beverages containing caffeine, but certainly the subtle (and sometimes not so subtle) stimulant effects of the caffeine present in these drinks have had some social influence.

These beverages have become integrated into social customs and ceremonies and recognized as traditional drinks.

Today, drinks containing caffeine are consumed by many people with ritualistic devotion first thing in the morning, following every meal, and at frequent interludes throughout the day known as "coffee breaks" or "tea times." The immense popularity of these products is certainly a consequence of the stimulant actions of caffeine. Both the dependence on the 'jump-start" effect of caffeine and the avoidance of unpleasant withdrawal consequences in the frequent user ensure the continual popularity of these products.

Other Natural Caffeine Sources

Although coffee and tea are two of the most common sources of natural caffeine in the United States, other caffeine-containing beverages and food are popular in different parts of the world. Some of the most common include guarana from Brazil; mate from Argentina, Southern Brazil, and Paraguay; and kola nuts from West Africa, West Indies, and South America (Kihlman 1977).

Chocolate

Although chocolate contains small amounts of caffeine (see Table 10.4), the principal stimulant in chocolate is the alkaloid theobromine, named after the cocoa tree,-Theobroma cacao. (Theobroma is an Aztec word meaning "fruit of the gods.") The Aztecs thought very highly of the fruit and seed pods from the cacoa tree, and they used the beans as a medium of exchange in bartering. The Mayan Indians adopted the food and made a warm drink from the beans that they called chocolatl (meaning "warm drink"). The original chocolate drink was a very thick concoction that had to be eaten with a spoon. It was unsweetened because the Mayans apparendy did not know about sugar cane.

Hernando Cortes, the conqueror of Mexico, took some chocolate cakes back to Spain with him in 1528, but the method of preparing them remained a secret for nearly 100 years. It was not until 1828 that the Dutch worked out a process to remove much of the fat from the kernels to make a chocolate powder that was the forerunner of the cocoa we know today. The cocoa fat, or cocoa butter as it is called, was later mixed with sugar and pressed into bars. In 1847, the first chocolate bars appeared on the market. By 1876, the Swiss had developed milk chocolate, which is highly popular in today's confectioneries.

OTC Drugs Containing Caffeine

Although the consumption of beverages is by far the most common source of xanthines, a number of popular OTC products contain significant quantities of caffeine. For example, many OTC analgesic products contain approximately 30 milligrams of caffeine per tablet (Anacin). Higher doses of 100 to 200 milligrams per tablet, are included in stay-awake (NoDoz, Caffedrine) and "picker-upper" (Vivarin) products (Anderson and Nykamp 2004). The use of caffeine in these OTC drugs is highly controversial and has been criticized by clinicians who are unconvinced of caffeine's benefits. Some critics believe that the presence of caffeine in these OTC drugs is nothing more than a psychological gimmick to entice customers through mild euphoric effects provided by this stimulant. Caffeine is also included in so-called "energy drinks" sometimes advertised as a drug alternative, a dietary supplement, or a natural energy drink (Shute 2007). For example, such OTC products have been flagrantly marketed as "speed in a can," "Instant Rush," and "Liquid Cocaine" until the FDA declared the

company involved was marketing its products illegally (Rubinsky .2007; see "Here and Now" Energized Profits).

Despite this criticism, it is likely that caffeine has some analgesic (pain-relieving) properties of its own (Dunwiddie and Masino 2001). Recent studies suggest that 130 milligrams, but not 65 milligrams, of caffeine is superior to a placebo in relieving nonmigraine headaches. In addition, the presence of caffeine has been shown to enhance aspirin-medicated relief from surgical pain (such as tooth extraction). Based on such findings, more clinicians are recommending the use of caffeine in the management of some types of headaches and minor to moderate pains (Zhang 2001).

Physiological Effects of the Xanthines

The xanthines significantly influence several important body functions. Although the effects of these drugs are generally viewed as minor and short-term (Goldstein 1994), when used in high doses or by people who have severe medical problems, these drugs can be dangerous. The following sections summarize the responses of the major systems to xanthines.

Key Terms

cocaine babies
   infants born to women who used cocaine during their pregnancy

---

CNS Effects Among the common xanthines, caffeine has the most potent effect on the CNS, followed by theophylline; for most people, theobromine has relatively little influence. Although the CNS responses of users can vary considerably, in general 100 to 200 milligrams of caffeine enhances alertness, causes arousal, and diminishes fatigue (Wikipedia 2007a) . Caffeine is often used to block drowsiness and facilitate mental activity, such as when cramming for examinations into the early hours of the morning. In addition, caffeine stimulates the formation of thoughts but does not improve learning ability in the wide-awake student. The effects of caffeine are most pronounced in unstimulated, drowsy consumers (Goldstein 1994). The CNS effects of caffeine also diminish the sense of boredom (Wikipedia 2007a). Thus, people engaged in dull, repetitive tasks, such as assembly-line work, or nonstimulating and laborious exercises, such as listening to a boring professor, often consume caffeine beverages to help compensate for the tedium. Most certainly, xanthine drinks are popular because they cause these effects on brain activity.

Adverse CNS effects usually occur with doses greater than 300 milligrams per day, Some of these include insomnia, increased tension, anxiety, and initiation of muscle twitches. Doses over 500 milligrams can be dysphoric (unpleasant) and can cause panic sensations, chills, nausea, and clumsiness. Extremely high doses of caffeine, from 5 to 10 grams, frequently result in seizures, respiratory failure, and death (APA 2000).

Cardiovascular and Respiratory Effects Drugs that stimulate the brain usually stimulate the cardiovascular system as well. The response of the heart and blood vessels to xanthines is dependent on dose and previous experience with these mild stimulants. Tolerance to the cardiovascular effects occurs with frequent use (APA 2000). With low doses (100-200 milligrams), heart activity can either increase, decrease, or do nothing; at higher doses (more than 500 milligrams), the rate of contraction of the heart increases. Xanthines usually cause minor vasodilation in most of the body. In contrast, the cerebral blood vessels are

Key Terms

xanthines
   the family of drugs that includes caffeine

TABLE 4. Caffeine Content of Beverages and Chocolate

BEVERAGE	CAFFEINE CONTENT (MG/CUP)	AMOUNT
Brewed coffee	90-125	5 oz
Instant coffee	35-164	5 oz
Decaffeinated coffee	1-6	5 oz
Tea	25-125	5 oz
Cocoa	5-25	5 oz
Coca-Cola	H5	12 oz
Pepsi-Cola	38	12 oz
Mountain Dew	5H	12 oz
Chocolate bar	1-35	1 oz

vasoconstricted by the action of caffeine. In fact, cerebral vasoconstriction likely accounts for this drug's effectiveness in relieving some minor vascular headaches caused by vasodilation of the cerebral vessels.

Among the xanthines, theophylline has the greatest effect on the respiratory system, causing air passages to open and facilitate breathing. Because of this effect, tea has often been recommended to relieve breathing difficulties, and theophylline is frequently used to treat asthma-related respiratory problems.

Other Effects The methylxanthines have noteworthy— albeit mild — effects on other systems in the body. They cause a minor increase in the secretion of digestive juices in the stomach, which can be significant to individuals suffering from stomach ailments such as ulcers. These drugs also increase urine formation (as any heavy tea drinker undoubtedly knows).

Caffeine Intoxication

Consuming occasional low doses of the xanthines (equivalent of two to three cups of coffee per day) is relatively safe for most users (Kluger 2004). However, frequent use of high doses causes psychological as well as physical problems called caffeinism. This condition is found in about 10% of the adults who consume coffee (APA 2000; Heishman and Henningfield 1992).

The CNS components of caffeine intoxication are recognized as a "psychoactive substance-induced psychiatric disorder" in DSM-TV-TR criteria established by the American Psychiatric Association (2000). The essential features of this disorder are restlessness, nervousness, excitement, insomnia, flushed face, diuresis, muscle twitching, rambling thoughts and speech, and stomach complaints. These symptoms can occur in some sensitive people following a dose as low as 250 milligrams per day. Caffeine doses in excess of 1 gram per day may cause muscle twitching, rambling thoughts and speech, heart arrhythmias, and motor agitation. With higher doses, hearing ringing in the ears and seeing flashes of light can occur.

Some researchers suggest consuming large quantities of caffeine is associated with cancers of the bladder, ovaries, colon, and kidneys. These claims have not been reliably substantiated (Nawrot et al. 2003; Painter 2006).

One problem with many such studies is that they assess the effect of coffee consumption on cancers rather than the effect of caffeine itself. Because coffee contains so many different chemicals, it is impossible to determine specifically the effect of caffeine in such research (Gurin 1994). Other reports claim that caffeine promotes cyst formation in women's breasts. Although these conclusions have been challenged, many clinicians advise patients with breast cysts to avoid caffeine (Margen 1994). Finally, some reports indicate that very high doses of caffeine given to pregnant laboratory animals can cause stillbirths or offspring with low birthweights or limb deformities. Studies found that moderate consumption of caffeine (less than 300 milligrams per day) did not significantly affect human fetal development (Mills et al. 1993); however, intake of more than 300 milligrams per day during pregnancy has been associated with an increase in spontaneous fetal loss {ConsumerReports 1997). Expectant mothers are usually advised to avoid or at least reduce caffeine use during pregnancy (Margen 1994).

Based on the information available, no strong evidence exists to suggest that moderate use of caffeine leads to disease (Nawrot et al. 2003; Painter 2006). In fact, some recent research has suggested that moderate caffeine consumption may even reduce the risk of degenerative diseases of the brain such as Parkinson's disease and Alzheimer's disease (Fackelmann 2006; Painter 2006). There are, however, implications that people with existing severe medical problems — psychiatric disorders (such as severe anxiety, panic attacks, and schizophrenia), cardiovascular disease, and possibly breast cysts — are at greater risk when consuming caffeine. Realistically, other elements, such as alcohol and fat consumption and smoking, are much more likely to cause serious health problems (Gurin 1994).

Caffeine Dependence

Caffeine causes limited dependence, which, for most people, is relatively minor compared with that of the potent stimulants; thus, the abuse potential of caffeine is much lower and dependence is less likely to interfere with normal daily routines (Kluger 2004). Despite this, caffeine use

TABLE 5. Caffeine Withdrawal Syndrome

SYMPTOM	DURATION
Headache	Several days to 1 week
Decreased alertness	2 days
Decreased vigor	2 days
Fatigue and lethargy	2 days
Nervousness	2 days

Source: Based on Holtzman, S. "Caffeine as a Model Drug of Abuse." Trends in Pharmacological Sciences 11 (1990): 355-356.

TABLE 6. Common OTC Sympathomimetics

DRUG	OTC PRODUCT (FORM)
Ephedrine	Before removed, was used as a decongestant (oral, nasal spray, or drops)
Naphazoline	Decongestant (nasal spray or drops)
Oxymetazoline	Decongestant (nasal spray or drops)
Phenylephrine	Decongestant (oral, nasal spray, or drops, eyedrops)
Pseudoephedrine	Decongestant (oral)
Tetrahydrozoline	Decongestant (eye drops)

Source: Scolaro, K. "Disorders Related to Colds and Allergy." in Handbook of Nonprescription Drugs, 15th ed., 201-228. Washington, DC: American Pharmaceutical Association, 2001.

is thought to be able to produce a significant addiction (Biotech Week 2004). Consequently, 50% of those consuming one to three cups of coffee each day develop headaches when withdrawing and 10% become significantly depressed, anxious, or fatigued without their coffee. Some people experience elements of withdrawal every morning before their first cup and claim caffeine gives them an edge at work or in school (Shute 2007). However, caffeine is so readily available and socially accepted (almost expected) that the high quantity of consumption has produced many modestly dependent users. In fact, we are seeing younger and younger persons consuming more and more caffeine; from 2004 to 2007 the percentage of 18-24-year-olds who consumed caffeine daily went from 16% to 31% (Shute 2007; see "Here and Now" Caffeine Emergencies).

The degree of physical dependence on caffeine is highly variable but related to dose. With typical caffeine withdrawal, adverse effects can persist for several days (see Table 10.5). Although these symptoms are unpleasant, they usually are

---

Key Terms

caffeinism
   symptoms caused by taking high chronic doses of caffeine

---

not severe enough to prevent most people from giving up their coffee or cola drinks if motivated. It is noteworthy that two thirds of those patients who. are treated for caffeinism relapse into their caffeine-consuming habits (Heishman and Henningfield 1992).

Variability in Responses

Caffeine is eventually absorbed entirely from the gastrointestinal tract after oral consumption. In most users, 90% of the drug reaches the bloodstream within 20 minutes and is distributed into the brain and throughout the body very quickly (Sawynok and Yaksh 1993), The rate of absorption of caffeine from the stomach and intestines differs from person to person by as much as sixfold. Such wide variations in the rate at which caffeine enters the blood from the stomach likely account for much of the variability in responses to this drug.

Caffeine Emergencies

Because of the increased popularity of caffeine-containing products, especially with teenagers, poison control centers across the country are reporting increased numbers of people presenting at emergency rooms with rapid heart rates and nausea from caffeine overdose. Such was the case when a 14-year-old boy recently showed up at a Minneapolis emergency room having difficulty with breathing after washing down several caffeine pills with so-called "energy drinks" in order to continue playing video games all night. But instead of having a night of video recreation with friends, he spent the evening in an intensive care unit intubated until the caffeine cleared from his system and normal breathing was restored.

Source: Shute, N;"Americans Young and Old Crave High-Octane Fuel, and Doctors Are Jittery." IAS. News and World Report (29 April 2007): 58-68.

OTC Sympathomimetics

Although often overlooked, the sympathomimetic decongestant drugs included in OTC products such as cold, allergy, and diet aid medications have stimulant properties like those of caffeine (Appelt 1993). For most people, the CNS impact of these drugs is minor, but for those people who are very sensitive to these drugs, they can cause jitters and interfere with sleep. For such individuals, OTC products containing the sympathomimetics should be avoided before bedtime.

The common OTC sympathomimetics are shown in Table 10.6 and include ephedrine. In the past, OTC agents were packaged to look like amphetamines (called look-alike drugs) and legally sold on the street, usually to children or high school students. Although much less potent than amphetamines (even though they can be used as precursor chemicals to make methamphetamine), these minor stimulants can be abused and have caused deaths. Attempts to regulate look-alike drugs resulted in passage of the federal and state Imitation Controlled Substances Acts. These statutes prohibit the packaging of OTC sympathomimetics to look like amphetamines.

These laws have not resolved the problem, however. Other products containing the OTC sympathomimetics are promoted on the street as "harmless speed" and "OTC uppers." It is likely that use of such products can lead to the abuse of more potent stimulants.

As previously mentioned, some of the sympathomimetics that are included in cold medicines can be readily converted into methamphetamine. For this reason, as of 2006 federal statutes require these products be secured in a locked case behind the counter and sold in limited quantities (Baldauf 2006).

Herbal Stimulants

Some OTC sympathomimetics occur naturally and are also found in herbal stimulants or dietary supplements sold by mail and in novelty stores, beauty salons, health food stores, online, and sometimes by health professionals, including physicians (Fessenden and Drew 2003; Gugliotta 2000). These pills have been sold under names such as "Cloud 9," "Ultimate Xphoria," and "Herbal Ecstasy" and contained stimulants such as ephedrine, ephedra, or ma huang (Gugliotta 2000; Pharmacy Times 1996; Sprague et al. 1998). These products are promoted as natural highs to be used as diet aids, energy boosters, or performance enhancers for athletics (Legal Herbal Drugs 2007; Mihoces 2001). Excessive use of these products can cause seizures, heart attacks, and strokes (Gugliotta 2000). In fact, several deaths and many cases of severe reactions have been reported in the United States from excessive use of these products (Washington Times 2003). The death of a major league baseball player (see "Here and Now," Diet Pills Are Russian Roulette for Athletes) resulted in particularly strong pressure to ban OTC products, including dietary supplements, containing either the herb ephedra or the active ingredient ephedrine (Shipley 2003). In response to these pressures, the FDA banned the use of ephedrine or ephedra in OTC products; however, it will be difficult to actually remove herbal stimulants from the marketplace because of a 1994 federal law that prohibits such action until the FDA conclusively proves the dangers of these substances (Rubin 2003). There have been numerous lawsuits filed against herbal companies that manufactured products containing ma huang and the drug ephedrine. These legal actions claim that such products have caused serious illness and even death. Several of these lawsuits have been settled out of court reportedly for millions of dollars (Ephedrine News 2007). Even before the FDA ban, because ephedrine can be converted into methamphetamine, the Comprehensive Methamphetamine Act passed in 1996 regulated the amount of ephedrine that could be purchased or sold at one time (Sprague etal, 1998).

Tobacco Products and Nicotine Addiction

By Harold E Doweiko

Historians believe that the natives of the New World were familiar with tobacco at least 16,000 years B.C.E.[1] and that natives living in what is modern-day Peru and Equador have been actively cultivating it since 5000 B.C.E. (Burns, 2007). Tobacco-was used in religious and social ceremonies of the era, and when the smoke of the tobacco plant was delivered rectally it was thought to be a useful medicine (Burns, 2007).[2] The first written record of tobacco use in the New World is found in Mayan carvings that date back to approximately 600 B.C.E. (Schuckit, 2006). Then the first European explorers arrived in what would one day be called the Americas. The art of smoking was carried back across the Atlantic to Europe by these early explorers, many of whom had themselves adopted the habit of smoking tobacco during their time in the New World.

In Europe, the use of tobacco for smoking was received with some skepticism if not outright hostility. In Germany, public smoking was once punishable by death, while in Russia, castration was the sentence for the same crime (Hymowitz, 2005). In Asia, the use or distribution of tobacco was deemed a crime punishable by death, and smokers were executed as infidels in Turkey. In spite of these rather harsh measures, the practice of smoking became quite popular in Europe, and within a few decades of its introduction the use of tobacco had spread across Europe and moved into Asia (Schuckit, 2000).

Because of tobaccos ability to impact how the body functioned, European physicians in the 14th and 15th centuries viewed tobacco as a medicine, and like their New World counterparts saw it as a cure for numerous conditions. By the 19th and early 20th centuries, smoking was interpreted as a

---

[1] Which stands for Before Common Era.

[2] Although, as the author suggests, it is hard to imagine that practitioners of the era were enthusiastic about the use of this folk medicine (Burns, 2007). Burns also presented evidence that at least some tribal warriors in the New World would chew tobacco leaves so they might attempt to spit the expectorant into the eyes of their opponent, thus blinding him in the heat of battle.

mark of sophistication both in Europe and North America, but in the last half of the 20th century tobacco use came under fire as its addictive properties and the long-term consequences of its use became clear. In the first years of the 21st century, tobacco use is both widespread and the subject of much controversy. In this chapter, the history of tobacco use and the complications caused by using tobacco are reviewed.

History of Tobacco Use in the United States

Anthropological evidence suggests that a form of tobacco was cultivated in South America as early as 8,000 years ago (Burns, 2007; Walton, 2002). But todays tobacco is much different from the tobacco used centuries ago in the New World. The original strain of the tobacco plant used by the natives of the New World was possibly more potent and may have contained hallucinatory substances not found in the form of tobacco now in general use (Schuckit, 2006; Walton, 2002). This is because European tobacco users preferred the milder Nicotiana tahacum as opposed to the more potent Nicotina rustica used by the native peoples of what would come to be called the New World by early European explorers (Burns, 2007; Hilts, 1996).

Tobacco use was. quite common in England in the 15th and 16th centuries, and it can be argued that the English demand for tobacco fueled the early English settlement of what would become the thirteen original colonies and later the United States (Burns, 2007). Tobacco use was also popular in the colonies, usually in the form of pipe or cigar smoking, although the tobacco leaf was also used as a form of currency in some colonies. In spite of the prevalence of tobacco smoking in the colonies, a small number of nonconformists preferred to chew the leaf, either spitting out the expectorant, or, if they were of the upper classes,

swallowing it (Burns, 2007). No less a person than John Hancock was one of those who chose to chew the leaf, and he went on to prove that he was indeed a nonconformist when he became the first person to sign the Declaration of Independence in 1776.

By the 19th century, tobacco was well entrenched in American culture, but by mid-century several different forces combined to change the shape of tobacco use. First, new varieties of tobacco were planted, allowing for greater yields, while new methods of curing the leaf of the tobacco plant were found, speeding up the process by which the leaf might be prepared for use. Also, the advent of the industrial age brought with it machinery capable of manufacturing the cigarette, a smaller, less expensive, neater way to smoke than handmade cigars. Just one machine invented by James A. Bonsack could produce 120,000 mini-cigars, ox cigarettes, a day. The development of such machines greatly increased the number of cigarettes that could be produced while reducing the price. This made it possible for less affluent groups to afford tobacco products, and cigarettes soon became a favorite of the poor (Tate, 1989). By 1890, the price of domestic cigarettes had fallen to a nickel for a pack of 20 (Tate, 1989), making them affordable to all but the poorest smoker. But this rapid acceptance of cigarettes was not always welcomed; by 1909, no less than 10 different states had laws that prohibited the use of cigarettes, with little effect on the practice of smoking them.

The most common method of tobacco use in the 18th and 19th centuries was chewing. The practice of chewing tobacco, then spitting into the ever-present cuspidor, was found to contribute to the spread of tuberculosis and other diseases at the start of the 20th century (Brecher, 1972). Public health officials began to campaign against chewing tobacco after 1910, and in many cases they suggested cigarettes as a more sanitary and relatively inexpensive alternative to chewing tobacco. Unlike cigar or pipe smokers, cigarette smokers soon discovered that the cigarette smoke was also so mild that it could be inhaled (Burns, 1991). Cigarette smoking became the preferred method through which their nicotine addiction might be serviced, and the world has never been the same since.

Scope of the Problem

At the start of the 21st century, approximately 1 billion men and 250 million women around the world were smoking on a daily basis (Levitz, Bradley, & Golden, 2004; Rose et al., 2003). The global per capita cigarette consumption is estimated at 1,000 cigarettes for every man, woman, and child on earth, with 15 billion cigarettes being smoked each day on this planet (Sundaram, Shulman, & Fein, 2004). In the United States, the estimated 45 million active cigarette smokers consumed an estimated 378.6 billion cigarettes in 2005 (Kaufman, 2006). Although this figure is impressive, it is actually the lowest number of cigarettes consumed in this country in the past 21 years, according to Kaufman (2006). Approximately 20.9% of adults in the United States smoke cigarettes at this time ("Cigarette Smoking Among Adults," 2004).

While only a small minority of cigarette smokers abuse other chemicals, it is not uncommon for substance abusers to be heavy smokers. The prevalence rates for cigarette smoking among alcohol and drugdependent persons range from 71% to 100% (elGuebaly, Cathcart, Currie, Brown, & Gloster, 2002). These figures suggest that cigarette use is a significant problem for those who are addicted to other chemicals.

Although children are not often viewed as a major part of the smoking problem, researchers have found that they actually begin to form pro-smoking attitudes early in life, and then experiment with the use of cigarettes either in late childhood or early adolescence. One-third of 9-year-olds in the United States have taken at least one experimental "puff" on a cigarette (Hymowitz, 2005). The median age at which individuals begin to experiement with regular cigarette use is thought to be around 15 (Patkar, Vergare, Batra, Weinstein, & Leone, 2003). The fact that the roots of adult smoking are found in the childhood years has apparently not been lost on some cigarette manufacturers, who have developed flavored cigarettes that are apparently most attractive to younger individuals.

Pharmacology of Cigarette Smoking

The primary method by which tobacco is used is by smoking cigarettes (Schuckit, 2006), although chewing tobacco and cigar smoking are again becoming popular in some quarters. Chemically, cigar smoke is very similar to cigarette smoke, although it does contain a higher concentration of ammonia (Jacobs, Thun, & Apicella, 1999). For these reasons, the terms smoking, cigarette, and tobacco will be used interchangeably in this chapter, except when other forms of tobacco (such as tobacco prepared for chewing) are discussed.

The chemistry of tobacco smoke is influenced by a number of variables, including (a) the exact composition of the tobacco, (b) how densely the tobacco is packed, (c) the length of the column of tobacco (for cigarette or cigar smokers); (d) the characteristics of the filter being used (if any), (e) the paper being used (for cigarette smokers), and (f) the temperature at which the tobacco is burned (Jaffe, 1990). To further complicate matters, the cigarette of today is far different from the cigarette of 1900, or even the cigarette of 1950, with up to 40% of the typical cigarette being composed of "leftover stems, scraps and dust" (Hilts, 1996,

p. 44). In 1955, it took 2.6 pounds of tobacco leaves to produce a thousand cigarettes; today, the use of these fillers has reduced the amount of tobacco needed to produce a thousand cigarettes to 1.7 pounds (Hilts, 1996). This practice seems to account for why a pack of Marlboro cigarettes that sells for $3.15 yields a profit of $1.40 for the manufacturer, the Phillip Morris Tobacco Company— a profit margin of 44% per pack (Fonda, 2001). While the price of cigarettes might be higher, the profit margin is still the same.

Some 4,700 chemical compounds have been identified in cigarette smoke, of which some 2,550 come from the unprocessed tobacco itself (Fiore, 2006; Schmitz & Delaune, 2005; Stitzer, 2003). It has been estimated that perhaps as many as 100,000 other chemical compounds might also remain to be discovered in cigarette smoke (Schmitz & Delaune, 2005). Many of the compounds in cigarette smoke come from additives, pesticides, and a range of other organic or metallic compounds that either intentionally or unintentionally find their way into the cigarette tobacco. A partial list of the compounds found in tobacco smoke would include these: acetaldehyde, acetone, aceturitrile, acrolein, acrolein, acrylonitrile, ammonia, arsenic, benzeye, butylamine, carbon monoxide, carbon dioxide, cresols, crotononitrile, DDT, dimethylamine, endrin, ethylamine, formaldehyde, furfural hydroquinone, hydrogen cyanide (used in the gas chamber), hydrogen sulfide, lead, methacrolein, methyl alcohol, methylamine, nickel compounds, nicotine, nitric oxide, nitrogen dioxide, phenol, polonium210 (radioactive), pyridine, "tar" (burned plant resins) (Shipley & Rose, 2003, p. 83, heavy print in original deleted).

In addition to all of these compounds, various perfumes are added to the tobacco leaves to give the cigarette a distinctive aroma (Hilts, 1996). Dane, Havey, and Voohees (2006) found dangerous levels of pesticides classified as human carcinogens in the cigarettes that they

tested. Other compounds found in cigarettes or the paper wrapper include various forms of sugar, herbicides, fungicides, rodenticides, and manufacturing machine lubricants (which come into contact with the tobacco leaves and paper as these products move hrough machines used in the manufacturing process) (Glantz, Slade, Bero, Hanauer & Barnes, 1996). Although the smoker inhales these products when he or she smokes a cigarette, there has been virtually no research into the effects of these chemicals on the human body when they are smoked.

In an effort to combat the negative image of cigarette smoking, many tobacco companies introduced "light" or "ultra-light" brands of cigarettes in the 1960s. Unfortunately, research suggests that these brands do not bring about a significant reduction in the exposure to the toxins found in regular cigarettes, and they are just as addictive as regular cigarettes ("Light Cigarettes Just as Addictive,"2006; Hymowitz, 2005).

The concentrations of many of the chemicals found in cigarette smoke, such as carbon monoxide, are such that "uninterrupted exposure" (Burns, 1991, p. 633) would result in death. For example, Burns noted that the concentration of carbon monoxide found in cigarettes is "similar to that found in automobile exhaust" (p. 633), a known source of potentially dangerous concentrations of this chemical. There are at least 60 compounds found in cigarette smoke that are known carcinogens[3] (Levitz et al., 2004). When the individual smokes, radioactive compounds absorbed from the soil by the tobacco plant are also carried into the lungs along with the smoke. Over a year, the cumulative radiation exposure for a two-pack-a-day smoker is equal to what a person would receive if he or she had 250-300 chest x-rays (Evans, 1993). Further, cigarette

---

[3] See Glossary.

smoke is known to contain a small amount of arsenic, a known poison (Banerjee, 1990).

Nicotine. Nicotine was first isolated in 1828, and while this substance was known as early as 1889 to have an effect on nervous tissue, not until almost a century later was the mechanism by which nicotine affected neurons identified (Stitzer, 2003). As a result of legal action against tobacco companies, documents have come to light revealing that these companies knew for decades that nicotine was the major psychoactive agent in cigarettes, and that they view cigarettes as little more than a single-dose nicotine administration system (Benowitz & Henningfield, 1994; Glantz, Barnes, Bero, Hanauer, & Slade, 1995; Glantz et al., 1996; Hilts, 1996). Further, there is strong evidence that cigarette manufacturers increased the nicotine content of most major brands of cigarettes by almost 10% from 1998 to 2004 (R. Brown, 2006).

Although nicotine is well absorbed through the gastrointestinal tract, much of orally administered nicotine is rapidly biotransformed by the liver as a result of the "first-pass metabolism" effect, limiting its effect on the body (see Chapter 3). Cigarette smoking avoids this danger and is the ideal method of introducing nicotine into the body. Each "puff" on a cigarette introduces a small dose of nicotine into the circulation that reaches the brain in less than 10 seconds (Gwinnell & Adamec, 2006). Through this process, the typical tvvo-pack-a-day smoker self-administers approximately 400 doses of nicotine each day without the problem of first-pass metabolism (Gwinnell & Adamec, 2006; Jorenby, 1997; Parrott, 1999). The smoker "over-learns" the process of nicotine self-administration through hundreds of thousands or even millions of repetitions over his or her lifespan (Hughes, 2005).

The lethal dose of nicotine for the average adult is estimated to be approximately 60 mg (Stitzer, 2003). Atlhough the average cigarette contains approximately 10 milligrams (mg) of nicotine (Greydanus & Patel, 2005), only about 25% of this actually enters the smoker s bloodstream (Sadock & Sadock, 2003). Nicotine is not able to cross from the lungs to the blood very easily, and so the typical smoker actually absorbs only 1-3 mg of the available nicotine in each cigarette (Oncken & George, 2005; Stitzer, 2003). In terms of absolute toxicity, the typical smoker will receive between l/60th and 1 /24th of the estimated lethal dose of nicotine with each cigarette. Over the course of the typical day, the average smoker absorbs a cumulative dose of 20-40 mg of nicotine, a dosage level that, if not lethal to the smoker, is still quite toxic to his or her body (Henningfield, 1995).

Once in the body, nicotine is rapidly distributed to virtually every blood-rich tissue including the lungs, spleen, and especially the brain (Hymowitz, 2005). Nicotine is both water-soluble and lipid-soluble, and its lipid solubility allows it to cross over the blood-brain barrier into the brain very rapidly. This allows nicotine to accumulate, and the level of nicotine in the brain will be approximately twice as high as the level found in the blood (Fiore, Jorenby, Baker, & Kenford, 1992). Very little nicotine becomes protein bound in the blood (Hymowitz, 2005).

The nicotine molecule has a shape similar to that of the neurotransmitter acetylcholine, and it rapidly causes a cascade of neurochemical changes in the brain (Schmitz, & Delaune, 2005). One of the earliest of these changes involves the nicotine-induced release of the neurotransmitter epinephrine,[4] causing the smoker to feel stimulated or aroused (Gwinnell & Adamec, 2006). It also stimulates the release of the neurotransmitters acetylcholine and dopamine in the brain, the latter activating the brain's pleasure center and making the smoker feel relaxed (Gwinnell & Adamec, 2006). The impact of the dopamine

---

[4] Also known as adrenaline.

that is released is enhanced by nicotines ability to reduce the levels of monoamine oxidase β in the brain, which breaks down dopamine molecules after their release into the synapse. At the same time, nicotine stimulates the release of nitric oxide in the brain, which has the effect of slowing the process of dopamine reuptake (Fogarty, 2003).

Other neurochemical changes included in the nicotine-induced cascade include vasopressin, GABA, glutamate, beta endorphine (β-endorphin), and serotonin (Fogarty, 2003; Hymowitz, 2005; Schmitz & Delaune, 2005). Nicotine causes virtually a complete saturation of at least one subtype of acetylcholine receptor in the brain[5] (Brody et al., 2006). Long-term binding of nicotine to this acetylcholine receptor subtype causes these receptors to become desensitized, and when they are not occupied by nicotine molecules this might cause or exacerbate nicotine withdrawal symptoms, according to the authors.

Peak nicotine concentrations are reached in the first minutes after the cigarette is smoked, and then drop as the nicotine is redistributed to various body tissues. The biological half-life of nicotine is approximately 2 hours (J. R. Hughes, 2005; Stitzer, 2003). Since only 50% of the nicotine from one cigarette is biotransformed during the first half-life period, over the course of a day a reservoir of unmetabolized nicotine is established in the smoker's body. A limited degree of tolerance to nicotine s effects develops each day, but this acquired tolerance is lost just as rapidly during the night hours when the typical smoker abstains from cigarette use (J. R. Hughes, 2005). This is why many smokers find that the first cigarette of the day has such a strong effect.

Only 5% to 10% of the nicotine that enters the body is excreted unchanged (Hymowitz, 2005). The rest is biotransformed by the liver, with about 90% of the nicotine being biotransformed into cotinine, a metabolite of nicotine that in recent years has been shown to possibly have psychoactive effects of its own (Schmitz & Delaune, 2005). The other 10% of the nicotine is biotransformed into nicotine-N-oxide. These chemicals are then excreted from the body in the urine. Although it was once thought that cigarette smokers were able to biotransform nicotine more rapidly than nonsmokers, research has failed to support this belief (Benowitz & Jacob, 1993).

Acetaldehyde. In addition to nicotine, tobacco smoke also includes a small amount of acetaldehyde. By coincidence, this is also the first metabolite produced by the liver when the body biotransforms alcohol. Researchers now know that the acetaldehyde that forms as a result of cigarette smoking bonds with the saliva, which then allows the toxin a longer period of contact with oral tissues than the smoke allows, increasing the individuals risk of oral cancer (Melton, 2007).

Drug interactions between nicotine and other chemicals. Drug interactions between nicotine and various other therapeutic agents are well documented. Cigarette smokers, for example, will require more morphine for the control of pain (Bond, 1989; Jaffe, 1990). Smokers also achieve a lower blood plasma concentration of such compounds as propranolol, haloperidol, and doxepin at a given dosage level than do nonsmokers (J. R. Hughes, 2005). Tobacco smokers may experience less sedation from benzodiazepines than do nonsmokers (Barnhill, Ciraulo, Ciraulo, & Greene, 1995). Surprisingly, cigarette smokers appear to biotransform THC faster than nonsmokers, and thus the effects of marijuana do not last quite as long in the cigarette smoker as in the nonsmoker (Nelson, 2000).

Tobacco also interacts with many anticoagulants as well as the beta blocker propranol and caffeine (Bond, 1989). Women who use oral

---

[5] It is known as the $\alpha_4\beta_2$ nicotinic acetylcholine receptor subtype.

contraceptives and who smoke are more likely to experience strokes, myocardial infarction, and thromboembolism than their nonsmoking counterparts, according to Bond. There is an interaction between cigarette smoking and theophylline, and after the smoker stops smoking, he or she will experience a 36% rise in theophylline blood levels over the first week of abstinence. This seems to be caused by the effects of such chemicals as benzopyrene in the tobacco smoke (Henningfield, 1995). Also, the concentration of caffeine in the blood might increase by as much as 250% following smoking cessation, causing caffeine-induced anxiety symptoms. Anxiety is an early symptom of nicotine withdrawal, and smokers quickly learn to avoid this unpleasant experience by smoking another cigarette (Little, 2000). The result of this process is that the former smoker might interpret caffeine-related anxiety symptoms as a sign that he or she should have a cigarette.

Nicotine use has been found to decrease the blood levels of clozapine and the antipsychotic medication haloperidol by as much as 30% to 50% (American Psychiatric Association, 1996; Kavanagh, McGrath, Saunders, Dore, & Clark, 2002). It has also been found to increase the blood levels of medications such as clomipramine, and antidepressant medications such as desipramine, doxepin, and nortriptyline (American Psychiatric Association, 1996).

Scientists have discovered that between 70% (Enoch & Goldman, 2002) and 95% (Hughes, Rose, & Callas, 2000) of heavy drinkers also smoke, possibly because nicotine is more reinforcing for alcohol users than for nondrinkers.[6] There is also an emerging body of evidence based on animal research that suggests that nicotine addiction is mediated by many of the same genes that trigger alcohol dependence (Le et al., 2006). Cigarettes slow the process of gastric emptying, and thus the process of alcohol absorption, and this reinforces the tendency for the drinker to also smoke (Nelson, 2000). Further, the nicotine absorbed by the smoker seems to counteract some of the sedation seen with alcohol use.

While the list of potential interactions between nicotine and various pharmaceuticals reviewed in the last few paragraphs does not list every possible chemical that might interact with nicotine, it does highlight nicotine's very strong effect on the way other chemicals work in the body.[7]

The Effects of Nicotine Use

Nicotine causes a dose-dependent, biphasic response at the level of the individual neuron, especially those that utilize the neurotransmitter acetylcholine (Oncken & George, 2005; Ritz, 1999; Rose et al., 2003). The chemical structure of nicotine is very similar to that of acetylcholine, and nicotine initially stimulates these neurons, possibly contributing to the smoker s feeling of increased alertness. However, over longer periods of time nicotine blocks the acetylcholine receptor sites, reducing the rate at which those neurons "fire." This might be the mechanism by which cigarette smoking makes the individual feel relaxed. Further, the chronic use of nicotine results in an increase in the total number of nicotine receptors in the wall of the neurons, which might explain at least part of the craving that smokers experience initially after they stop smoking.

[6] The author has met a number of alcohol abusers, for example, who report that they smoke only when they are drinking. The author has never met somebody who has claimed the opposite, however.

[7] To avoid potentially dangerous interactions between medications and cigarettes, the individual is advised to consult a physician or pharmacist before using a pharmaceutical and then smoking.

Nicotine is quite toxic, and the estimated lethal oral dose is thought to be between 40 and 60 mg (Hymowitz, 2005). Symptoms of nicotine toxicity include nausea, vomiting, diarrhea, abdominal pain, headache, sweating, and pallor (Hymowitz, 2005).[88] These symptoms seem to account for reports that first-time smokers often experience a sense of nausea and may possibly even vomit (Restak, 1991). However, if the individual persists in his or her attempts to smoke, the stimulation of the neurotransmitter systems outlined above will eventually result in an association between smoking and the nicotine-induced pleasurable sensations, as the smoker "over-learns" the association between smoking and the drug-induced subjective experience of pleasure as the neurotransmitters norepinephrine and dopamine are released within the brain.

For much of the latter part of the 20th century, tobacco companies argued that since nicotine does not produce the pattern of intoxication seen with alcohol or barbiturate abuse, it was not addicting in the traditional sense of the word (Stitzer, 2003).[9] However, as the brain mechanisms involved in addiction have become more clearly defined, it has become evident that nicotine is indeed an addictive substance in every sense of the word (Stitzer, 2003). Unfortunately, scientists still do not fully understand the mechanism by which nicotine causes the smoker to become addicted (Rose et al., 2003).

Outside of the brain, nicotine stimulates the release of acetylcholine, which is involved in controlling many of the body's muscle functions. Nicotine-induced acetylcholine release in the body seems to account, at least in part, for nicotine s immediate effects on the cardiovascular system, such as an increase in heart rate and blood pressure, as well as an increase in the strength of heart contractions (Jorenby, 1997). At the same time, the heart rate is increased, as nicotine causes the blood vessels in the outer regions of the body to constrict, causing a reduction in peripheral blood flow (Schuckit, 2000). In addition, nicotine causes a decrease in the strength of stomach contractions (Schuckit, 2000), while the cigarette smoke can cause irritation of the tissues of the lungs and pulmonary system. The process of smoking deposits potentially harmful chemicals in the lungs and causes a decrease in the motion of the cilia[10] in the lungs. These features of cigarette smoking are thought to contribute to the development of pulmonary problems in long-term smokers.

Nicotine Addiction

Sometime in the early 1960s, researchers for various tobacco companies discovered that nicotine, which is the chemical in cigarettes that makes smoking rewarding, was also highly addictive. This research was apparently suppressed by the tobacco industry for many years (Hurt & Robertson, 1998; Slade, Bero, Hanauer, Barnes, & Glantz, 1995). Indeed, one memo from 1963, cited by Slade et al., illustrates that the tobacco industry knew it was "in the business of selling nicotine, an addictive drug" (p. 228), to smokers. However,

---

[8] In extreme cases, oral doses of nicotine might also cause dizziness, weakness, confusion, coma, and possible death from respiratory paralysis. Unfortunately small children who ingest tobacco are exceptionally vulnerable to a nicotine overdose, which might result in death for the child.

[9] In an intesting twist, the tobacco industry has also switched tactics from a blanket denial that smoking is bad for your health to blaming the victims of tobacco-related illness, pointing to the federally mandated warnings on cigarette packages as evidence that they had warned consumers about the dangers of cigarette use ("Tobacco Company Tactics," 2007).

---

[10] See Glossary.

not until 1997 did a major tobacco company in the United States, the Liggett Group, admit in court that tobacco was addictive (Solomon, Rogers, Katel, & Lach 1997):

Nicotine, like other addictive compounds, is able to activate the mesolimbic dopaminergic pathways that make up part of the reward system in the brain (Zubieta et al., 2005). The addictive potential of cigarettes would seem to be significantly greater than that of cocaine: Only 3% to 20% of those who try cocaine once go on to become addicted to it (Musto, 1991), but 33% to 50% of those who experiment with smoking will become addicted (Henningfield, 1995; Oncken & George, 2005; Pomerleau, Collins, Shiftman, & Pomerleau, 1993). Further, like the other drugs of abuse, the greater the individual's level of exposure to cigarette smoking, the greater are his or her chances of becoming addicted.

As another reflection of the strength of nicotine addiction, scientists have discovered neurochemical, changes in the brain after even a few cigarettes, suggesting that even a limited exposure to nicotine may initiate the addiction process (Mansvelder, Keath, & McGehee, 2002). This might explain why children who smoke just four or more cigarettes stand a 94% chance of continuing to smoke (Walker, 1993).

Given its addictive potential, it is surprising that a small minority (perhaps 5%-10%) of those who smoke cigarettes are not addicted to nicotine (Jarvik & Schneider, 1992; Shiffmari, Fischer, Zettler-Segal, & Benowitz, 1990). These individuals, who demonstrate an episodic pattern of nicotine use, are classified as "chippers" As a group, chippers do not appear to smoke in response to social pressures, and they do not seem to smoke to avoid the symptoms of withdrawal (Shiftman,Fischer, ZettlerSegal, & Benowitz, 1990). Unfortunately, very little is known about the phenomenon of tobacco "chipping," and researchers still do not understand what personality or biological characteristics separate those who "chip" from those who go on to become addicted to cigarette smoking.

But 90% to 95% of those who smoke are addicted to nicotine and demonstrate all of the characteristics typically seen in necessary drug addiction: (a) tolerance, (b) a withdrawal syndrome, and (c) drug-seeking behaviors (Rustin, 1988, 1992). Further, like drug abusers, tobacco users develop highly individual drug-using rituals that seem to provide the individual with a sense of security and contribute to the person's tendency to engage in smoking behaviors when he or she is anxious. It has been observed that cigarette smokers tend to smoke in such a way as to regulate the nicotine level in their blood (Oncken & George, 2005). When given cigarettes of a high nicotine content, smokers will use fewer cigarettes; the reverse is true when a smoker is given low-nicotine cigarettes (Benowitz, 1992; Djordjevic, Hoffmann, & Hoffmann, 1997; Jaffe, 1990). Smokers using "low tar" brands have been found to inhale more deeply and to hold the smoke in their lungs longer than do smokers of traditional cigarettes (Djordjevic et al., 1997). This difference in smoking pattern may account for the increased incidence of certain forms of cancer found in the lungs of some smokers. Obviously, there is a need for more research into how the "tar" content of a cigarette affects the way a smoker smokes.

Nicotine withdrawal Withdrawal symptoms usually begin within 2 hours of the last use of tobacco, peak within 24 hours (Oncken & George, 2005), then gradually decline over the next 10 days to several weeks (Hughes, 1992; Jaffe, 1989). The exact nature of the withdrawal symptoms varies from person to person. Surprisingly, in light of the horror stories often heard about the agony of giving up cigarette smoking, research has found that approximately one-quarter of those who quit cigarettes report no significant withdrawal symptoms at all (Benowitz, 1992).

Some symptoms of nicotine withdrawal include sleep disturbance, irritability, impatience, difficulties in concentration, lightheadedness, restlessness, fatigue and/or drowsiness, strong craving for tobacco, hunger, gastrointestinal upset and/or constipation, headache, and increased coughing (Fiore et al., 1992; Jarvik & Schneider, 1992; Oncken & George, 2005). Although many cigarette smokers report that the act of smoking a cigarette helps to calm them down, evidence now suggests that nicotine can induce or exacerbate anxiety symptoms in individuals who suffer from a panic disorder (Isensee, Hans-Ulrich, Stein, Hofler, & Lieb, 2003; Parrott, 1999; West & Hajek, 1997). The subjective distress caused by the cigarette withdrawal syndrome will gradually decrease over the first 2 weeks after the individual's last cigarette. However, some withdrawal discomfort and craving for cigarettes will continue for at least 6 months after the last cigarette (Hughes, Gust, Skoog, Keenan, & Fenwick, 1991).

Complications of the Chronic Use of Tobacco

Tobacco use is associated with increased mortality; this has now been established beyond question. Globally, the smoking of tobacco products is thought to cause 21% of all cancer deaths, while in areas with a long tradition of smoking this figure increases to 40% of deaths caused by cancer (Ezzati, Henley, Lopez, & Thun, 2005). In the United States, 87% of all cases of cancer of the lung, 75% of all cases of esophageal cancer, 30% to 40% of all bladder cancers, and 30% of the cases of cancer of the pancreas are thought to be attributable to cigarette smoking (World Health Organization, 2006; Hymowitz, 2005; Sherman 1991).

In the United States, the average male smoker is thought to lose 13.2 years of his life because of smoking-related illness, and the average female smoker is thought to lose 14.5 years of potential life (Carmona, 2004; Sundaram et al., 2004). Scientists believe that tobacco use is the cause of 19% of the annual deaths in the United States, or an estimated 440,000 premature deaths (Fiore, 2006; Hymowitz, 2005). This number includes 15,000 nonsmokers who are estimated to die each year in the United States from what is known as passive, environmental tobacco smoke (ETS) or secondhand smoke (which will be discussed, below).

It is difficult to state the risks associated with cigarette smoking strongly enough. Wadland and Ferenchick (2004) estimated that one of every six deaths in the United States might be traced to cigarette smoking. Table 19.1 identifies the various causes of death associated with cigarette smoking.

One of the mechanisms by which cigarette smoking is thought to cause death is by exacerbating, if not causing, the development of cancer in the smoker s body. The carcinogenic potential is clearly seen in the fact that researchers have found abnormal bronchial cells in 98% of current smokers, as opposed to just 26% of nonsmokers (Wadland & Ferenchick, 2004). In addition to the cancer-related deaths, each year in the United States, cigarette smoking is thought to cause (J. R. Hughes, 2005; Miller, 1999)

- 17%—30% of the deaths caused by cardiovascular disease
- 24% of deaths caused by pneumonia and/or influenza
- 10% of infant deaths

The direct annual cost of health care problems caused by cigarette smoking is estimated at $75 billion in the United States alone, with an additional $82 billion a year in lost productivity from smoking-related illness (Carmona, 2004). For each person who dies from smoking-related

TABLE 1. Tobacco-Related Causes of Death

Condition	Percentage of smoking-related deaths	If annual death toll from smoking is 430,000 people a year in the U.S.	If annual death toll from smoking is 450,000 people a year in the U.S.
Smoking-induced lung cancer	28%	120,000	126,000
Smoking-induced coronary heart disease	23%	98,900	103,500
Smoking-induced chronic lung diseases other than lung cancer	17%	73,100	76,500
Other forms of smoking induced cancer	7%	30,100	31,500
Smoking-related strokes	6%	25,800	27,000
All other forms of smokinginduced illness	19%	81,700	85,500

illness, 20 people are thought to be living with a tobacco-related disorder (Carmona, 2004). The cost of cigarette smoking to society (in terms of lost productivity, medical care, and premature death) is estimated at $3,000 per smoker per year (Centers for Disease Control, 2004).[11] Smoking is a known risk factor for residential fires, causing an estimated 187,000 smokingrelated fires that result in an estimated loss of $550 million in property damage each year in the United States alone (Bhandari., Sylvester, & Rigotti, 1996).

There is hardly a body system that is not affected bycigarette smoking. What follows is just a short list of the various conditions known or strongly suspected to be a result of cigarette smoking.

The mouth, throat, and pulmonary system. Chronic smokers are at increased risk for sleep-related respiratory problems (Wetter, Young, Bidwell, Badr, & Palta, 1994). The authors examined data from 811 adults who were observed at the sleep disorders program at the University of Wisconsin-Madison medical center and found that current smokers were at greater risk than nonsmokers for such sleep breathing disorders as snoring and sleep apnea. The relationship between smoking and sleep disorders is so strong that Wetter et al. (1994) recommended that smoking cessation be considered one of the treatment -interventions for a patient with a sleep-related breathing disorder.

In spite of the tobacco industry's refusal to admit to the evidence, the research data strongly support a firm link between smoking and lung cancer (Carmona, 2004). Researchers believe that cigarette smokers are 10-15 times (1,000%-1,500%) more likely to develop lung cancer than are nonsmokers (Kuper et al., 2002). Fully 24% of male cigarette smokers in the United States can expect to develop lung cancer (World Health

---

[11] Many smokers argue that since they are forced to pay taxes on the cigarettes that they purchase, they are contributing their fair share to the government's income. However, even the most dedicated smoker does not pay $3,000 per year in taxes for the amount of cigarettes he or she consumed, and thus this argument is not valid.

Organization, 2006). Cigarette smokers are also 10-15 times (Kuper, Boffetta & Adami, 2002) to 27 times (World Health Organization, 2006) more likely to develop laryngeal cancer than nonsmokers, with the degree of risk increasing with greater cigarette consumption. In addition to the increased risk for cancer, cigarette smokers have higher rates for chronic bronchitis, pneumonia, and-chronic obstructive pulmonary disease (COPD) such as emphysema, compared to nonsmokers (Carmona, 2004). Indeed, it has been estimated that 90% of all deaths from COPD might be traced to cigarette smoking (Anczak & Nogler, 2003).

One often forgotten aspect of the problem of cigarette smoking is that approximately 10% of individuals over the age of 65 continue to smoke cigarettes (Gwinnell & Adamec, 2006). Many of these people mistakenly believe that since they have been smoking for so long, the damage to their bodies is already irrevocable and so there is no sense in quitting at their age. In reality there are benefits to quitting even for the elderly. For example, 3 months after giving up cigarettes, lung function improves by about one-third, an issue of some importance for many older individuals with chronic obstructive pulmonary disease (COPD) (Gwinnell & Adamec, 2006). Thus, smoking cessation has benefits even for older smokers.

The digestive tract. Cigarette smoking is the cause of approximately half of all cases of tooth loss and gum disease (Centers for Disease Control, 2004). Smokers are also at greater risk for oral cancers than nonsmokers (Carmona, 2004). This risk is compounded by the effects of alcohol, if the smoker is also an alcohol abuser (Garro, Espin, & Lieber, 1992). Heavy drinkers have almost a sixfold greater chance of developing cancer in the mouth and pharynx than nondrinkers, while cigarette smokers have a sevenfold increased risk of mouth or pharynx cancer over nonsmokers. However, alcoholics who also smoke have a 38-fold greater risk for cancer of the mouth or pharynx than do nonsmoking nondrinkers ("Alcohol and Tobacco," 1998).

For reasons that are not entirely clear, the use of tobacco products is thought to contribute to the formation of peptic ulcers (Carmona, 2004; Jarvik & Schneider, 1992; Lee & D'Alonzo, 1993) and cancer of the stomach (Carmona, 2004), and contributes to the development of cancer of the pancreas (Carmona, 2004). For reasons that are not clear, regular smoking also places the smoker at increased risk for developing diabetes (Rimm, Chan, Stampfer, Colditz, & Willett, 1995).

The cardiovascular system. The negative impact of cigarettes is so great that even a single cigarette has been shown to cause the heart to alter its regular rhythm (McClain, 2006). Chronic cigarette smoking has been identified as the "single most important preventable risk factor for cardiovascular disease" (Tresch & Aronow, 1996, p. 24). Smoking is thought to be the cause of 30% of the annual death toll from coronary heart disease deaths in the United States, with smokers being at greater risk for such problems as hypertension, aortic aneurysms, and atherosclerotic peripheral vascular disease than nonsmokers.

Smoking is also a known risk factor for leukemia (Carmona, 2004), with approximately 14% of all cases of adult-onset leukemia in the United States thought to be caused by cigarette smoking (Brownson, Novotony, & Perry, 1993). Cigarette smokers are at increased risk for cerebrovascular diseases such as cerebral infarction or a cerebral hemorrhage (a stroke or CVA) (Carmona, , 2004; Robbins, Manson, Lee, Satterfield, & Hennekens, 1994; Sherman, 1991). Cigarette smoking is thought to be the cause of 60,000 strokes a year in the United States alone (Sacco, 1995), of which an estimated 26,000 are fatal (Carpenter, 2001).

One way that cigarette smoking impacts the cardiovascular system is by causing the coronary arteries to constrict briefly. Fifteen years ago,

Moliterno et al. (1994) measured the diameters of the coronary arteries of 42 cigarette smokers who were being evaluated for complaints of chest pain. The authors found a temporary 7% decrease in coronary artery diameter for those without identified coronary artery disease who had recently smoked a cigarette. Since the coronary arteries are the primary source of blood for the heart, anything that causes a reduction in the amount of blood flow through the coronary arteries, even if for a short period of time, holds the potential to cause damage to the heart itself. Thus, the short-term reduction in coronary artery diameter brought on by cigarette smoking may ultimately contribute to cardiovascular problems for the smoker.

In addition to causing a reduction in coronary artery diameter, cigarette smoking introduces large amounts of carbon monoxide into the circulation. The blood of a cigarette smoker might lose as much as 15% of its oxygen-carrying capacity, as the carbon 'monoxide binds to the hemoglobin in the blood and blocks the transportation of oxygen to the body's cells (Parrott, Morinan, Moss, & Scholey, 2004; Tresch & Aronow, 1996).

The skin. Smoking contributes to the welldocumented process of premature aging of the skin noted in chronic cigarette smokers (Parrott et al., 2004). Drawing on the results of a study involving 82 subjects aged 22-91 years of age, Hefrich etal. (2007) attempted to develop an objective scale to assess skin aging in adults and in the process observed that cigarette smoking does seem to be associated with changes in the skin normally seen with simple aging. Further, the authors identified evidence that these changes were not just limited to the facial regions or to body parts normally exposed to sunlight, but that they occurred across the entire skin surface, which scientists had not suspected. Further, the authors found that there was a strong correlation between the amount of cigarette smoking by the research subjects and the level of changes in the skin.

The visual system. In addition to cigarette-induced cancer, smokers may experience other, nonfatal forms of illness as well. Cigarette smoking appears to be associated with a higher risk of cataract formation (Centers for Disease Control, 2004; Christensen et al., 1992; Hankinson et al., 1992). Although the exact mechanism for cataract formation was not clear, male smokers who used 20 or more cigarettes a day were twice as likely to form cataracts as were nonsmokers (Christensen et al., 1992). Former female smokers were found to be at increased risk for cataract formation, even if they had quit smoking a decade earlier (Hankinson.et al., 1992). The findings from these two studies reveal that cigaretteinduced disease is far more extensive than previously believed, and that at least some of the physical damage caused by cigarette smoking does not reverse itself if the smoker quits.

The reproductive system. The chemicals introduced into the body by smoking reach every body system, including the reproductive system. Smoking has been identified as a cause of reduced fertility in women and as a causal factor for fetal death/stillbirth (Carmona, 2004; Reichert et al., 2005). Cigarette smoking has been identified as a risk factor for the development of cervical cancer (Carmona, 2004; Reichert, Selzcr, Efferen, & Kohn, 2005; World Health Organization, 2006). Fortunately when a woman stops smoking, her risk of cervical cancer slowly declines; and in many cases stopping smoking might even contribute to a reduction in the size of a cancerous growth that has already developed (Szarewskietal., 1996).

Male smokers are also at increased risk for reproductive system dysfunctions as a result of cigarette smoking. There is a significant body of evidence that cigarette snioking is a cause of erectile dysfunction for men, possibly through smoking-induced circulatory damage to Wood vessels involved in the erectile response (Bach, Wincze & Barlow, 2001). Surprisingly, men who smoke do not appear to be at increased risk for cancer of the prostate, although they suffer from a higher mortality rate than nonsmokers when this form of cancer develops (Carmona, 2004).

Other complications caused by cigarette smoking. For reasons that remain unclear, cigarette smoking is thought to be a risk factor for the development of psoriasis (Baughman, 1993). Cigarette smokers are known to suffer from higher rates of cancer of the kidneys than nonsmokers, and there appears to be a relationship between cigarette smoking and a thyroid condition known as Graves' disease (Carmona, 2004). There is a relationship between cigarette smoking and bone density reduction in postmenopausal women (Carmona, 2004). Further, as a group, older women who smoke were found to be physically weaker and had less coordination than did nonsmoking women of the same age (Nelson, Nevitt, Scott, Stone, & Cummings, 1994). The mechanism by which cigarette smoking might interfere with neuromuscular performance in women smokers is not known.

Finally, there is evidence that smoking can alter brain function, possibly for many years after the individual stops (Sherman, 1994). There is a measurable decline in mental abilities that begins about 4 hours after the last cigarette, and many former smokers report that they have never felt "right" for as long as 9 years after their last cigarette. While there has been no research into the long-term effects of cigarette abstinence on cognitive function (Sherman, 1994), these reports are quite suggestive.

The degrees of risk. There is no such thing as a "safe" cigarette, and smoking cessation is the only proven way to reduce or avoid these known smoking-related problems (Carmona, 2004). "Low tar" cigarettes were found to present the same degree of risk as regular cigarettes (Carmona, 2004).

The passive smoker. Many nonsmokers are exposed to the toxins found in cigarette smoke by inhaling cigarette smoke exhaled by others. This is called "environmental tobacco smoke," "secondhand smoke," or "passive smoking," and it would appear to be a common problem. For example, research has shown that more than almost 88% of nonsmokers have cotinine[12] in their blood, suggesting that passive exposure to cigarette smoke in the United States is quite common (Pirkle et al., 1996).

In light of all of the toxins found in cigarettes, it would be natural to expect that nonsmokers would also suffer from the toxic effects of cigarette smoke. After all, these toxins do not disappear when the smoker exhales.

This is supported by studies that suggest that 3,000-8,000 people die from lung cancer each year as a result of exposure to environmental tobacco smoke (Fiore, 2006). It is also thought that secondhand smoke causes 22,700 to 69,000 cases of fatal heart disease in nonsmokers in the United States each year (Fiore, 2006). The coronary arteries of nonsmokers who are exposed to secondhand smoke become constricted, just as happens in cigarette smokers, reducing the blood flow to the heart (Otsuka et al., 2001). Exposure to ETS is now thought to increase the speed at which atherosclerotic plaque forms by 20%, as compared to 50% faster for the smoker (Howard et al., 1998).

Children are especially vulnerable to secondhand tobacco smoke. Mannino, Moorman, Kingsley, Rose, and Repace (2001) found that 85% of the children studied were exposed to tobacco smoke at least once in the 6 days preceeding their study. Environmental tobacco smoke exposure has been identified as the cause of approximately 6,100 childhood deaths per year in the United States and thousands of nonfatal bouts of such conditions as acute otitis media (Aligne & Stoddard, 1997) or respiratory disease

_____

[12] A metabolite of nicotine.

in the United States alone (Bartecchi, MacKenzie, & Schrier, 1994a). Children who are exposed to secondhand tobacco smoke are at increased risk for asthma (Guilbert & Krawiec, 2003), and it has been estimated that secondhand smoke causes 202,000 childhood asthma attacks and 789,000 middle ear infections in children each year in this country (Fiore, 2006). Finally, there is emerging evidence that children exposed to environmental tobacco smoke are significantly more likely to begin to smoke themselves than are children who are not exposed to secondhand smoke (Becklake, Ghezzo, & Ernst, 2005).

By the start of the 21st century, ETS remains the third most common preventable cause of death in the United States, and only active smoking and alcohol use result in a greater number of preventable deaths in this country (Werner & Pearson, 1998). However, in spite of these facts, what is loosely called "the tobacco industry" (Glantz & Parmley, 2001, p. 462) attempts to dispute research findings suggesting that secondhand cigarette smoke is dangerous (Glantz & Parmley, 2001), possibly to limit the movement to allow cigarette smoking only in designated areas.

The initiative to limit cigarette smoking to specific areas is supported by research findings such as the apparent precancerous changes in the lung tissue of nonsmokers who live with smokers (Trichopoulos et al., 1992) and the finding that nonsmoking women who were exposed to secondhand smoke have a 30% greater chance of developing lung cancer than nonsmokers who do not live with a smoker (Fontham et al., 1994). Nonsmoking women who are exposed to cigarette smoke have also been found to have a higher incidence of breast cancer (Morabia, Bernstein, Heritier, & Khatchatrian, 1996), and there is evidence of a relationship between secondhand smoke and sudden infant death syndrome (SIDS) (Klonoff-Cohen etal., 1995).

In response to these studies and the EPA's decision to classify environmental smoke as a carcinogen, several scientists were paid by the tobacco industry to write letters or papers questioning these conclusions (Hanners, 1998). The tobacco industry paid some $156,000 to 13 scientists to write challenges to the EPA's ruling and reviewed their work before it was submitted for editorial review for possible publication. In some cases the letters or articles were actually written by-the staff of law firms that represented the tobacco industry and only signed by the scientists in question (Hanners, 1998). Most certainly, these actions underscore the length that the tobacco industry is willing to go to in order to keep their product on the market with as few restrictions as possible.

Complications caused by chewing tobacco. There are three types of "smokeless" tobacco: moist snuff, dry snuff, and chewing tobacco (Westman, 1995). Chewing tobacco is also known as "spit tobacco" (Bell, Spangler, & Quandt, 2000). Of these three forms of smokeless tobacco, chewing tobacco is the most common, although even then it is quite rare. Only 5.6% of men, and 0.6% of the adult women in the United States use smokeless tobacco, although there are regional variations in the frequency with which people use chewing tobacco (Bell, Spangler, & Quandt, 2000).

Many of those who use chewing tobacco mistakenly believe that the use of oral tobacco is safer than cigarette smoking, or that it will expose them to lower levels of nicotine. Research has shown that using smokeless tobacco 8-10 times a day will expose the user to as much nicotine as if he or she had smoked 30-40 cigarettes (Shipley & Rose, 2003). Further, at least three compounds in smokeless tobacco are capable of causing hypertension: nicotine, sodium, and licorice (Westman, 1995). Research has also shown that there are 16 known carcinogens in the typical sample of chewing tobacco, placing individuals who use oral forms of tobacco at increased risk for cancer of the mouth and throat (Hecht & Hatsukami, 2005). Research has demonstrated that 60%—78% of those who use smokeless tobacco products on a regular basis were found to have some kind of oral lesion (Sundaram et al., 2004). Other possible consequences that seem to be caused by the use of smokeless tobacco include damage to the tissues of the gums, staining of the teeth, and damage to the teeth (Spangler & Salisbury, 1995). Surprisingly, former smokers who switched to chewing tobacco were found to suffer a 46% higher incidence of lung cancer than their nonusing peers, suggesting that chewed tobacco is still associated with an increased incidence of lung cancers (Henley etal, 2007).

It is not clear whether tobacco chewers experience the same degree of risk for coronary artery disease as cigarette smokers, but they are known to have a greater incidence of coronary artery disease than individuals who do not use tobacco. Further, smokeless tobacco can contribute to problems with the control of the individual's blood pressure (Westman, 1995). Thus, while smokeless tobacco is often viewed as "the lesser of two evils," it is certainly not without an element of risk.

Recovery from risk When a cigarette smoker stops the use of all tobacco products, his or her body will begin the process of recovery from smoking-related damage. It has been estimated, for example, that the impact of smoking cessation is at least as powerful a treatment for coronary artery disease as are the effects of the cholesterol-lowering agents, aspirin, and angiotensin-converting enzyme inhibitors (ACE) combined (Critchley & Capewell, 2003). The Centers for Disease Control (2004) identified some of the benefits of quitting smoking:

Stroke/CVA: Within 5-15 years of the last cigarette, the former smoker's risk of a CVA is about that of a person who never smoked.

Cancer of mouth, throat, and esophagus: These are 50% less likely to develop after 5 years of abstinence from smoking.

Coronary artery disease (CAD): The former smoker's risk of CAD is cut in half after 1 year of abstinence, and is virtually the same as a person who never smoked after 15 years of abstinence.

Lung cancer: This is 50% less likely to develop in the former smoker who abstains for 10 years.

A recent findings by Jatoi, Jerrard-Dunne, Feely, and Mahmud (2007) found that there was a relationship between the amount of cigarette smoking that the individual had engaged in over the course of his or her lifetime and the stiffness of the walls of the body's arteries. This in turn affects the workload imposed on the individual's heart, with the greater workload being associated with the highest degree of arterial wall stiffness. However, the authors also found that smoking cessation was associated with a linear improvement in arterial wall flexibility over the first decade after the individual's last cigarette.

Other improvements in the ex-smoker's health status include a slowing of peripheral vascular disease and an improved sense of taste and smell, according to Lee and D'Alonzo (1993). In addition, Grover, Gray-Donald, Joseph, Abrahamowicz, and Coupal (1994) found that former cigarette smokers as a group added between 2.5 and 4.5 years to their life expectancy when they stopped smoking. The authors found that cessation of cigarette use was several times as powerful a force in prolonging life as was changing one's dietary habits. Finally, as a group, former smokers show less cardiac impairment and lower rates of reinfarction than do smokers who continue to smoke after having a heart attack. As these findings suggest, there are very real benefits to giving up cigarette smoking.

Smoking Cessation

In spite of the health advantages noted in the last section, it is difficult to quit smoking. J. R. Hughes

(2005) suggested that only 19% of cigarette smokers have never tried to quit, which means that more than 80% of cigarette smokers will try to quit smoking at least once. The success rate for smoking cessation is quite low, with only 30% of those who try to quit remaining smoke-free for as long as 48 hours, and only 5%-10% achieving long-term abstinence (J. R. Hughes, 2005). The typical smoker requires 5-10 attempts before being able to stop smoking, although 50% of smokers will eventually be able to stop (J. R. Hughes, 2005). In the United States, the number of former smokers is now larger than the number of current smokers (Fiore, Hatsukami, & Baker, 2002). There is cause for optimism, but it is difficult for the smoker to stop smoking cigarettes. (See Table 19.2.)

The process of smoking cessation is quite complex and surprisingly includes the smoker's dietary choices (McClemon, Westman, Rose, & Lutz, 2007). The authors found that cigarette smokers as a group said that foods such as meat, coffee, and alcohol tended to enhance their pleasure from cigarettes, while diary products and some vegetables such as celery tended to reduce the subjective pleasure from cigarette use. Thus, individuals who wish to quit smoking need to review their dietary habits and change their food intake patterns at least on a temporary basis to enhance their chances of quitting cigarettes.

The most common and least effective method of smoking cessation is going "cold turkey" (Patkar et al., 2003). The sudden discontinuation of cigarettes tends to result in the highest relapse rates; those methods that utilize a nicotine replacement therapy combined with psychosocial support have higher success rates (Patkar et al., 2003). The various methods of nicotine replacement are discussed in Chapter 33.

Former smokers are vulnerable to relapse "triggers," the most important of which is being around people, who are still smoking. Watching others smoke cigarettes, going through their smoking rituals, and expressing satisfaction at being able to smoke obviously would make it difficult for the individual to quit, while the smell of cigarette smoke from other people would add an olfactory relapse trigger to the individual at a time of vulnerability. Such situations appear to be factors in more than 50% of the cases when a former smoker relapses (Ciraulo, Piechniczek-Buczek, & Iscan, 2003). As with other forms of drug addiction, smokers who want to quit will have to avoid contact with friends who continue to use cigarettes.

There is a poorly understood relationship between cigarette smoking and depression. Evidence suggests that individuals who are depressed experience more reinforcement from cigarette smoking than nondepressed individuals, while persons with a history of depression seem vulnerable to a recurrence of this disorder after giving up cigarette use (Patkar et al., 2003). Cigarette smoking seems to precede the development of depression in teenagers (Goodman & Capitman, 2000). These findings suggest that cigarette smoking and depression are separate conditions that

TABLE 2. The Stages of Smoking Cessation

Precontemplation phase	Contemplation phase	Action phase	Maintenance phase
Smoker is not considering an attempt to stop smoking. Smoker is still actively smoking.	Smoker is now seriously thinking about trying to give up smoking in the next 6 months.	Day to stop smoking is selected. The individual initiates his or her program to stop smoking.	Having been smoke free for 6 months, the ex-smoker works to remain smoke free.

may be influenced by the same genetic factors (Breslau, Kilbey, & Andreski, 1993; Glassman, 1993). For this reason, individuals who wish to quit smoking and who have experienced past depressive episodes should be warned about the possibility that depression might trigger thoughts of returning to cigarette smoking.

In addition to depression, some cigarette smokers have come to rely on cigarette smoking as a way to deal with such negative emotional states as anxiety, boredom, and sadness (Sherman, 1994). Because nicotine is an easily administered, quick method for coping with these feelings, the smoker soon learns that he or she can control such negative emotional states through the use of cigarettes. Unless the smoker-learns alternative methods for coping with these painful emotional states, he or she is unlikely to be able to give up reliance on cigarette smoking as a way to deal with the emotional stresses of everyday life.

Cigarette smoking and Alzheimers disease? In the early 1990s, researchers found a "negative association" (Brenner et al., 1993, p. 293) between cigarette smoking and the later development of Alzheimer's disease. However, subsequent research failed to support the theory that cigarette smoking somehow protected the individual from Alzheimer's. Indeed, later studies found that cigarette smokers were[13] at increased risk for developing some form of dementia in later life (Ott et al., 1998; Sundram etal., 1998).

Cigarette smoking cessation and weight gain. Many cigarette smokers justify their continued use of cigarettes because of stories they have heard about former smokers gaining weight after they quit smoking. Admittedly, about 80% of former smokers will gain some weight after they quit, but this statistic is misleading: 57% of cigarette smokers also gain weight during the same period of life (Centers for Disease Control, 2004). Still, it is known that following smoking cessation, the average smoker increases his or her daily caloric intake by 200 calories a day, a factor that over time will contribute to weight gain (Stitzer, 2003).

Another factor that contributes to weight gain following smoking cessation is the impact of nicotine on the smoker's metabolism. Regular use of nicotine raises the individual's metabolism by about 10%, which means that he or she burns off weight faster when smoking (Stitzer, 2003). Finally, most smokers are underweight for their sex/age/body frame so that postcessation weight gain tends to reflect the body's attempt to "catch up" to its normal weight level (Stitzer, 2003). But a smoker also tends to retain less fluid compared to a nonsmoker, and some of the weight gain noted after a person stops smoking might reflect fluid weight gain.

Following smoking cessation, the average individual gains about 5 pounds (Centers for Disease Control, 2004). Ten percent of men and 13 % of women who stop smoking experience a larger weight gain of 13 kilograms (28.6 pounds) following their last cigarette. On the positive side, those who gain weight following smoking cessation seem more likely to remain abstinent from cigarettes (Hughes et al, 1991; Shipley & Rose, 2003). Klesges et al. (1997) found that former smokers who remained abstinent for an entire year averaged a 13-pound (5.90-kg) weight gain, while smokers who had "slipped" during the initial year had a smaller average weight gain of 6.7 pounds (3.04 kg). Also, although the initial weight gain is often distressing to the former smoker, there is strong evidence that the individual's weight will return "to precessation levels

---

[13] The initial research finding was apparently the result of flawed methodology, which failed to take into account the many complications of cigarette smoking that would have caused the death of many of those individuals who had the potential to develop a neurodegenerative disease like Alzheimer's before they could actually develop symptoms of the disease.

at 6 months [following his or her last cigarette]" (Hughes etal, 1991, p. 57).

Although obesity is a known risk factor for cardiovascular disease, the health benefits obtained by giving up cigarette use far outweigh the potential risks associated with post-smoking weight gain (Eisen, Lyons, Goldberg, & True, 1993). A former smoker would have to gain 50-100 pounds after giving up cigarettes before the health risks of the extra weight came close to those from cigarette smoking (Brunton, Henningfield, & Solberg, 1994).

Summary

Tobacco use, once limited to the New World, was first introduced to Europe by Columbus's men. Once the practice of smoking or chewing tobacco reached Europe, tobacco use rapidly spread. Following the introduction of the cigarette around the turn of the century, smoking became more common, rapidly replacing tobacco chewing as the accepted method of tobacco use.

The active psychoactive agent of tobacco, nicotine, has an addiction potential similar to that of cocaine or narcotics. Each year, 34% of people who smoke attempt to quit, but only 2.5% are ultimately successful in this endeavor (McRae, Brady, & Sonne, 2001). More comprehensive treatment programs have been suggested for nicotine addiction/smoking cessation. These comprehensive programs are patterned after alcohol addiction treatment programs but have not demonstrated a significantly improved cure rate for cigarette smoking. It has been suggested that such formal treatment programs might be of value for those individuals whose tobacco use has placed them at risk for tobaccorelated illness.

Factors Influencing Openness to Future Smoking Among Nonsmoking Adolescents*

By Dong-Chul Seo, PhD, Mohammad R. Torabi, PhD, Amy E. Weaver, MPH

BACKGROUND: *To investigate the correlates of youth tobacco use in terms of nonsmoking adolescents' openness to future smoking, a secondary analysis of the 2000 and 2004 Indiana Youth Tobacco Survey (IYTS) was conducted.*

METHODS: *A representative sample of 1416 public high school students in grades 9-12 and 1516 public middle school students in grades 6-8 (71.44% and 72.53% response rates, respectively) were surveyed in 2000, and 3433 public high school students and 1990 public middle school students (63.04% and 65.44% response rates, respectively) were surveyed in 2004.*

RESULTS: *Seventy-four percent of students in 2000 were not open to future smoking and 77% were not open in 2004. The adolescent cohort in 2004 became more exposed to antitobacco messages and less exposed to protobacco messages and environmental tobacco smoke (ETS) compared with their counterpart in 2000. Whereas gender, grade, race/ ethnicity, and exposure to antitobacco messages were insignificant predictors for openness to future smoking, exposure to ETS either in homes or in cars was a strong predictor for openness to future smoking (the higher the exposure to ETS, the more open to future smoking) in both unadjusted and adjusted multivariate models. Exposure to protobacco messages had a greater effect on openness to future smoking than exposure to antitobacco messages. The rate of transition from openness to future smoking to tobacco use initiation is higher among white adolescents than among minority adolescents.*

CONCLUSIONS: *More efforts should be made to reduce adolescents' exposure to ETS and protobacco messages.*

Keywords: *adolescents; youth tobacco survey; smoking.*

Dong-Chul Seo, Mohammad R. Torabi, & Amy E. Weaver, "Factors Influencing Openness to Future Smoking Among Nonsmoking Adolescents," *Journal of School Health*, vol. 78, no. 6, pp. 328-336. Copyright © 2008 by John Wiley & Sons, Inc. Reprinted with permission.

Although the vast majority of morbidity and mortality caused by tobacco use occurs in adulthood, the initiation of tobacco use and the development of addiction typically occur during adolescence.[1-3] More than 80% of adult tobacco users started their smoking regularly before they reached age 18.[1] Study findings indicate that nicotine can produce addiction as powerful as heroin and cocaine.[4-6] This is affirmed by Anthony et al[7] and McNeill[8] who suggest that 32-50% of people who have tried cigarettes show addictive patterns of use, whereas a smaller percentage of people who have tried cocaine or heroin do. In addition to a host of negative health consequences for adolescents who smoke, smoking is associated with several other risk behaviors such as increased use of illicit drugs, fighting, and engaging in unprotected sex.[9]

The evidence from these aforementioned findings warrants serious inquiry into prevention strategies of youth tobacco initiation. Thus, it is critically important to have a thorough understanding of correlates of youth tobacco initiation and use as well as to monitor changes related to youth tobacco use over time.

Although the association of youth tobacco use with race/ethnicity,[10-13] peer influence,[14-20] tobacco advertisements,[21-29] and acceptance of tobacco marketing promotional items[30-32] is well established, less is known about other moderators and mediators of youth tobacco use such as exposure to antitobacco messages and information, exposure to environmental tobacco smoke (ETS) either in home or in cars, perceived benefit of smoking, and perceived peer acceptance to smoking. Also, few studies have examined whether these factors may affect nonsmoking adolescents' openness to future smoking. In addition, considering that adolescents' behavior is rapidly evolving and variable due to the biological, cognitive, psychological, and sociocultural factors that define their developmental stage,[33] there is a need to closely monitor changes related to youth tobacco use in terms of correlates as well as prevalence.

Understanding the factors that are related to openness to future smoking is imperative to plan effective prevention strategies during the critical time in adolescence before the initiation of tobacco use. A recent study[34] that examined the progression to established smoking among US youths suggested that interventions should be focused on youths open to future smoking (susceptible never smokers) to prevent adolescents from progressing to established smoking. Exposure to ETS has recently been shown to predict adolescent smoking, even when controlling for sex, socioeconomic status of parents, a crowding index, and the numbers at home of siblings, adult smokers, and cigarettes smoked.[35] Further inquiry into the risk factors for tobacco uptake among never-smoking adolescents is still needed.

This study aimed to examine correlates of openness to future smoking among nonsmoking adolescents in grades 6-12 by analyzing the Indiana Youth Tobacco Survey (IYTS) data of 2000 and 2004. It was hypothesized that after controlling for demographic variables such as gender, grade, and race/ethnicity, nonsmoking adolescents' openness to future smoking would be predicted by exposure to protobacco or tobacco coun- termarketing messages, exposure to information about health consequences of tobacco use, exposure to secondhand smoke in homes and/or cars, perceived benefit of smoking, and perceived peer acceptance toward smoking.

METHODS

Sampling

The 2000 and 2004 IYTS data collection protocol was designed by the Centers for Disease Control and Prevention (CDC). A 2-stage cluster sample design was used to produce a representative sample. All public schools containing grades 6-12 were included in the sampling frame. Schools were selected with probability proportional to school enrollment size. Then, classes were chosen using systematic equal probability sampling from each school that participated in the survey.

2000 IYTS Sample. Data were obtained from 2932 students at 80 schools across the state (1516 in grades 6-8 and 1416 in grades 9-12; 48% female). Thirty-eight of 47 selected middle schools participated (80.85% school response rate) and 1516 of 1690 middle school students completed usable questionnaires (89.7% student response rate), resulting in an overall response rate of 72.53%. Of the high schools, 42 of 50 selected high schools participated (84.0%) and 1416 of 1665 students completed usable questionnaires (85.05%), resulting in an overall response rate of 71.44%.

2004 IYTS Sample. The sample in 2004 was considerably larger than in 2000, with a sample of 5423 students in 92 schools across the state (1990 in grades 6-8 and 3433 in grades 9-12; 48% female). Forty-seven of 60 selected middle schools participated (78.33% school response rate) and 1990 of 2382 middle school students completed usable questionnaires (83.54% student response rate), resulting in an overall response rate of 65.44%. Of the high schools, 45 of 57 selected high schools participated (78.95%) and 3433 of 4299 students completed usable questionnaires (79.86%), resulting in an overall response rate of 63.04%.

Procedures

The IYTS is a state-level survey, beginning in 2000, whose protocol is similar to the National Youth Tobacco Survey, a nationwide initiative to track and understand youth tobacco usage over a series of years.[34,36] The IYTS questionnaire was developed by CDC and included questions about tobacco use, familiarity with pro- and antitobacco media messages, exposure to ETS, minors' ability to purchase or obtain tobacco products, and general knowledge, attitudes, and beliefs about tobacco. Each IYTS was an anonymous, school-based, self-administered paper-and-pencil survey. Each questionnaire took about 25 minutes to complete.

Measures

Several key variables of interest were generated using the operational definitions provided by Indiana Tobacco Prevention and Cessation. Openness to future smoking is the primary outcome variable in this analysis. The students who were open to future smoking were those respondents who had never smoked, not even a few puffs, but who answered "definitely yes," "probably yes," or "probably no" to the question about smoking in the future: (1) "Do you think you will smoke a cigarette at anytime during the next year?" or (2) "If one of your best friends offered you a cigarette, would you smoke it?"[34]

Six items were used to measure respondents' exposure to protobacco messages and advertisements through various media including TV, movies, Internet, convenience stores, or a racing event. These 6 items were summated and the score was categorized into low, medium, and high exposure. Two items that measured respondents' exposure to tobacco countermarket- ing through various media were also summated and categorized into low, medium, and high exposure. A dichotomous variable was generated to indicate respondents' exposure to information about health consequences of tobacco use based upon reported exposure to the messages received from their parents, doctors, dentists, schoolteachers, or peers. Respondents' exposure to secondhand smoke was measured by 2 separate questions: (1)

"During the past 7 days, on how many days were you in the same room with someone who was smoking cigarettes?" and (2) "During the past 7 days, on how many days did you ride in a car with someone who was smoking cigarettes?" Perceived benefit of smoking was measured by a summated scale of 5 variables: "having more friends," "looking cool" "helping relaxation," "feeling more comfortable in social situations," and "helping keep weight down." Finally, respondents' perceived peer acceptance to smoking was measured by the question "Do most people of your age think it is okay to smoke?" The response options included "definitely yes," "probably yes," "probably not," and "definitely not."

Data Analysis

For each year, middle school and high school data were combined and primary sampling unit was recoded using sequential numbers. Then, all the variables were renamed for easy identification and consistency between 2000 and 2004 data sets especially given the inconsistencies in the variable names in the original data sets. Small frequency categories were collapsed to compute reliable estimates in bivariate and multivariate data analyses. For example, in IYTS 2000, the age categories "18 years old" and "19+ years old" were merged into "18+ years old" because the frequency for "19+ years old" was too small (n = 6).

The statistical package SUDAAN (Research Triangle Institute, Research Triangle Park, NC) was used to estimate sampling variances and standard errors, which takes into account the complex sample design of IYTS. Sampling weights were used to adjust for unequal probabilities of selection, nonresponse, and disproportionate selection of different population groups. After bivariate relationships were examined using chi-square tests and standard logistic analyses, adjusted odds ratios of each of the significant predictors

of openness to future smoking were computed, controlling for gender, grade, and race/ethnicity.

RESULTS

Descriptive Results

Descriptive frequencies and weighted percentages for each category of variables are shown in Table 1. Whereas 74% of students in 2000 were not open to future smoking, 77% were not open in 2004 (z = 2.63, p < .01). The proportion of students who had been highly exposed to antitobacco messages increased from 7% to 15% (z = 10.96, p < .0001) and those exposed to information about health consequences of tobacco use from their parents, doctors, dentists, schoolteachers, or peers increased significantly from 84% to 89% (z = 5.68, p < .0001). Consistent with these desirable changes, students' exposure to ETS was reduced both in homes and in cars. Whereas 30% of students were in the same room everyday with someone who smoked during the past 7 days in 2000, 24% did in 2004 (z = 4.05, p < .0001). Also, whereas 45% of students did not ride in a car with someone who smoked during the past 7 days in 2000, 53% did not in 2004 (z = 5.40, p < .0001). In terms of students' exposure to protobacco messages and advertisements on TV, movies, Internet, convenience stores, or racing events, the proportion of students who were moderately exposed to such messages significantly decreased from 65% in 2000 to 59% in 2004 (z = 5.98, p < .0001), although the proportion of highly exposed students did not differ significantly between 2 years.

Bivariate and Multivariate Analyses

As shown in Tables 2 and 3, gender, grade, race/ethnicity, and exposure to pro- or antitobacco messages and information were insignificant or

TABLE 1. Demographic Characteristics and Descriptive Results, IYTS

	2000			2004		
	Unweighted Frequency	Weighted Percent	Standard Error	Unweighted Frequency	Weighted Percent	Standard Error
Gender						
Female	1438	48342	1.42	2712	48.19	1.24
Male	1488	51.58	1.42	2682	51.81	1.24
Grade						
6th	434	15.40	3.81	343	15.09	4.22
7th	492	15.01	3.06	898	14.54	336
8th	579	14.39	2.88	719	15.28	2.99
9th	301	15.49	3.09	989	16.02	297
10th	435	14.26	2.52	1044	1430	218
11th	344	13.05	2.54	832	12.72	2.06
12th	325	12.39	2.32	516	12.04	2.06
Race/ethnicity						
White	2345	84.57	1.86	38.25	76.08	2.02
Black	316	8.88	1.66	921	13.57	1.70
Hispanic	100	2.71	0.54	342	5.26	0.71
Other	128	3.83	0.44	244	5.09	0.47
Exposure to protobacco message						
Low	819	26.96	1.23	1740	36.36	1.00
Moderate	1780	65.16	1.17	2772	58.93	0.96
High	133	4.87	0.47	226	4.71	0.45
Exposure to antitobacco message						
Low	720	25.67	1.20	1754	34.33	1.28
Moderate	1879	67.43	1.17	2603	50.86	1.23
High	203	6.90	0.54	755	14.81	0.77
Exposure to information about health consequences of tobacco use						
No exposure	459	16.27	0.84	597	10.94	0.99
Exposed	2421	83.73	0.84	4592	89.06	0.99
Exposure to ETS in homes (days)						
0	943	31.65	1.74	1863	35.95	1.36
1 or 2	642	22.52	0.90	1166	23.16	0.85
3 or 4	301	10.58	0.57	543	9.95	0.50
5 or 6	169	5.72	0.49	330	6.46	0.42
7	820	29.53	1.51	1256	24.49	1.07
Exposure to ETS in cars (days)						
0	1327	45.13	1.67	2728	53.21	1.41

1 or 2	542	18.98	0.80	873	16.73	0.67
3 or 4	320	11.40	0.76	524	10.20	0.62
5 or 6	150	5.20	0.52	300	5.73	0.31
7	535	19.29	1.06	731	14.13	0.79
Perceived benefit of smoking*						
High perceived benefit				599	11.24	0.64
Moderate perceived benefit				1878	33.34	1.40
Low perceived benefit				2886	55.42	1.68
Perceived peer acceptance to smoking*						
Definitely yes				1118	19.94	1.19
Probably yes				2113	37.85	1.65
Probably not				1427	29.40	1.79
Definitely not				616	12.81	1.15
Open to future smoking among those who never smoked						
Not open to smoking	997	73.67	1.41	2087	76.72	1.04
Open to smoking	357	26.33	1.41	649	23.28	1.04

*These variables were measured only for 2004.

weak predictors for openness to future smoking (hereafter OFS). Only in 2004, students who experienced a high level and a moderate level of exposure to protobacco messages were more likely than those with a low level of exposure to such messages to be open to future smoking by a factor of 2.85 and 1.40, respectively, controlling for the 3 demographic variables.

For both years, students' exposure to ETS was significantly associated with OFS. Students who were in the same room every day with someone who smoked during the past 7 days were more likely than those who were not in any of the past 7 days to be open to future smoking by a factor of 2.18 (95% confidence interval [CI]: 1.54-3.10) in 2000 and 1.88 (95% CI: 1.31-2.70) in 2004, controlling for the 3 demographic variables. Students who rode in a car with someone who smoked 1 or 2 days in the past 7 days were more likely than those who did not in any of the past 7 days to be open to future smoking by a factor of 1.91 (95% CI: 1.32-2.76) in 2000 and 1.73 (95% CI: 1.30-2.31) in 2004 in the adjusted model.

Perceived benefit of smoking ($v^2 = 55.56$, p < .0001) and perceived peer acceptance to smoking ($v^2 = 16.14$, p < .002), measured only in 2004, were also significantly associated with OFS. Students with high and moderate perceived benefit of smoking were more likely than those with low perceived benefit to be open to future smoking by a factor of 3.97 (95% CI: 2.63-5.98) and 2.56 (95% CI: 2.06-3.17), respectively, in the adjusted model. Students who answered "definitely yes," "probably yes," and "probably not" to the question "Do most people of your age think it is okay to smoke?" were more likely than those who answered "definitely not" to be open to future smoking by a factor of 4.18 (95% CI: 2.34-7.47), 1.99 (95% CI: 1.34-2.95), and 1.62 (95% CI: 1.17-2.24), respectively, in the adjusted model.

DISCUSSION

Findings of this study indicate that desirable changes occurred between 2000 and 2004 in

TABLE 2. Bivariate Association for OFS, IYTS

	2000			2004		
	Unweighted Frequency	Weighted Percent	χ^2 (P Value)	Unweighted Frequency	Weighted Percent	χ^2 (P Value)
Gender			2.25 (.1386)			0.08 (.7751)
Female	191	54.74		342	49.36	
Male	166	45.26		306	50.64	
Grade			5.45 (.4947)			13.79 (.0423)
6th	77	22.74		46	15.89	
7th	78	20.10		144	19.18	
8th	87	17.91		117	21.33	
9th	38	16.63		139	18.35	
10th	31	8.68		92	10.14	
11th	29	8.67		65	7.94	
12th	17	5.28		38	7.16	
Race/ethnicity			2.84 (.4243)			4.29 (.2401)
White	292	86.88		464	77.01	
Black	34	7.54		98	11.56	
Hispanic	13	3.09		43	5.44	
Other	11	2.50		35	6.00	
Exposure to protobacco message			4.11 (.1370)			8.58 (.0169)
Low	110	31.64		221	34.47	
Moderate	214	64.20		336	60.84	
High	13	4.16		23	4.69	
Exposure to antitobacco message			0.23 (.8924)			5.08 (.0851)
Low	93	27.31		236	39.46	
Moderate	238	66.93		309	48.53	
High	20	5.75		69	12.01	
Exposure to information about health consequences of tobacco use			1.71 (.1961)			0.00 (1.000)
No exposure	61	16.98		70	9.84	
Exposed	293	83.02		560	90.16	

Exposure to ETS in homes (days)			23.50 (.0005)			16.61 (.0041)
0	121	33.04		270	40.55	
1 or 2	99	29.44		148	26.36	
3 or 4	37	9.89		56	7.97	
5 or 6	24	6.78		30	3.93	
7	73	20.85		122	21.18	
Exposure to ETS in cars (days)			22.99 (.0006)			15.73 (.0057)
0	184	51.36		396	60.33	
1 or 2	75	21.89		108	18.35	
3 or 4	38	10.29		42	7.06	
5 or 6	16	4.86		25	4.30	
7	41	11.59		56	9.97	
Perceived benefit of smoking*						55.56 (<.0001)
High perceived benefit				60	9.42	
Moderate perceived benefit				249	39.01	
Low perceived benefit				338	51.57	
Perceived peer acceptance to smoking*						16.14 (.0020)
Definitely yes				127	20.24	
Probably yes				239	34.39	
Probably not				206	34.93	
Definitely not				68	10.44	

*These variables were measured only for 2004.

adolescents' smoking-related environmental factors. The adolescent cohort in 2004 became more exposed to antitobacco messages and less exposed to protobacco messages and ETS compared with their counterpart in 2000. During the same time frame, the proportion of nonsmoking adolescents who were not open to future smoking significantly increased. Although no valid causal inference can be made from this repeated cross-sectional data analysis, this finding is indicative of a possible impact of environmental factors on adolescents' intention to smoke. Future studies are warranted to examine temporal trends of OFS among comparable adolescent cohorts especially with regard to the changes in smoking-related environmental factors.

The finding that the proportion of students who were highly exposed to antitobacco messages was only 15 % in 2004 might imply that there is still an increased need for concerted efforts by

TABLE 3. Logistic Regression of OFS, IYTS

	2000				2004			
	OR	95% CI	AOR	95% CI	OR	95% CI	AOR	95% CI
Gender								
Female	1.21	0.94-1.57			1.03	0.82-1.30		
Male	1.00	Reference			1.00	Reference		
Grade								
6th	0.72	0.41-1.25			0.56	0.37-0.85		
7th	0.82	0.49-1.37			0.88	0.66-1.16		
8th	0.91	0.57-1.47			1.17	0.77-1.78		
9th	1.00	Reference			1.00	Reference		
10th	0.68	0.39-1.19			0.65	0.46-0.92		
11th	0.68	0.37-1.25			0.60	0.42-0.86		
12th	0.58	0.29-1.16			0.71	0.42-1.22		
Race/ethnicity								
White	1.00	Reference			1.00	Reference		
Black	0.93	0.62-1.41			1.02	0.76-1.36		
Hispanic	2.00	1.02-3.91			1.48	0.98-2.23		
Other	0.90	0.46-1.77			1.32	0.74-2.35		
Exposure to protobacco message								
Low	1.00	Reference	1.00	Reference	1.00	Reference	1.00	Reference
Moderate	1.23	0.91-1.64	1.24	0.92-1.66	1.41	1.14-1.74	1.40	1.13-1.74
High	1.97	0.90-0.31	2.04	0.95-4.39	2.62	1.05-6.51	2.85	1.09-7.42
Exposure to antitobacco message								
Low	1.03	0.52-2.01	1.03	0.53-2.02	1.29	0.84-1.98	1.28	0.82-2.00
Moderate	1.10	0.55-2.17	1.10	0.55-2.16	0.98	0.66-1.45	0.97	0.63-1.49
High	1.00	Reference	1.00	Reference	1.00	Reference	1.00	Reference
Exposure to information about health consequences of tobacco use								
No exposure	1.23	0.90-1.67	1.28	0.93-1.76	1.00	0.73-1.37	1.00	0.72-1.40
Exposed	1.00	Reference	1.00	Reference	1.00	Reference	1.00	Reference
Exposure to ETS in homes (days)								
0	1.00	Reference	1.00	Reference	1.00	Reference	1.00	Reference
1 or 2	2.08	1.40-3.10	2.11	1.40-3.17	1.20	0.88-1.63	1.21	0.87-1.67
3 or 4	1.99	1.29-3.05	2.00	1.30-3.07	1.20	0.76-1.89	1.16	0.75-1.79
5 or 6	3.44	1.78-6.65	3.65	1.87-7.13	0.99	0.57-1.72	0.96	0.54-1.70
7	2.15	1.51-3.05	2.18	1.54-3.10	1.91	1.41-2.60	1.88	1.31-2.70
Exposure to ETS in cars (days)								
0	1.00	Reference	1.00	Reference	1.00	Reference	1.00	Reference
1 or 2	7 8	1.31-2.67	1.91	1.32-2.76	1.71	1.29-2.26	1.73	1.30-2.31

	OR	95% CI	AOR	95% CI	OR	95% CI	AOR	95% CI
3 or 4	2.10	1.30-3.40	2.09	1.28-3.41	1.06	0.76-1.47	1.04	0.74-1.45
5 or 6	2.15	1.03-4.52	2.18	1.03-4.62	8 6	0.81-3.51	1.81	0.88-3.75
7	1.97	1.30-2.98	2.00	1.35-2.97	1.94	1.38-2.73	1.77	1.29-2.45
Perceived benefit of smoking*								
High perceived benefit					4.25	2.87-6.31	3.97	2.63-5.98
Moderate perceived benefit					2.61	2.15-3.16	2.56	2.06-3.17
Low perceived benefit					1.00	Reference	1.00	Reference
Perceived peer acceptance to smoking								
Definitely yes					3.82	2.23-6.53	4.18	2.34-7.47
Probably yes					7 8	1.23-2.86	1.99	1.34-2.95
Probably not					1.76	1.26-2.45	1.62	1.17-2.24
Definitely not					1.00	Reference	1.00	Reference

OR, odds ratio; AOR, adjusted odds ratio.
*These variables were measured only for 2004.

state and local governments and tobacco control and prevention coalitions. However, exposure to antitobacco messages was not predictive of lack of OFS in the adjusted model. This is contrary to previous studies that have indicated that antitobacco messages seem to have the desired effect on adolescents' perceptions of tobacco[31,37] and help deter tobacco use initiation.[37,38] This can be interpreted in a few different ways. First, although frequencies of counter tobacco marketing and resulting students' exposure to these antitobacco messages might have increased significantly, the actual impact of these messages on students' intention to smoke might be intrinsically minimal, that is, a low effect size. The magnitude and enduring psychological impact of the antitobacco messages might not be strong enough to combat protobacco messages. Second, the study population may have received different messages or the quality of the messages may have been different. Third, given the different study designs and operational definitions of key variables among different studies, any delayed or concurrent effects of environmental factors on students' OFS could be captured differently. Related to this finding, it

is noteworthy that students who experienced a moderate or high level of exposure to protobacco messages were more likely than those with a low level of exposure to such messages to be open to future smoking both in the unadjusted and in the adjusted models in 2004. This association was marginally significant in 2000, primarily due to the small cell size. These findings converge on the idea that it might be more important to make efforts to reduce students' exposure to protobacco messages than to increase their exposure to antitobacco messages. Future studies are desirable to examine various strategies of counter tobacco marketing in terms of their relative impact on student's intentions to smoke or actual tobacco use initiation.

Another important finding of this study was a strong impact of exposure to ETS either in homes or in cars on adolescents' OFS in both years. This finding is not surprising given the finding that parental smok

ing has previously been linked with persistence of offspring smoking.[39] This is likely to indicate both genetic and environmental influence,[39] which could offset any positive counter tobacco efforts. An effective, preventive antismoking initiative or intervention program, including enactment of a law that bans smoking in a car when minors are riding the car, would be necessary that targets nonsmoking adolescents whose parents or caretakers are smokers.

The findings of this study support the inclusion of items in IYTS 2004 that measured perceived peer acceptance to smoking as they were significantly associated with OFS. This is in line with the previous finding of a significant association between youth tobacco use and peer influence.[14-20] However, contrary to the previous finding where youth tobacco use was significantly associated with race/ethnicity (ie, white students are more likely than black and Hispanic students to report current cigarette use),[10-13] race/ethnicity was not associated with OFS in this study. This could be interpreted in 2 ways. First, this implies that OFS does not always lead to actual smoking behavior. Students' attitudes and perceptions toward tobacco smoking could change over time. Second, this finding indicates that the rate of transition from OFS to actual tobacco use initiation is higher among white students than among minority students. Future studies are necessary to investigate the determinants of the differential rates in their transition from OFS to tobacco use initiation among different racial/ethnic groups.

The findings of this study are subject to limitations. One limitation is the findings were based on self- report of the students, as opposed to more objective methods of measurement. However, self-report is commonly used for measurement in youth tobacco research and is relied upon by the CDC as an accepted method of national youth tobacco surveillance.[11,12,36] Second, causal relationships should not be inferred from the present findings as the data were collected using a cross-sectional survey design, although the consistent patterns observed across the 2 different years of surveys shed added light on possible causal links such as the linkbetween exposure to ETS and OFS. Third, the findings apply only to the students who attended a public middle school or high school. Fourth, if the nonres- pondents had different perceptions from those who participated in the survey, the findings might have reduced external validity, although the response rates were high. Despite these limitations, this study provides valuable information about the factors affecting nonsmoking adolescents' openness to tobacco use.

CONCLUSIONS

Results from this study show that desirable changes occurred between 2000 and 2004 in terms of exposure to anti- or protobacco messages, exposure to ETS, and the proportion of nonsmoking adolescents who were not open to future smoking among Indiana adolescents. Adolescents' OFS is strongly associated with exposure to ETS, exposure to protobacco messages, perceived peer acceptance to smoking, and perceived benefit of smoking. Thus, it may help prevent adolescents from initiating tobacco use to adopt policies to reduce adolescents' exposure to ETS such as a smoking ban in a car when minors are riding in the car. Also, findings of this study suggest that more efforts should be made to reduce adolescents' exposure to proto- bacco messages than to increase their exposure to antitobacco messages. Results also suggest that the rate of transition from OFS to tobacco use initiation is higher among white adolescents than among minority adolescents. It may therefore be beneficial to examine the determinants of the differential rates in their transition from OFS to tobacco use initiation among different racial/ethnic groups.

REFERENCES

1. US Department of Health and Human Services. Preventing Tobacco Use Among Young People. A Report of the Surgeon General. Atlanta, Ga: Centers for Disease Control and Prevention, National Center for Chronic Disease Prevention and Health Promotion, Office on Smoking and Health;1994.

2. Chassin L, Presson CC, Rose JS, Sherman SJ. The natural history of cigarette smoking from adolescence to adulthood: demographic predictors of continuity and change. Health Psychol. 1996;15(6):478-484.

3. Orlando M, Tucker JS, Ellickson PL, Klein DJ. Developmental trajectories of cigarette smoking and their correlates from early adolescence to young adulthood. J Consult Clin Psychol. 2004; 72(3):400-410.

4. Henningfield JE, Clayton R, PollinW. The involvement of tobacco in alcoholism and illicit drug use. Br J Addict. 1990;85:279-292.

5. Henningfield JE, Cohen C, Slade JD. Is nicotine more addictive than cocaine? Br J Addict. 1991;86:565-569.

6. US Department of Health and Human Services. The Health Consequences of Smoking: Nicotine Addiction—A Report of the Surgeon General. Washington, DC: US Government Printing Office; 1988. DHHS Publication No. CDC 88-8406.

7. Anthony JC, Warner LA, Kessler RC. Comparative epidemiology of dependence on tobacco, alcohol, controlled substances, and inhalants: basic findings from the National Co-morbidity Survey. Exp Clin Psychopharmacol. 1994;2:244-268.

8. McNeill AD. The development of dependence on smoking in children. Br J Addict. 1991;86:589-592.

9. Milton MH, Maule CO, Yee SL, Backinger C, Malarcher AM, Husten CG. Youth Tobacco Cessation: A Guide for Making Informed Decisions. Atlanta, Ga: US Department of Health and Human Services, Centers for Disease Control and Prevention; 2004.

10. US Centers for Disease Control and Prevention. Tobacco Use Among U.S. Racial/Ethnic Minority Groups. Atlanta, Ga: National Center for Chronic Disease Prevention and Health Promotion, Office on Smoking and Health;1998.

11. US Centers for Disease Control and Prevention. Trends in cigarette smoking among high school students—United States, 19912001. MMWR Morb Mortal Wkly Rep. 2002;51:409-428.

12. US Centers for Disease Control and Prevention. Tobacco use among middle and high school students—United States, 2002. MMWR Morb Mortal Wkly Rep. 2003;52:1093-1116.

13. Wills TA, Cleary SD. The validity of self-reports of smoking: analyses by race/ethnicity in a school sample of urban adolescents. Am J Public Health. 1997;87:56-61.

14. Ennett ST, Bauman E. The contribution of influence and selection to adolescent peer group homogeneity: the case of adolescent cigarette smoking. JPers SocPsychol. 1994;67:653-663.

15. Engels RCME, Knibbe RA, Drop MJ, De Haan YT. Homogeneity of cigarette smoking within peer groups: influence or selection? Health Educ Behav. 1997;24:801-811.

16. Engels RCME, Knibbe RA, De Vries H, Drop MJ, Van Breukelen GJP. Influences of parental and best friends' smoking and drinking on adolescent use: a longitudinal study. J Appl Soc Psychol. 1999;29:338-362.

17. Engels RCME, Knibbe RA, Drop MJ. Predictability of smoking in adolescence: between optimism and pessimism. Addiction. 1999; 94:115-124.

18. Urberg KA, Degirmencioglu SM, Pilgrim C. Close friend and group influence on adolescent cigarette smoking and alcohol use. Dev Psychol. 1997;33:834-844.

19. De Vries H, Engels RCME, Kremers S, Wetzels J, Mudde A. Parents' and friends' smoking status as predictors of smoking onset: findings from six European countries. Health Educ Res. 2003;18: 617-632.

20. Chassin L, Presson CC, Sherman SJ. Social-psychological antecedents and consequences of adolescent tobacco use. In: Wal- lander JL, Siegel

LJ, eds. Adolescent Health Problems: Behavioral Perspectives Advances in Pediatric Psychology. New York, NY: Guilford Press;1995: 141-159.

21. Santana Y, Gonzalez B, Pinilla J, Calvo JR, Barber P. Young adolescents, tobacco advertising, and smoking. J Drug Educ. 2003;33:427-444.

22. Braverman MT, Aaro LE. Adolescent smoking and exposure to tobacco marketing under a tobacco advertising ban: findings from 2 Norwegian national sampling. Am J Public Health. 2004;94: 1230-1238.

23. Distefan JM, Pierce JP, Gilpin EA. Do favorite movie stars influence adolescent smoking initiation? Am J Public Health. 2004;94: 1239-1244.

24. Gutschoven K, Van den Bulck J. Television viewing and smoking volume in adolescent smokers. PrevMed. 2004;39:1093-1098.

25. Difranza JR, Richards JW, Paulman PM, et al. RJR Nasbisco's cartoon camel promotes Camel cigarettes to children. JAMA. 1991;266:3149-3153.

26. US Centers for Disease Control and Prevention. Changes in the cigarette brand preferences of adolescent smokers—United States, 1989-1993. MMWR Morb Mortal Wkly Rep. 1994;43:577-581.

27. Sargent JD, Dalton M, Beach M, Bernhardt A, Heatherton T, Stevens M. Effect of cigarette promotions on smoking uptake among adolescents. Prev Med. 2000;30:320-327.

28. Rombouts K, Fauconnier G. What is learnt early is learn well? A study of the influence of tobacco advertising on adolescents. J Health Commun. 1988;3:303-322.

29. Pierce JP, Gilpin EA, Burns DM, et al. Does tobacco advertising target young people to start smoking? Evidence from California. JAMA. 1991;266:3154-3158.

30. Pierce JP, Choi WS, Gilpin EA, Farkas AJ, Berry CC. Tobacco industry promotion of cigarettes and adolescent smoking. JAMA. 1998;279:511-515.

31. BeinerLB, SeigalM. Tobacco marketing and adolescent smoking: more support for causal inference. Am J Public Health. 2000;90: 407-411.

32. Kaufman NJ, Castrucci BC, Mowery PD, Gerlach KK, Emont S, Orleans CT. Predictors of change on the smoking uptake continuum among adolescents. Arch Pediatr Adolesc Med. 2002;156: 581-587.

33. Lerner RM, Galambos NL. Adolescent development: challenges and opportunities for research, programs, and policies. Annu Rev Psychol. 1998;49:413-446.

34. Mowery PD, Farrelly MC, Haviland L, Gable JM, Wells HE. Progression to established smoking among US youths. Am J Public Health. 2004;94:331-337.

35. Becklake MR, Ghezzo H, Ernst P. Childhood predictors of smoking in adolescence: a follow-up study of Montreal school children. CMAJ. 2005;173(4):377-379.

36. Evans WD, Powers A, Hersey J, Renaud J. The influence of social environment and social image on adolescent smoking. Health Psychol. 2006;25(1):26-33.

37. Hersey JC, Niederdeppe J, Evans WD, etal. The effects of state coun- terindustry media campaigns on beliefs, attitudes, and smoking status among teens and young adults. Prev Med. 2003;37:544-552.

38. Reinert B, Carver V, Range LM. Anti-tobacco messages from different sources make a difference with secondary school students. J Public Health Manag Pract. 2004;10(6):518-523.

39. White VM, Hopper JL, Wearing AJ, Hill DJ. The role of genes in tobacco smoking during adolescence and young adulthood: a multi-variate behaviour genetic investigation. Addiction. 2003;98:1087-1100.

The Price of Smoking

Frank A. Sloan, Jan Ostermann, Christopher Conover, Donald H. Taylor Jr., and Gabriel Picone

Reviewed by Shyam Biswal

Heart attacks, several forms of cancer, and chronic obstructive pulmonary diseases due to cigarette smoking remain among the major causes of mortality and morbidity in the United States and other countries. In spite of this, 50 million Americans continue to smoke, which makes it impossible to tackle this highly preventable cause of death. Freedom of choice has always been the major reason for keeping cigarettes flowing in our society. But using freedom of choice and self- inflicted injury as arguments for justifying continued cigarette consumption loses validity when smoking becomes an overhead that society must find a way to pay for. Health economics is a major factor in framing public health policy and legislation. So, what is the price of smoking? How much does the individual smoker pay, and what is the financial burden on others in society, including those exposed to the effects of secondhand smoke and faced with the resultant rising costs to Medicare, Medicaid, and Social Security?

Frank Sloan and his coauthors, Jan Ostermann, Christopher Conover, Donald H. Taylor Jr., and Gabriel Picone have undertaken a thorough and systematic analysis of the health economics of lifetime smoking. While most previous studies have taken a cross-sectional approach, The price of smoking is based on a longitudinal study — the 1998 Health and Retirement Study — conducted by the University of Michigan and the Assets and Health Dynamics among the Oldest Old (AHEAD) and on the 1998 National Health Interview Survey.

The data in this book are based on present value of loss for men and women who are smokers at the age of 24. One factor that is distinct in this study is the calculation of "quasi-external cost," which the authors define as the cost of freedom of choice to the family members of smokers, including children who are nonsmokers. In their longitudinal analysis of lifetime smoking, the authors estimate that the social cost of smoking, which is a sum of purely private, quasi-external, and external costs (the latter determined by excise tax) for a 24-year-old person turns out to be $39.66 per pack of cigarettes. The cost to Medicare, Medicaid, and Social Security is substantial. The quasi-external cost of smoking to the spouse of a 24-year-old who smokes comes to a staggering $28 billion. After considering these numbers and the amount of people who turn 24 each year and smoke, the authors of this book have predicted that the national external and quasi-external lifetime cost per year is $13.8 billion for females and $32.8 billion for males. Thus, with each new cohort of 24-year-old smokers in the United States there is an additional $204 billion of lifetime costs. These staggering expenses in light of the high number of smokers in the country make a convincing argument for rethinking the issue of public health policy making. Federal and state cigarette excise taxes have increased dramatically over the years. The calculations made by Sloan and his coauthors provide an analytical reason for such increases.

Readers should be cautioned that the monetary estimates in similar but different studies on the cost of smoking vary greatly. The approximations presented by Sloan and his coauthors are likely to cause some controversy, because the cost effect on Medicaid and Medicare is estimated to be relatively small in this compared with other studies.

The book ends with a strong message: both smokers and society will face a huge financial expense. The young smokers are unaware of this when they start smoking. Individuals who decide to smoke will have to live with the fact that smoking is not only cutting into their personal finances but will also have a huge impact on the national expenditure.

The book makes an excellent reference for researchers and workers in health economics, tobacco control legislation, and public policy. Even though the major part of the book deals with economics, it is enjoyable for social scientists and lay readers interested in learning about the social cost of smoking. Dissemination of such information in real dollar amounts (even though not precise) may be a creative way of discouraging the initiation of smoking.

Methamphetamine

Stimulant of the 1990s?

By Robert W. Derlet, MD and Bruce Heischober, MD

During the past several years, the use of a smokable form of methamphetamine hydrochloride called "ice" has increased rapidly. The heaviest use has occurred on the West Coast and in Hawaii. Many regional emergency departments treat more methamphetamine users than cocaine-intoxicated patients. The ease of synthesis from inexpensive and readily available chemicals makes possible the rampant abuse of a dangerous drug that can produce a euphoria similar to that induced by cocaine. Clinicians should be familiar with the medical effects and treatment of acute methamphetamine toxicity.

A dramatic increase has occurred in the illicit production and use of methamphetamine hydrochloride (HC1) over the past several years (M. Glover, "State Production of Speed Worries U.S. Drug Officials," Sacramento Bee, October 10,1988, pi).[1-3] Endemic areas for this increase include the Pacific Coast states and Hawaii.[4] In 1987 in San Diego County, California, methamphetamine intoxication played a role in 40% of all drug-related homicides.[5] This represents a 52% increase in methamphetamine involvement in serious crime over the previous year. In San Bernardino County, California, the number of coroners' cases involving methamphetamine use has been twice that of cocaine.[6] At present, this epidemic appears confined to the West Coast where in some emergency departments, the number of visits resulting from methamphetamine intoxication exceeds that necessitated by cocaine use.[6,7] Although data from the National Institute on Drug Abuse indicate that cocaine abuse is still greater than that of methamphetamine, the new trend is of great concern.[8]

Methamphetamine provides a euphoria similar to that of cocaine.[9] Studies in animals have shown that methamphetamine and cocaine induce similar behavior.[10] The smokable form of methamphetamine ("ice") can bring on an immediate euphoria with effects that may last many times longer than those of cocaine.[4] Methamphetamine abuse involves a wide age range, and epidemic methamphetamine abuse has recently been described in adolescents. In one inpatient adolescent drug treatment unit, methamphetamine was listed as the drug of choice by about 80% of patients recently admitted.[1] The reasons given for this preference include availability, low cost, and a longer duration of action compared with cocaine. Both oral and intravenous use are well documented, but the use of smokable methamphetamine has received little attention in medical literature.

History

Amphetamine was introduced in the 1930s in the form of inhalers for treating rhinitis and asthma.[11] The stimulant, euphoriant, and anorectic effects of amphetamine were quickly recognized, leading to its abuse. A report in 1937 stating that amphetamine could enhance intellectual performance through enhanced wakefulness further contributed to amphetamine abuse.[12] Amphetamine was used by some foreign armies during the Second World War, allegedly to increase wakefulness and attention.[13] After the mid- 19408, epidemics of amphetamine abuse occurred in several countries, most notably Japan and Sweden. Initial federal controls were enacted in the late 1950s, but amphetamine continued to be abused by some students, athletes, shift workers, and truck drivers into the next decade.[14] The Controlled Substance Act of 1970 stringently regulated the manufacturing of amphetamine. As a result, the availability of dextroamphetamine sulfate (Dexedrine) and

other pharmaceutical amphetamines decreased. Despite the declining availability of pharmaceutical synthesized amphetamines, methamphetamine use has increased notably.

Illicit Production

Unlike d-amphetamine, methamphetamine is easy to synthesize in a crude laboratory.[15] Like other sympathomimetic drugs, both are derivatives of phenylethylamine. Structurally, the substances differ in that a methyl group attaches to the terminal nitrogen of methamphetamine. Although some states have enacted laws decreasing the availability of necessary precursor chemicals,[16] these agents may still be obtainable in neighboring states.

One common method of synthesis begins with L-ephedrine, which is reduced to methamphetamine using hydriodic acid and red phosphorus.[17] Variations on this process include using a different acid or catalyst or a substituted ephedrine such as chloroephedrine or methyl-ephedrine. The product is pure d-methamphetamine, which is several times more active than the l form. The ephedrine reduction process is responsible for more than 90% of the methamphetamine produced in southern California (P. Gregory, Drug Enforcement Administration, Sacramento, California, oral communication, November 1988). The methamphetamine produced is a lipid-soluble pure base form, which is volatile and evaporates if left exposed to room air. The producer, therefore, uses hydrochloride to convert it to the water-soluble form, methamphetamine-HC1 powder. This substance has traditionally been sold on the street as "speed," "crank," "go," "crystal," or metham- phetamine, and it is highly water soluble.

Other stimulants such as cocaine, phenylpropanolamine hydrochloride, d-amphetamine, ephedrine, or pseudo- ephedrine have been mixed

---

Abbreviations Used In Text

CNS = central nervous system

HCl = hydrochloride

MDMA = methylenedioxymethamphetamine

with or substituted for meth- amphetamine. Several years ago, street methamphetamine was highly impure and found in only 40% of the street-purchased drug.[18] More recent information from law enforcement laboratories suggests that the methamphetamine available now is nearly pure.[6] Some clandestine chemists purposely produce other stimulants with toxicity of their own, which may be sold as methamphetamine. These stimulants structurally resemble methamphetamine and include methylenedioxymethamphetamine (MDMA), methylenedioxyamphetamine (MDA), 2,5-dimethoxy-4- methylamphetamine (DOM), and bromodom (DOB) and have been referred to as "designer drugs."[19] The routine toxicologic screen may not detect many of the new congeners, such as MDMA, and the drugs may produce symptoms indistinguishable from those induced by methamphetamine.[20,21] Illicitly synthesized methamphetamine may be contaminated by non-stimulant organic or inorganic substances. Lead poisoning and exposure to carcinogenic material have been reported.[22] Street methamphetamine may be mixed with cocaine, and studies show that 8% to 20% of street-available stimulants contain both drugs.[18] In a recent report on cocaine intoxication, 7% of patients sought medical help because of the concurrent use of cocaine and amphetamines.[23]

Ice

The term "ice" originated in the Far East as the result of synthesizing large crystals of methamphetamine through the ephedrine-reduction method (M. Corwin, "Potent Form of Speed Could Be the Drug of '90s," Los Angeles Times, October 8, 1989, pi). Once the methamphetamine HC1 is produced, making ice involves a process analogous to making rock candy out of sugar. The methamphetamine HC1 is slowly added to water, heated to 80°C to 100°C until a supersaturated solution is obtained, and the slurry is then cooled. The pure HC1 salt of methamphetamine, also known as ice, precipitates from this. Isopropanol has been used as the solvent in place of water. The many variations of this process result in an unreliable removal of impurities. Many physical characteristics of the final product depend on the quality of the reagents and on the contaminants. Unlike cocaine HC1, methamphetamine HC1 is volatile and can be smoked.[24] For cocaine to be smoked, it must be converted to pure cocaine alkaloid, commonly called crack (Table 1).

The popularity of smoked methamphetamine is due to the immediate clinical effects of a euphoria resulting from the drug's rapid absorption from the lungs. Thus, the effect of intravenous use can be achieved without using needles. For several years, patients of one of us (B.H.) have described smoking methamphetamine-HCl powder or crystals by first placing the substance in a piece of metal foil molded into the shape of a bowl and then heating it over the flame of a cigarette lighter. The fumes then can be inhaled through a straw. Because of a more rapid and intense drug effect, these patients described a "high" distinct from that produced by snorting or ingesting methamphetamine. They also reported that smoking the drug produced a high lasting a shorter time than that experienced with other routes of ingestion. As would be expected when methamphetamine is smoked, the duration of action is similar to that produced with intravenous injection.

Clinical Pharmacology

Methamphetamine causes central nervous system (CNS) stimulation that may induce euphoria, increase alertness, intensify emotions, alter self-esteem, and allegedly increase sexuality.[9] At the cellular level, dopamine is displaced from specific nerve terminals, causing hyperstim- ulation of dopaminergic receptor neurons in the synaptic cleft.[25,26] These hyperstimulated neurons in turn stimulate various CNS pathways and the sympathetic nervous system. Direct peripheral and organ stimulation by methamphetamine may also occur. The half-life of amphetamines ranges from 10 to 30 hours, depending on urine pH.[27,28] Methamphetamine has greater CNS efficacy compared with d-amphetamine, presumably because of increased CNS penetration.[29]

The euphoric effects produced by methamphetamine, cocaine, and various designer amphetamines are similar and may be difficult to differentiate clinically. The findings from many studies in animals and humans support these observations. A distinguishing clinical feature is the longer half-life of methamphetamine, which may be as much as ten times longer than the half-life of cocaine.[16-30] Nevertheless, more recent studies in animals with d-amphetamine and cocaine suggest differences in underlying CNS mechanisms between the two types of stimulants.[31-33]

Because methamphetamine is purchased illicitly and may be mixed with both inert and other toxic substances, the clinical observation of toxic effects is more relevant than an estimate of ingested dose. In addition, tachyphylaxis occurs with methamphetamine use, and long-term users tolerate higher doses with fewer symptoms. Fatalities have been reported after ingestions as low as 1.5 mg per kg of methamphetamine,[34] whereas long-time abusers in whom tolerance to the drug develops may use as much as 5,000 to 15,000 mg per day.

Toxic Effects

In toxic doses, methamphetamine induces unpleasant CNS symptoms such as agitation, anxiety, hallucinations, delirium, and seizures; death can occur.[16,35-37] Cardiovascular symptoms such as chest pain, palpitations, or dyspnea can also develop. There is evidence that high doses of methamphetamine induce irreversible CNS-destructive changes.[38-39]

Methamphetamine can both induce an acute toxic psychosis in previously healthy persons and precipitate a psychotic episode in those with psychiatric illness.[40] Nearly all patients presenting to emergency departments with toxic effects require referral to a psychiatric center. In the past, psychiatric disorders were diagnosed before addiction in many amphetamine users. This has not been the case recently, however.[41] An acute and dramatic choreoathetoid disorder can also be triggered by amphetamines.[42] Hyperthermia may result from CNS-induced abnormalities, seizures, or muscular hyperactivity. Rhabdomyolysis may occur secondarily.[15]

TABLE 1. Comparison of Methamphetamine and Cocaine

Common Street Name	Chemical Description	Characteristics
Cocaine		
Coke, snow.....	D-Cocaine HC1 and cutting impurities	Not volatile; administered through nasal or intravenous route
Crack, rock, free base......	Pure alkaloid cocaine	Volatile; can be smoked
Methamphetamine		
Crank, speed......	D-, L-, or D/L-Methamphetamine HC1 and impurities	Volatility dependent on impurities
Ice, crystal......	D-Methamphetamine HCI (high purity, uncut)	Volatile; can be smoked

HCI = hydrochloride

Cardiovascular manifestations of amphetamine toxicity include hypertension, tachycardia, atrial and ventricular arrhythmias, and myocardial ischemia.[43-44] Chest pain has been reported in some persons but usually without electrocardiographic changes. The incidence of toxicity-induced cardiovascular symptoms is less than with cocaine.

Patients who are unconscious on arrival at an emergency department or who have been found unresponsive may have used methamphetamine. In some of these persons, lack of responsiveness may be due to the use of other drugs such as opiates. Other patients may be unresponsive because of intravenous methamphetamine use. Hypothesized reasons for this effect include seizure, hypotension, a reaction to a contaminant, or undescribed effects of intravenous amphetamine. Other disorders that have been described include cerebrovascular accident due to hemorrhage or vasospasm.[45-46]

Treatment

Despite methamphetamine's ability to induce significant CNS and cardiovascular stimulation, relatively few patients who present to emergency departments for acute intoxication require pharmacologic intervention.[7] In many emergency departments, patients are not treated for agitation unless they could harm themselves while jerking or tearing at their restraints. These hyperactive or agitated persons can be treated with haloperidol or diazepam, and all appear to respond well to treatment with either drug.

Central Nervous System Toxicity

Haloperidol and diazepam are well-established agents that antagonize CNS symptoms. Haloperidol, a dopamine-2 blocking agent, can specifically antagonize the central effects of methamphetamine. Studies in animals have shown the superiority of haloperidol to diazepam in protecting against death.[33] Multiple clinical reports attest to the efficacy of haloperidol.[7-14,15] In addition, on receiving intravenous haloperidol, patients who sustain the acute choreoathetoid syndrome may have symptoms quickly resolve. Haloperidol has an advantage over diazepam in that it can be given intravenously or intramuscularly. Recommended doses are 2.0 to 5.0 mg initially, with additional dosing titrated to clinical response.

Diazepam, a benzodiazepine that enhances 7-aminobu- tvric acid neurotransmission, affects methamphetamine intoxication through a nonspecific sedative action. Diazepam is highly effective in antagonizing the stimulant toxic effects of cocaine but not amphetamines in animals.[31-33] Despite this observation, diazepam is used successfully to control clinical symptoms.

Cardiovascular Effects

Many antihypertensive agents and 0-blockers are effective in reversing methamphetamine-induced cardiovascular symptoms. For treating an amphetamine-induced hypertensive crisis, agents such as phentolamine or nitroprusside provide efficacy. Blood pressures may also respond indirectly to the sedating effects of haloperidol. Calcium channel blockers have been used successfully in some emergency departments.

Many cases of methamphetamine toxicity can be managed conservatively. The clinician should confirm suspected amphetamine use through a urine toxicologic analysis. Other conditions that may produce symptoms—such as infections, metabolic disorders, or use of other drugs- should be excluded. Patients should receive volume replacement as determined by hydration status. In past studies, as few as 10% of the patients presenting to emergency departments required admission, and those who were admitted to hospital were generally discharged within two days. In the past, vital signs were thought to be an indicator of the severity of intoxication, with a temperature above 40°C being a poor prognostic sign. In one series, however, there was no significant difference in vital signs between those admitted and those not admitted.

Summary

In conclusion, methamphetamine is a dangerous drug that matches or supersedes cocaine in inducing symptoms of euphoria. The volatility of methamphetamine appears similar to that of crack cocaine, and thus it can compete with cocaine for use by long-term or recreational users wanting a rapid high through inhalation. Unlike that of cocaine, the half-life of methamphetamine may produce exceptionally long-lasting toxic effects. Clinicians should consider the possibility of methamphetamine use or abuse in any patient presenting with psychosis, violence, seizures, or cardiovascular abnormalities.

References

1. Heischober B, Derlet RW: Update on amphetamine abuse. West J Med 1989; 151:70-71

2. Dixon SD: Effects of transplacental esqjosure to cocaine and methamphetamine on the neonate. West J Med 1989; 150:436-442

3. Rangel C (D-NY): Chair Select Committee on Narcotics Abuse and Control. Washington, DC, Methamphetamine hearing, Oct. 24, 1989

4. Jackson JG: The hazards of smokable methamphetamine (Letter). N Engl J Med 1989; 321:907

5. Bailey DN, Shaw RF: Cocaine and methamphetamine-related deaths in San Diego County (1987): Homicides and accidental overdoses. J Forensic Sci 1989; 34:407-422

6. Puder KS, Kagan DV, Morgan JP: Illicit methamphetamine: Analysis, synthesis, and availability. Am J Drug Alcohol Abuse 1988; 14:463-473 (erratum 1989; 15:353)

7. Derlet RW, Rice P, Horowitz BZ, Lord RV: Amphetamine toxicity: Experience with 127 cases. J Emerg Med 1989; 7:157-161

8. US Department of Health and Human Services (Public Health Service): National Institute on Drug Abuse Statistical Series Annual Data 1988 Series 1, No. 8. Rockville, Md, National Institute on Drug Abuse, Division of Epidemiology and Prevention Research, 1989, p 26

9. Gawin FH, Ellinwood EH: Cocaine and other stimulants: Actions, abuse, and treatment. N Engl J Med 1988; 318:1173-1182

10. Schechter MD, Glennon RA: Cathinone, cocaine and methamphetamine: Similarity of behavioral effects. Pharmacol Biochem Behav 1985; 22:913-916

11. Snyder SH: Drugs and the Brain. New York, NY, Scientific American Books, 1986, pp 130-131

12. Myerson A: Effect of benzedrine sulphate on mood and fatigue in normal and in neurotic persons. Arch Neurol Psychiatry 1936; 36:816-822

13. Litovitz T: Amphetamines, In Haddad LM, Winchester JF (Eds): Clinical Management of Poisoning and Drug Overdose. Philadelphia, Pa, WB Saunders, 1983, pp 469-470

14. Segar DL: Substances of abuse. Topics Emerg Med 1985; 7:18-30

15. Allen A, Cantrell T: Synthetic reductions in clandestine amphetamine and methamphetamine labs. J Forensic Sci 1989; 42:183-199

16. Cal Health & Safety Code §§ 11055, 11100, 11383, 11400 (1988)

17. Allen AC, Kiser WO: Methamphetamine from ephedrine: I. Chloroephe- drines and aziridines. J Forensic Sci 1987; 32:953-962

18. Klatt EC, Montgomery S, Namiki T, Noguchi TT: Misrepresentation of stimulant street drugs: A decade of experience in an analysis program. J Toxicol Clin Toxicol 1986; 24:441-450

19. Buchanan JF, Brown CR: 'Designer drugs'—A problem in clinical toxicology. Med Toxicol Adverse Drug Exp 1988; 3:1-17

20. Brown C, Osterloh J: Multiple severe complications from recreational ingestion of MDMA ('ecstasy'). JAMA 1987; 258:780-781

21. Dowling GP, McDonough ET 3d, Bost RO: 'Eve' and 'Ecstasy'—A report of five deaths associated with the use of MDEA and MDMA. JAMA 1987; 257:1615-1617

22. Allcott JV III, Barnhart RA, Mooney LA: Acute lead poisoning in two users of illicit methamphetamine. JAMA 1987; 258:510-511

23. Derlet RW, Albertson TE: Emergency department presentation of cocaine intoxication. Ann Emerg Med 1989; 18:182-186

24. Chiang N, Hawks R: Pyrolysis studies—Cocaine, PCP, Heroin, Methamphetamine—Technical Review. Rockville, Md, National Institute on Drug Abuse, June 23, 1989

25. Pitts DK, Marwah J: Cocaine and central monoaminergic neurotransmission: A review of electrophysiological studies and comparison to amphetamine and antidepressants. Life Sci 1988; 42:949-968

26. Scheel-Kruger J: Behavioral and biochemical comparison of amphetamine derivatives, cocaine, benztropine and tricyclic anti-depressant drugs. Eur J Pharmacol 1972; 18:63-73

27. Bryson PD (Ed): Comprehensive Review in Toxicology, 2nd Ed. Rockville, Md, Aspen Publications, 1989, pp 370-372

28. Beckett AH, Rowland M: Urinary excretion kinetics of amphetamine in man. J Pharm Pharmacol 1965; 17:628-639

29. Lake C, Quirk R: Stimulants and look-alike drugs. Psychiatr Clin North Am 1984; 7:689-701

30. Byck R, Van Dyke C, Jatlow P, Barash P: Clinical pharmacology of cocaine, In Jeri FR (Ed): Cocaine 1980—Proceedings of the Interamerican Seminar on Medical and Sociological Aspects of Coca and Cocaine. Luna, Peru, Pacific Press, 1980, pp 250-256

31. Derlet RW, Albertson TE: Diazepam in the prevention of seizures and death in cocaine intoxicated rats. Ann Emerg Med 1989; 18:542-546

32. Derlet RW, Albertson TE, Rice P: The effect of haloperidol in cocaine and amphetamine intoxication. J Emerg Med 1989; 7:633-637

33. Derlet RW, Albertson TE, Rice P: Protection against D-amphetamine toxicity. Am J Emerg Med 1990; 8:105-108

34. Zalis EG, Parmley LF: Fatal amphetamine poisoning. Arch Intern Med 1963; 112:822-826

35. Kramer JC, Fischman VS, Littlefield DC: Amphetamine abuse: Pattern and effects of high doses taken intravenously. JAMA 1967; 201:305-309

36. Zalis EG, Lundberg GD, Knutson RA: The pathophysiology of acute amphetamine poisoning with pathologic correlation. J Pharmacol Exp Ther 1967;

37. Conci F, D'Angelo V, Tampieri D, Vecchi G: Intracerebral hemorrhage and angiographic beading following amphetamine abuse. Ital J Neurol Sci 1988; 9:77-81

38. Woolverton WL, Ricaurte GA, Forno LS, Seiden LS: Long-term effects of chronic methamphetamine administration in rhesus monkeys. Brain Res 1989' 486:73-78

39. Konradi C, Manzino L, Sonsalla PK, et al: Modification of methampheta- mine-induced neurotoxicity in mice, In Abstracts: Society for Neuroscience— 19th Annual Meeting, Phoenix, Ariz, 1989, p 140

40. Ellinwood H Jr: Amphetamine psychosis: A multidimensional process. Semin Psychiatry 1969; 1:208-226

41. Kalant O (Ed): The Amphetamine Toxicity and Addiction, 2nd Ed. Toronto, Canada, University of Toronto Press, 1973, pp 69-76

42. Rhee K, Albertson T, Douglas J: A choreoathetoid movement disorder associated with intravenous amphetamine use. Am J Emerg Med 1988; 6:131-133

43. Lam D, Goldschlager N: Myocardial injury associated with poly substance abuse. Am Heart J 1988; 115:675-680

44. Lucas PB, Gardner DL, Wolkowitz OM, Tucker EE, Cowdry RW: Methyl- phenidate-induced

cardiac arrhythmias (Letter). N Engl J Med 1986; 315:1485

45. Chyun KY: Acute subarachnoid hemorrhage. JAMA 1975; 233:55-56

46. Salanova V, Taubner R: Intracerebral hemorrhage and vasculitis secondary to amphetamine use. Postgrad Med J 1984; 60:429-430

Moral Panic Over Meth

By Edward G. Armstrong

In the last few years., 'meth' (methampbetamine) has become a major concern for law enforcement officials in rural America. Meth is the label given to a homemade substance that is manufactured (typically) in rural labs using fertilizers, cold tablets, and household acids. The ama teur na ture of the production process separates meth from its commercially produced equivalents, the stim ulant medica tions that are the first-line therapy agents for attention-deficitlhyperactivity disorder and narcolepsy and that are authorized by the United States Air Force as fatigue countermeasures. A way to understand the social construction of the meth-scare is to apply the moral panic conceptual framework. A moral panic, is a social condition that becomes defined as a threat to community values and whose nature is presented in a stereotypical fashion by the mass media. The official reaction to the social condition is out of all proportion to the alleged threat. Reporting about a moral crisis involves a continuous exaggeration of the problematic aspects of the social condition and an ongoing repetition of fallacies. Discussions of meth tend to obscure its nature while heightening horrors that immediately promote a limited and inaccurate notion of the nature of meth. The emergence of the idea that meth is something, new has activated a particular set of social responses that have a harsh impact on those designated as meth users. The meth scare is blinding people to the plight of white, underclass, rural, poor people.

Keywords: *Meth; Moral Panic; Amphetamines; Methamphetamines; Ritalin; Meth Babies*

Edward G. Armstrong, "Moral Panic Over Meth," *Contemporary Justice Review*, vol. 10, no. 4, pp. 427-442. Copyright © 2007 by Taylor & Francis Group LLC. Reprinted with permission.

Introduction

In the last few years, meth (methamphetamine) has become a major concern for law enforcement officials in rural America. A way to understand the social construction of the meth scare is to apply the moral panic conceptual framework. A moral panic is a social condition that becomes defined as a threat to community values and whose 'nature is presented in a stylized and stereotypical fashion by the mass media' (Cohen, 1972, p. 9). The official reaction to the social condition is 'out of all proportion' to the alleged threat (Hall, Critcher, Jefferson, Clarke, & Roberts, 1978, p. 16). Reporting about a moral crisis involves a continuous exaggeration of the problematic- aspects of the social condition and an ongoing repetition of fallacies.

Before I deal with the moral panic criteria and apply this framework to the meth scare, I suggest we first answer the question: What is meth? Discussions of meth tend to obscure its nature while heightening horrors that immediately promote a limited and inaccurate notion of the nature of meth. The emergence of the idea that meth is something new has activated a particular set of social responses that have a harsh impact on those designated as meth users.

What is Meth?

On February 6, 2005, an article appeared in the New York Times Magazine that made a commonly held point—meth is 'a new drug' (Sheff, 2005, p. 45). It isn't. Meth is simply an amphetamine. Illegally produced meth, methamphetamines, and other amphetamines are all the same. The constant focus on meth and the use of the term 'meth' itself, as if a new drug has appeared on the scene, ignores the essential equivalence of methamphetamine and other amphetamines. As Time magazine recognizes, pharmaceutically-produced meth is approved for the treatment of obesity and attention-deficit disorder (Kirn, 1998). Scientific research concurs. The differences between methamphetamine and amphetamine have thus far 'evaded researchers' (Shoblock, Sullivan, Maisonneuve, & Glick, 2003, p. 360). Methamphetamines have the same stimulant effect as any other amphetamine. Perhaps more to the point: 'There are no known neurobiological differences in action between the two drugs' (Shoblock et al, 2003, p. 359). Defining meth as somehow unique fails to demonstrate that the constituent species (meth/other amphetamines) of the genus exclude one another. At least two government agencies agree. '

For Medline, whose sponsoring agencies are the National Library of Medicine and the National Institutes of Health, meth is just a kind, of amphetamine. In Medline (2003) under the rubric 'amphetamines' are found amphetamines, dextroamphetamines, and methamphetamines. For children of six years of age or older with attention-deficit hyperactivity disorder, the recommended dosage for the oral extended release meth tablet is 20-25 mg a day.

For the National Survey on Drug Use and Health (NSDUH), which is sponsored by the Substance Abuse and Mental Health Services Administration (SAMHSA), an agency of the U.S. Public Health Service and a part of the Department of Health and Human Services (DHHS), meth is just a kind of stimulant, simply listed under 'stimu-. lants' (SAMHSA, 2004, p. 11). Specifically, the NSDUH survey operationally defined stimulants as follows:

> Feeder question: 'These next questions are about the use of drugs such as amphetamines that are known as stimulants, uppers, or speed. People sometimes take these drugs to lose weight, to stay awake, or for attention deficit disorders.'

.,... The following prescription stimulants were listed on Pill Card C (Stimulants): (1) Methamphetamine (crank, crystal, ice, or speed) (no picture), Desoxyn", or Methedrine (no picture); (2) Amphetamines (no picture), Benzedrine", Biphetamine^, Fasting or Phentermine; (3) Ritalin[0*] or Methylphenidate; (4) Cylert^; (5) Dexedrine[00]; (6) Dextroamphetamine (no picture); (7) Didrexv; (8) Eskatrolv; (9) lonamin[0""]; (10); (11) Mazanor[®]; (11) Obedrin-LAv (no picture); (12) Plegine[®]; (13) Preludin"; (14) Sanorex'"; and (15) Tenuate[®]. (SAMHSA, 2004, p. 143)

Ritalin, the most popular brand-name methylphenidate (MPH) used in the treatment of attention deficit (hyperactivity) disorders, is third on the list. Chemists developed Ritalin in an attempt to diminish the 'unpleasant cardiovascular effects[5] of amphetamines. But Ritalin has the same 'pharmacological actions' (Klerman & Paykel, 1969, p. 189). Writing on the Holistic Children's Health website, a physician states: 'Ritalin is an amphetamine ... speed' (Whitaker, n.d., para. 1). The Christian Science Monitor paraphrases a DEA spokesperson: 'Ritalin is interchangeable with amphetamine and methamphetamine' (Marks, 2000, p. 9). Ritalin is an 'amphetamine-based chemical' (Mailer & Lynch-German, 2001, para. 17); its properties are'the 'same as those of amphetamines' (Ghodse, 1999, p. 265). According to the DEA, U.S. physicians wrote more than nine million MPH prescriptions during 1998 (Knickerbocker, 1999). Today 6-10 million Americans take Ritalin (Wenske, 2005).

The vision that meth is something new, different from other drugs, is fundamentally flawed. Although chemically synthesized in 1887, the medical uses of amphetamines did not begin until

1927. The commercial marketing of the product started in 1932 (Brecher, 1972a). Certainly, sociologists are aware that meth 'has been used for decades' (Akers, 1991, p. 778). Typically the term 'meth' is applied to a homemade substance that is manufactured in rural labs using fertilizers, cold tablets, and household acids. Only the amateur nature of the production process separates meth from its commercially produced equivalents. But that is not how meth is portrayed.

Moral Panic

Goode and Ben-Yehuda (1994a) catalog five criteria that are essential to moral panics. First, there is a heightened level of concern over certain behavior. Next, there is hostility linked to the category of people responsible for the threatening behavior. The targeted individuals are seen as evil. Third, there is public consensus that the threat is real. Fourth, there is disproportionality—the perceived threat is far removed from any objective measure of seriousness. Finally, there is volatility. Moral panics erupt suddenly and subside just as quickly. The meth scare encompasses all of these dimensions.

Concern

The first sign of a moral panic is a heightened level of concern about an issue. On the national level, members of the Senate [S. 103] introduced the Combat Meth Act on January 23, 2005, and a day later, House members [H.R. 314] proposed identical legislation (The Orator, 2005a, 2005b). Presently, at least 28 states are considering similar legislation (Rosario, 2005).

Three other state examples should suffice. First, on September 1, 2004, the State of Tennessee issued the final report of the Governor's Task Force on Methamphetamine Abuse. The 'severity of the [meth] problem in Tennessee' required just such a report (State of Tennessee, 2004, p. 4), which said that a 'proliferation' of meth labs existed (p. 3) that posed a 'serious threat to children' (p. 2). Second, on September 30, 2004, the Kentucky Attorney General Greg Stembo announced that he was reorganizing the Kentucky Bureau of Investigation to focus on meth use because it was a 'terrible problem ... in Kentucky' (quoted in Yetter, 2004, p. Al). Finally, on November 12, 2003, a North Carolina prosecutor, with the backing of a state senator, appealed against a judge's decision that meth was not a weapon of mass destruction (Sparks, 2003).

The volume of articles on InfoTrac and LexisNexis supports the importance of meth as a social threat. Both databases show a large jump in the number of articles with 'meth' in their titles/headlines from 2000 to 2004. Table 1 shows the number of articles in 2000, 2002, and 2004, and the percentage increase.

Another way of demonstrating the heightened concern is to compare a set of InfoTrac and LexisNexis articles with a government survey, the DAWN Report. The Drug Abuse Warning Network (DAWN) is a 'national surveillance system that collects data on drug abuse-related visits to emergency departments (EDs)' (DAWN, 2003,

p. 8); the U.S. Department of Health and Human Services is the sponsoring agency. Table 2 presents a comparison of the DAWN figures for ED visits for meth, as a percentage of the total drug-related ED visits, and the percentage of InfoTrac and LexisNexis articles concerned with meth from 1994 to 2002. One striking point is that in both 1996 and 2001, ED mentions of methf comprised 1.2% of the total drug-related ED mentions. In 1996 meth was a topic of only 6% of the InfoTrac articles and only 3% of the LexisNexis articles. In 2001, the percentages increased to 27% of the InfoTrac articles and 17% of the LexisNexis articles.

Hostility

The distinction between who uses meth as opposed to who uses amphetamines is predicated on a presupposed distinction serving the interests of the definer. Thus we find answers such as 'methamphetamines until recent years were generally confined to motorcycle gangs in California[5] (Gerth, 2002, p. B3). The proper question, therefore, is: Who uses amphetamines? Besides children diagnosed with ADHD, individuals with sleep disorders consume the drug. United States Air Force pilots do so as well. At least since 1961, the U.S.A.F. has authorized the use of amphetamines 'to sustain the performance of sleep-deprived pilots' (Caldwell & Brown, 2003, p. 8). The U.S. Army Aeromedical Research Laboratory (USAARL) determined that the so- called 'Go Pills' have proven their effectiveness in sleep-deprived personnel, sustaining 'the flight, performance of pilots even after 60 hours of continuous 'wakefulness' (Caldwell & Brown, 2003, p. 9).

In 2003, a bombing error in Afghanistan drew attention to the use of Go Pills. According to a neuroscientist quoted in the New York Times, amphetamines bring the performance of fatigued

TABLE 1. Appearance of the Word 'Meth' in Headlines of Database Articles[a]

Database	Year	n	Percentage increase
InfoTrac[b]	2000	10	
	2002	24	140%
	2004	175	630%
LexisNexis[c]	2000	258	
	2002	323	25%
	2004	466	40%

[a]*March 21, 2005;* [b]*'meth' in the title limiter and 'methamphetamine' in the text word limiter;* [c]*'meth' in the headline/lead paragraph limiter and 'methamphetamine' in the full text limiter.*

TABLE 2. Percentages of Total Drug-Related ED Mentions that Mention Meth and Percentages of Headlines of the Database Articles with the Word "Meth"

Year	ED mentions	InfoTrac (n = 79)	LexisNexis (n = 1283)
1994	1.9	1	0
1995	1.7	0	1
1996	1.2	6	3
1997	1.8	0	5
1998	1.1	9	11
1999	1.0	14	17
2000	1.2	13	20
2001	1.2	27	17
2002	1.4	30	25

individuals 'back up to baseline'[5] (Shanker & Duenwald, 2003, p. 14). .So the substance is good for pilots, but bad for other users. Besides the pilots, some rather famous folks have found amphetamines beneficial. A physician injected John F. Kennedy with amphetamines before his historic debates with Richard Nixon, and Jean-Paul Sartre used them when he wrote Critique of Dialectical Reason (Courtwright, 2001). In baseball, Pete Rose got all of his 4,256 record-setting hits with the aid of amphetamines (Chass, 2002). Writing in 2003, then New York Yankees pitcher David Wells observed that a lot of baseball players have a stockpile of hundreds and hundreds of amphetamines (Daly, 2003). Who else?

In 2005, McCabe, Knight, Teter, and Wechsler (2005) reported the results of their survey concerning the non-medical use of prescription stimulants among US college students: 'The present study found that the population of US college students reporting life-time non-medical use of prescription stimulants was 6.9%, past year use was 4.1% and past month use was 2.1%[5] (p. 102). According to the most recent figures available, 16,334,134 individuals are attending college in the US (National Center for Educational Statistics, 2004, p. 220). Apparently, the 1,127,055

law-breakers have gone unnoticed. A particular group of students is drawn to non-medical amphetamine use. Survey results reveal that medical students' use of amphetamines ranges from 7-54% (McAuliffe et al, 1984). On campuses Ritalin goes by the nickname Vitamin R' (Healy, 2004).

The media interpretation of meth users is far removed from children, pilots, politicians, philosophers, athletes, and students. According to Manderson (1995), the 'compelling quality of drugs as objects, as emotional images, and as symbols leads us to fixate upon them' (p. 800). Like the vision of Chinese smoking opium in San Francisco, meth has become something strange, 'an all-encompassing sensation of dirtiness' (Manderson, 1995, p. 802). The language that describes meth users distances them from normal citizens and places them outside the boundaries of middle-class propriety.

Meth users are racially, geographically, and economically coded. The alleged relationship between meth and rural poverty has two different time orders. First, rural poverty precedes the meth use in time. The SA.MHSA experts 'say meth has become the drug of choice among poorly educated people who have stayed behind as others migrated to urban areas' ('Midwestern Rural Areas,' 2004, p.

2). Second, meth is temporally prior to rural poverty. As the Tennessee governor's task force report directly states: 'Methamphetamine abuse leads to ... poverty' (State of Tennessee, 2004, p. 1). Either way, meth is often labeled the 'poor man's cocaine' (LexisNexis, n = 134, March 27, 2005).

Other less popular descriptors include 'redneck cocaine[5] (Longa, 1998), 'redneck crack[5] (Lane, 2001), the 'trailer trash drug' (Poole, 2004), and the 'new moonshine[5] ('You Take the High Road,' 2003). The term 'redneck' is an 'expletive, carrying both regional and racial slurs simultaneously.' Often it is the 'semantic equivalent of "white trash"' (Rodgers, 1981, p. 72). The history of the use of the term 'white trash' is linked to a social ideology that reads the structure of social classes onto nature. White trash are inherently inferior and notoriously lazy. They are a dangerous class in need of monitoring. This labeling process facilitated the introduction of 'regulatory mechanisms into rural areas' (Rafter, 1988, p. 49). In case the redneck rhetoric fails in its evocative intent, other terminology is applied. First, a 'meth head' is a 'redneck whose teeth had fallen out' (Poole, 2004, p. 18). Next, the 'meth heads' bible' is Secrets of Methamphetamine Manufacture (Jubera, 2003, para. 14). Finally, the meth heads' preferred method for making meth is the 'Nazi method.' (Hathaway, 2002a, para. 8).

Consensus

The source of this consensus is the print media. In 1996, Democratic Senator Tom Harkin proposed that Iowa be designated a 'High-Intensity Drug Trafficking Area' because of its meth epidemic. Harkin requested seven million dollars. In explaining the need for the funds, Tom Gorton, Senator Harkin's spokesman, stated: 'Methamphetamine is a major issue in Iowa; it's been all over the newspapers out there[5] (quoted in 'Strange Bedfellows,' 1996, p. 3). Alligood (2004) demonstrated the power of the media by linking news reports to the 31 separate meth-related bills Tennessee legislators proposed for consideration during 2004.

Consensus is achieved further by the declarations that meth production is a threat to the environment, and that meth use victimizes children. After all, everyone cares about the environment and everyone is concerned with child welfare.

According to Reinarman (2000, p. 155), American moral entrepreneurs continually blame 'new chemical bogeymen' for society's ills. A unique aspect of the meth threat is that a chemical bogeyman actually is seen as posing a threat to the environment. I assume that there is nothing nice about dumping chemical waste from meth labs. But environmental threats can only be judged in terms of their relative place in the full range of ecological horrors.

What is a meth lab? One would think that meth labs are places marked by one common characteristic—meth making. But that is only part of the definition. Meth labs are 'labs where the drug is made, abandoned labs, ingredient and equipment stockpiles and meth-related dump sites' (Rowden, 2004, para. 7). The so-called labs are usually mobile and small—a lab can be carried in a suitcase (Bier, 2004). In Indiana during 2002, for example, an individual was arrested for making meth on his motorcycle (Hefting, 2002). It turns out that these smaller labs are the more dangerous labs. George Cazenavette of the DEA offered this testimony before the U.S. House Judiciary Committee's Subcommittee on Crime: 'The smaller labs are usually more dangerous than the larger operations because the cooks are generally less experienced chemists who often have little regard for the safety issues that arise when dealing with explosive and poisonous chemicals' (quoted in Whitsett, 2001, para. 38).

According to the Office of National Drug Control Policy, meth labs pose both immediate and long-term environmental risks. 'For each pound of "meth" produced, five to six pounds of hazardous waste are generated' (U.S. Department of State, 2003, para. 14). But as a Texas sheriff department captain observes, the labs 'are pretty much what we call mom and pop operations' (Ken Ariola, quoted in Bier, 2004, para. 6). These homemade facilities produce an ounce or less of the drug ('Meth Seizures,' 2002). A standard lab produces five to six ounces of hazardous waste. According to the DEA, in 2004 law enforcement made 16,800 meth-related seizures. These meth-related seizures supposedly correspond to the discovery of nearly 17,000 meth labs (Plummer, 2005). Ignoring the all-inclusive nature of the definition of a meth lab, let's assume, for argument's sake, that every lab actually produced meth. at least once. Doing the meth math, the labs produced approximately 6,300 pounds of toxic waste. According to the U.S. Environmental Protection Agency, the U.S. livestock industry produces 2,700,000,000,000 tons of waste each year (McCauley, 2002), with 2,000 pounds to the ton. The EPA also estimates that livestock herds account for 25% of the anthropogenic emissions of methane, and that waste lagoons from factory-farm operations emit an additional 5% of human-induced methane (Worldwatch Institute, 1998). Obviously, every little bit of pollution counts. Nevertheless, my conservative conclusion is that methane emissions are a bigger environmental problem than meth labs.

The attacks on meth are also framed by a concern for child welfare. Medical and social service workers have compared children whose parents were arrested for meth with other neglected children. The former were more likely to be sexually abused, to be violent, to have more lice, and to have rotten teeth (Ko, 2001). According to a Washington state liaison between Child Protective Services and law-enforcement authorities, the majority of meth households have high levels of domestic violence, sex, and pornography, and lots of junk food. And when the children are taken into care, they have 'caked-on dirt' (quoted in Ko, 2001, para. 10). In this regard, People Weekly quotes an Arkansas caseworker: 'Mom or Dad or both are so strung out that they can't provide proper care for the children. In one house there was dog feces all over' (quoted in Hewitt, 2004, p. 98). As a captain in the King County (WA) Sheriffs Office concludes, 'Meth is a wretched drug when it comes to caring for kids' (quoted in Ko, 2001, para. 15). Oddly, sometimes experts present an alternative viewpoint. What remains the same is the problematic aspect of meth use. The statement: 'Experts and users say the drug [meth] appeals to women because it ... gives them energy, to take care of their children or feel more efficient in everything they do' ('Meth Use,' 2002, p. 6).

According to child welfare officials, children with prenatal exposure to meth often suffer 'medical and behavioral problems' ('Meth Abuse,' 2003, p. 8). Specifically, one 'meth baby' was born with 'an arm growing out of the neck' and another 'meth baby' was 'missing a femur' (McCann, 2004, p. M17). As everyone knows, the notion of 'crack babies' is mythical in nature (Goode & Ben-Yehuda, 1994b). Likewise, the so- called 'meth baby' has 'no basis in science.' Based on 'what we now know from medical and psychological research,' we should 'eliminate' the terms 'crack baby' and 'meth baby' from our usage (Lewis, 2004, p. 8). Amazingly, however, journalists notice the similarity between 'crack babies'and'meth babies.'

Although research on "crack babies" began more than a decade ago, Hathaway (2004, para. 54) observes, scientists 'still are trying to determine to what extent fetuses exposed to cocaine are likely to develop physical and behavioral disabilities.' But even less is known about meth babies and childhood exposure to meth ingredients. Months before Hathaway's analogy between "crack babies" and "meth babies", the Los Angeles Times editorialized: "'Meth babies" have not set off the public frenzy that crack babies did 15 years ago. But the less publicized methamphetamine epidemic is proving just as devastating' ('Editorial,' 2003, para. 1). The editorial referred to a mother whose infant died apparently after, consuming meth and did not mention the issue of prenatal exposure to meth. Indeed, a Los Angeles area judge sentenced a woman to 'life in prison for murdering her infant son by allowing him to ingest a lethal dose of methampheta mine' (Pugmire, 2003, para. 1). However, the crack baby syndrome concerned babies born to mothers who used crack during pregnancy. Poisoning one's child is different.

Disproportionality

Meth is seen as an epidemic.. To begin, ED mentions of meth can be compared to ED mentions of some other drug. It appears that other drugs cause

TABLE 3. Total Drug-Related ED Visits in 2002

Alcohol	207,395
Cocaine	199,198
Anxiolytics, sedatives, hypnotics	137,350
Marijuana	119,472
Opiates/opioids	119,185
Heroin	93,5.19
Antidepressants	62,635
Other substances	5.1,333
Acetaminophen	36,086
Nonsteroidal anti-inflammatory agents (ibuprofen, naproxen)	21,414
Antipsychotics	20,221
Meth	17,696
Anticonvulsants	16,681
Muscle relaxants	13,259

Note: Adapted from Drug Abuse Warning Network (2003).

more problems for ED staff. Table 3 lists some of the numbers concerning drugs and ED visits.

A Lexis-Nexis search-(March 24, 2005) using the 'headline, lead paragraph' limiter for the word 'meth' and the 'full text[5] limiter for the word 'epidemic' found 202 newspapers articles referring to meth as an epidemic. An InfoTrac search (March .23, 2005) using the 'keyword[5] limiter 'meth[5] and the 'text word[5] limiter 'epidemic' found 85 periodical articles that did likewise. The extent of the meth problem appears agreed upon by numerous experts. Table 4 provides some expert testimony in this regard.

Meth may well be a problem for some people, but other problems are far more pervasive. For example, a November 2003 report issued by DAWN of the U.S. Department of Health and Human. Services ascertained that emergency department mentions of meth have been 'stable—Meth mentions represented 2.5% of the 'major substances of abuse' category for 2002. The percentages of alcohol (30%), cocaine (29%), marijuana (17%), and heroin (17%) were considerably higher (DAWN, 2003, p. 2). DAWN also provides mortality data. Meth was one of the top 10 drugs contributing to death in only 11 of the 31 metropolitan areas surveyed. In 88% of the cases, the ED mentioned at least one other drug in combination with meth, EDs listed only 59 deaths specifying meth alone (U.S. Department of Health & Human Services, 2004). While every death is tragic, the totals of some other drug-related deaths are far more significant: tobacco = 400,000+; alcohol = 100,000+; and prescription drug deaths in hospitals = 100,000+ ('US Recreational Drug Deaths,' 2002). Further, the lives of 18,900 babies would be saved if the U.S. infant mortality rate was number one in the world instead of number 42 (Kristof, 2005). Another 18,000 working age adults die annually because they lack health insurance and cannot afford operations (Kristof, 2005). Nevertheless, meth is seen as an epidemic caused by a killing

TABLE 4. Views of Experts on the Meth Problem

The statement	The expert	Source
'Right now, we're just inundated with meth'	Ron Gravitt, California Department of Justice	Sanchez (2001, para. 11)
'Meth is the overwhelming drug of choice among ... murderers'	Carol Cummings, King County (WA) Sheriffs Office	Ko (2001, para. 28)
'Meth. is the number one cause of crime'	Rep. Brian Baird (D-Washington)	Brogan (2001, p. 13A)
States are 'literally drowning in meth activity'	Asa Hutchinson, DEA Director	Sink (2002, para. 6)
'Now everybody is cooking meth'	Travis Blankenship, Franklin County (MO) Police	Pierre (2003, para. 4)
'Everyone is doing it [meth]'	Mike Szypeski, Narcotics Unit, Newport Beach (CA) Police	Lobdell and Tran (2003, para. 18)
'Perhaps more than any other drug, methamphetamine puts all of us—users and nonusers alike—at risk'	Armand McClintock, agent in charge of the DEA's Indianapolis district office	Peck (2004, para. 22)

chemical wrapped inside a wasting disease that eats up brain cells and transforms people into monsters. Table 5 provides some of the statements that make the case for meth's uniqueness.

The National Institute on Drug Abuse (NIDA) considers meth 'a potent, highly addictive form of amphetamine' (Mathias, 1998, p. '2). The alleged addictive quality of meth is a central element of the disproportionality of the claims. An advertisement for an educational video entitled Methamphetamin.es: The Icy Death notes: Ice [meth] is more devastating than cocaine, more addictive than crack, and stronger than LSD.... [I]t can be addictive or lethal after only one use" (NIMCO, 2002, p. 43). People Weekly described meth as 'fiendishly addictive' ("How Meth Destroys,' 2004, p. 98). Rolling Stone called it 'insuperably addictive' (Solotaroff, 2003, p. 49). The Tennessee governor's task force report notes that 'as many as 90% of methamphetamine addicts will return to the drug versus much lower rates for other substances' (State of Tennessee, 2004, p. 8).

Elsewhere, law-enforcement experts attest that only 1 % of meth users can overcome their addiction (Layton, 2005). Oddly, a government spokesperson inadvertently challenged the 'highly addictive' accusation. In 2003, John C. Horton, an associate deputy director of the White House Office of National Drug Control Policy, reported some statistics to a congressional hearing. According to Horton, nearly 10 million U.S. residents had used meth at least once in their lifetime and between 650,000 and 700,000 people were monthly users ('Analysis,' 2004). It seems that if the addictive accusations were true, there would be 10 million daily users.

Meth is as addicting as amphetamines because meth is critically isomorphic with amphetamines. In 1963, the American Medical Association found that compulsive abuse of amphetamines constitutes a 'small problem' (Brecher, 1972b, para. 1). Medical researchers appear unified in their opinion that amphetamines do not cause 'physical dependence' (Meyer, 1969, p. 381).

TABLE 5. Claims about the Nature of Meth

The statement	The expert	Source
Meth is associated with, 'brain damage, memory loss, psychotic-like behavior, heart damage, hepatitis, and HIV transmission'	Alan L Leshner, NIDA director	Mathias (1998, p. 2)
'Methamphetamine is a chronic wasting disease'	William Wasley, Director of the U.S. Forest Service's law enforcement division	Hathaway (2002b, para. 44)
It's the most insidious drug.... It eats up [users'] brain cells'	Bill Renton, DEA head, Midwest office (St. Louis)	Bryan (2002, p. Bl)
'It's a killing chemical'.	Carl Skelton, Wayne County (TN) Sheriff.	Alligood (2003, p. 7B)
'[Meth is] the worst drug ever to hit America'	Barry McCaffrey, President Clinton's 'drug czar'	'You Take the High Road' (2003, p. 30)
Meth turns a user 'into a monster'	Carey Pouse, an Oklahoma drug task force director	'.Meth and Murder' (2004, p. 95)

A groundbreaking survey found that the label 'abuser' applied to less than a tenth, of 1% of amphetamine users (Brecher, 1972c; Goldberg, 1968).

Recent research appears to cast additional doubts on meth's addictive properties. The 'stimulant sensitization hypothesis' predicting that stimulant-treated children have an increased sensitization to young adult stimulant exposure is rejected (Barkley, Fischer, Smallish, & Fletcher, 2003, p. 99). As mentioned, to treat ADHD, physicians prescribe stimulants (methylphenidate or amphetamine). A meta-analysis of the results of six studies found that pharmacotherapy with stimulants for ADHD is inversely related to young adult drug abuse (Wilens, Faraone, Biederman, & Gunawardene, 2003). A 13- year prospective study determined that duration of stimulant treatment was not significantly associated with frequency of stimulant use by young adulthood (Barkley et al., 2003). Given the pervasive prescribing of stimulants, if the addictive properties of meth were in any way comparable to media portrayals, meth labs would appear on every block in the USA.

As Akers (1991) notes, 'all drugs to which some become addicted have been controlled and used non-habitually by most of those who have tried them' (p. 779). In a scholarly study of meth users (as .opposed the media's collections of sensationalized anecdotes), the majority of respondents used the substance less than once a week and none reported daily use (Halkitis, Parsons, & Wilton, 2003). Here the respondents. used meth 'for a variety of reason, to cope with life experiences' (Halkitis et al., 2003, p. 425). These life experiences encompassed both unpleasant emotions and pleasant times with others.

Volatility

'The element of volatility indicates that moral panic erupts suddenly then subsides' (Welch, Price, & Yankey, 2002, p. 18). As is evident, a meth panic has recently erupted. However, this is a third coming. The first meth moral panic began in 1962 when individuals started to inject amphetamines. Worse still,.drug users mixed amphetamines with heroin and. injected both substances. Amphetamines replaced cocaine in the so- called 'speedball.' Habitual users of injectable amphetamines became known as 'speed freaks' (Brecher, 1972b). Jenkins (1994) details the dimensions of the next meth panic, which he called 'the Ice Age'—'ice' being a synonym for meth. His study considered a chronology of media accounts of meth from 1989 to 1991. Media attention focused primarily on Hawaii. But, as Jenkins (1994) concluded, 'The ice danger, however, did not materialize as a national crisis, and the prospective "plague" faded rapidly in early 1990' (p. 20). At that time, federal officials backed away from their claims about the ominous meth plague and the grave warnings about the forthcoming drug crisis (Lauderback & Waldorf, 1993).

Conclusion

The meth scare is blinding people to the plight of white, underclass, rural, poor people. The force of corporate agribusiness causes the abandonment of individually-owned farms. In the majority of family farms, the farmer, spouse, or both work off the farm ('Facts Help,' 2004). Farm jobs in rural areas in Alabama, Kentucky, and Tennessee 'declined by 8.6% from 1990 to 2000, and manufacturing jobs were down 2.2% in rural areas during the same period' ('Study: Farm, Factory Jobs,' 2004, p. B2). Jobs in the service industry have increased, while manufacturing jobs have been shipped overseas. Corporate agribusiness has turned farmers into 'little more than serfs' (Schlosser, 2002, p. 139). The result is the creation of 'rural ghettos in the American heartland' (Schlosser, 2002, p. 149). Surplus populations become society's scapegoats (Koski, 1999). Just like crack, meth has become a class code word.

The fear of crack translated into 'an irrational fear of inner city black men, at a time when the doors of opportunity in the society were simultaneously being closed to that same group' (Angeli, 1997, p. 1223). Changes in the urban economy, particularly the disappearance of industrial jobs that did not require higher levels of education, resulted in urban dwellers being permanently locked out of the mainstream of the American occupational system (Wilson, 1987). This 'jobless ghetto' lacked 'basic opportunities and resources' (Wilson, 1996, p. 23). The crack crisis invited people to ignore these economic transformations and 'the ways that cuts to social services and governmental transfer payments left working-class families scrambling' (Ortiz & Briggs, 2003, p. 46). In the logic of the crack scare, 'whatever economic and social troubles these people have suffered were due largely to drug use' (Reinarman & Levine, 1997, p. 66). The meth scare, just like the crack scare, has 'blinded people to the social sources of many social problems' (Reinarman & Levine, 1997, p. 66).

Over 10 years ago, Jenkins (1994) discerned the similarities between media approaches to crack and media approaches to meth. He explained the similarities in terms of a rhetorical process called convergence. Basically, the recent experience of crack made it easy for the media to represent meth as part of the same problem. Further, Jenkins saw that the political frameworks and bureaucracies that resulted from the intense focus on crack already existed when meth came along. As previously mentioned, 'poverty and unemployment—or underemployment—essentially set the stage for the cultural milieu in which drug selling takes place' (Koski, 1999, p. 302). I see poverty and unemployment—or underemployment—essentially setting the stage for a cultural milieu in which the media facilitate the operation of an inherently corrupt economic system by ongoing victim-blaming. After all, why should anyone care about these drug-addicted dregs that are destroying their communities and irreparably harming their own children?

References

Akers, R. L. (1991). Addiction: The troublesome concept. Journal of Drug Issues, 21, 777-793.

Alligood, L. (2003, September 7). Midstate meth labs using fertilizer for deadly mix. The Tennessecm, pp. 113,78.

Alligood, L. (2004, February 29). Attacking the meth trade. The Tennessecm, pp. 19A-20A.

Analysis: Meth focus of new laws, research. (2004, January 27). United Press International Retrieved February 28, 2004, from http://infotrac-college.thomsonlearning.com (Item A112595563).

Angeli, D. H. (1997). A 'second look' at crack cocaine sentencing policies. American Criminal Law Review, 34, 1211-1241.

Barkley, R. A., Fischer, M, Smallish L, & Fletcher, K. (2003). Does the treatment of attention-deficit/hyperactivity disorder with stimulants contribute to drug use/abuse? A 13-year prospective study. Pediatrics, III, 97-109.

Bier, C. (2004, August 19). Police fight meth labs in county. Houston Chronicle. Retrieved October 22, 2004, from http://web.lexis-nexis.com

Brecher, E. M. (1972a). The amphetamines. In The Consumer Union report on licit and illicit drugs. Boston, MA: Little, Brown and Company. Retrieved April 2, 2004, from http:// ww\v.druglib rary.org/schaffer/library/studies/cu/cu36.html

Brecher, E. M. (1972b). Enter the 'speed freak'. In The Consumer Union report on licit and illicit drugs. Boston, MA: Little, Brown and Company. Retrieved April 2, 2004, from http:// mvw.driiglibrary.org/schaffer/library/studies/cu/cu37.html

Brecher, E. M. (1972c). The Swedish experience,. In The Consumer Union report on licit and illicit drugs. Boston, MA: Little, Brown and. Company.

Retrieved April 2, 2004, from http:// www.druglibraiy.org/schaffer/library/studies/cii/cu39.html

Brogan, P. (2001, December 16). Meth bout continues with more funding. The Tennessean, p. 13A.

Bryan, B. (2002, November 11). New DEA head here will tackle the meth scourge. St. Louis Post-Dispatch, pp. B1-B2.

Caldwell, J. A., & Brown, C. L. (2003). Running on empty? Flying Safety, 59(3), 4-11.

Chass, M. (2002, May 31). On baseball. The.New York Times, p. D4.

Cohen, S. (1972). Folk devils and moral panic. London:. MacGibbon & Kee..

Courtwright, D. T. (2001). Forces of habit. Cambridge, MA: Harvard University Press.

Daly, D. (2003, March 12). A. strange tale of two 'authors'. Washington Times, p. CI. Retrieved March 27, 2005, from http://web.lexis-nexis.com

Drug Abuse Warning Network. (2003, November). Trends in drug-rejated emergency department visits, 1994-2002 at a glance. In The DAWN Report Rockville, MI): U.S. Department of Health 8c Human Services.

Editorial: The life and meth of babies. (2003, October 19). Los Angeles Times, p. M4. Retrieved March 1, 2004, from http://proquest.umi.com (ID 425335421)

Facts help. (2004). Farm Aid Information Center. Retrieved March 20, 2004, from http://www.farmaid.org/site/pageserver?pagename=info_facts_help

Gerth, J. (2002, June 6). Methamphetamine use, production increasing. Courier-Journal, pp. Bl, B3.

Ghodse, A. H. (1999). Dramatic increase in methylphenidate consumption. Current Opinion in Psychiatry, 12, 265-268.

Goldberg, L. (1968). Drug abuse in Sweden. Bulletin on Narcotics, h 1-31. Retrieved March 27, 2005, from http://www.unodc.org/unodc/en/bulletin/bulletin_1968-01-01_l_page002.html

Goode, E., & Ben-Yehuda, N. (1994a). Moral panics: Culture, politics, and social construction. Annual Review of Sociology, 20, 149-171.

Goode, E., & Ben-Yehuda, N. (1994b). Moral panics: The social construction of deviance. Cambridge, MA: BlackwelL

Halkitis, P. N., Parsons, J. T., & Wilton, L. (2003). An exploratory study of contextual and situational factors related to methamphetamine use among gay and bisexual men in New York City. Journal of Drug Issues, 33, 413-432.

Hall, S., Critcher, C, Jefferson, T., Clarke, J., & Roberts, B. (1978). Policing the crisis: Mugging, the state and law and order. New York:. Holmes & Meiser..

Hathaway, M. (2002a, May 9). Latest meth bust may slow other drug manufacturers. St. Louis Post-Dispatch. Retrieved March 24, 2005, from http://web.lexis-nexis.com

Hathaway, M. (2002b, July 1). Rise in meth labs in Mark Twain National Forest. KnightRidder/Tribime News Service. Retrieved March. 5, 2004, from http://infotrac-college.thomsonlearning.com (Item CJ88158631)

Hathaway, M. (2004, January 25). Police in meth belt scramble to keep up. St. Loins Post-Dispatch, p. AL Retrieved January 28, 2004, from http://web.lexis-nexis.com

Healy, M. (2004, December 20).. Sharper minds. Los Angeles Times, p. Fl. Retrieved January 5, 2005, from http://proquest.umi.com (ID 768533781).

Hefling, K. (2002, July 14). Cooking on road raiscs danger. Paducah Sun, pp. IOC, 12C.

Hewitt, B. (2004, February 16). Dying for crystal. People Weekly, 61(6), 92-98.

How meth destroys body and mind. (2004, February 16). People Weekly, 61 (6), 98.

Jenkins, P. (1994). 'The Ice Age': The social construction of a drug panic. Justice Quarterly, 11, 7-31.

Jubera, D. (2003, February 9). Moonshine country overrun by meth. Atlanta Journal-Constitution. Retrieved March-27, 2005, from http://web.lexis-nexis.com Kirn, W. (1998, June 22). Crank. Time, 151, 25-32.

Klerman, G. L., & Paykel, E. S. (1969). Clinical use of antidepressant drugs. In P. Black (Ed.), Drugs and the brain (pp. 185-201). Baltimore:. Johns Hopkins University Press..

Knickerbocker, B. (1999, May 19). Child rearing by prescription is becoming pervasive: Using drugs to rein in boys. Christian Science Monitor, pp. 1,4.

Ko, M. (2001, October 3). Meth labs take cruelest toll on kids. Knight Ridder/Tribune News Service. Retrieved February 29, 2004, from http://infotrac-college.thorasonlearning.com (item CJ78878656).

Koski, D. D. (1999). A critical perspective on drug selling in the United States. Contemporary Drug Problems, 26,289-329.

Kristof, N. D. (2005, January 12). Health care? Ask Cuba. The New York Times, p. A21.

Lane, M. B. (2001, March 25). Outlaw drug labs rapidly take root. Columbus Dispatch, p. 1A. Retrieved March 27, 2005, from http://web.lexis-nexis.com

Lauderback, D., & Waldorf, D. (1993). Whatever happened to ice? Journal of Drug Issues, 23, 597-613.

Layton, D. C. (2005, February 7). Meth makes no sense. Drug Topics, 149(3). Retrieved March 24, 2005, from http://www.drugtopics.com/drugtopics/article/articledetail.jsp?id= 145835

Lewis, D. C. (2004). Stop perpetuating the 'crack baby' myth. Brown University Digest of Addiction Theory and Application, 23(8), 8.

Lobdell, W., & Trail, M. (2003, October 12). California: Upscale, but within meth's grasp. Los Angeles Times, p. BL Retrieved March 1, 2004, from http://proquest.umi.com (ID 422859781).

Longa, L. (1998, February 28). Atlanta crawls in 'redneck cocaine'. Atlanta Journal-Constitution. Retrieved February 28, 1998, from http://www.accessatlanta.com/news/1998/02/28/. cocaine_fiill.html

Mailer, P., & Lynch-German, L. (2001, February 8). Ritalin high attracts adults in Wisconsin.

Milwaukee Journal-Sentinel. Retrieved March 24, 2005, from http://web.lexis-nexis.com

Manderson, D. (1995). Metamorphoses: Clashing symbols in the social construction of drugs Journal of Drug Issues, 25, 799-816.

Marks, A. (2000, October 31). Schoolyard hustlers' new drug: Ritalin. Christian Science Monitor, pp. 1,9.

Mathias, R. (1998). NIDA initiative tackles methamphetamine use. NIDA Notes, 13(1), 1-3.

McAuliffe, W. E., Rohman, M. P., Fishman, P., Friedman, R„ Wechsler, H., Soboroff, S. H., 8cToth, D. (1984). Psychoactive drug use by young and future physicians. Journal of Health and Social Behavior, 25, 34-54.

McCabe, S. E., Knight, I. R., Teter, C, 8c Wechsler, Ii. (2005). Non-medical use of prescription stimulants among US college students. Addiction, 100, 96-106.

McCann, S. (2004, November 17). Meth ravages lives-in northern counties: Drug makes messy life for innocent children. Star Tribune, pp. Nl, N17.

McCauley, M. A. (2002, April 19). Factory farms. Oxfam America. Retrieved March 3, 2004, from http://w\v\v.oxfamamerica.org/advocacy/art2566.html

Medline. (2003). Amphetamines, MedlinePlus drug information. U.S. National Library of Medicine 8c the National Institutes of Health. Retrieved February 29, 2004, from http://www.nlm.nih.gov/medlinephis/dmginfo/uspdi/202031.html

Meth abuse increases burden on Idaho foster care system, (2003, August 25). Alcoholism and Drug Abuse Weekly, 15(32), 8.

Meth and murder. (2004, February 16). People Weekly, 61 (6), 95.

Meth seizures cause concern. (2002, August 3i). Courier-Journal, p. B7.

Meth use growing among U.S. women. (2002, June 17). Alcoholism and Drug Abuse Weekly, 24(24), 6.

Meyer, R. E. (1969). The widening challenge of drug abuse: The non-opiates., In P. Black (Ed.), Drugs and the brain (pp. 379-390). Baltimore:. Johns Hopkins University Press.

Midwestern rural areas take brunt of meth epidemic. (2004, January 8). Drug Detection Report, 14(1),2.

National Center for Educational Statistics. (2004, December 31). Digest of educational statistics (NCES Publication 2005025). Retrieved March 27, 2005, from http://nces.ed.gov/programs/ digest/d03/tables/dtl 72.asp

NIMCO. (2002). Violence prevention, law enforcement and corrections [Brochure]. Calhoun, KY: Author.

The Orator. (2005a). S. 103. Retrieved March 24, 2005, from http://www.theorator.com/billsl09/ sl03.html

The Orator. (2005b). H. R. 314. Retrieved March 24, 2005, from http://wwv.theorator.com/billsl09/hr314.html

Ortiz, A. T., 8c .Briggs, L. (2003). The culture of poverty, crack babies, and welfare cheats. Social Text, 2/(3), 39-57.

Peck, C (2004, August 1). Got meth? Beef. Retrieved March 27, 2005, from, http://beef-mag.com/ma.g/beef_meth/

Pierre, R. E. (2003, June 17). In Missouri, an uphill battle against meth. Washington Post, p. A3. Retrieved October 22, 2004, from http://web.lexis-nexis.com

Poole, O. (2004, February 28). The trailer trash drug takes hold, of Hollywood worldwide. Daily Telegraph, p. 18. Retrieved October 22, 2004, from http://web.lexis-nexis.com

Plummer, D. (2005, February 22). Meth lab's residue casts pall. Atlanta Journal-Constitution, p. Bl. Retrieved March 27, 2005, from http://web.lexis-nexis.com

Pugmire, L. (2003, October 31). Woman whose baby died of meth' gets life. Los Angeles Times, p. Bl. Retrieved March 1, 2004, from http://proquest.umi.com (ID 43583035).

Rafter, N. H. (1988). White trash: Eugenics as social ideology. Society, 26(1), 43-49.

Reinarman, C. (2000). The social construction of drug scares. In P. A. Adler 8c P. Adler (Eds.), Constructions of deviance (3rd ed., pp. 147-158). Belmont, CA: Wadsworth..

Reinarman, C, 8c Levine, H. G. (1997). The crack attack. In C. Reinarman 8c H. G. Levine (Eds.), Crack in America (pp. 51-68). Berkeley:. University of California Press..

Rodgers, R. S. (1981). Images of rednecks in country music. Journal of Regional Cultures, 1, 71-81.

Rosario, R. (2005, February 21). Anti-meth. measures are sailing through legislature. St. Paul Pioneer-Press, pp. IB, 4B.

All Arounders

By Darryl S. Inaba and William E. Cohen

Marijuana & The Cannabinoids

"More than 250 marijuana plants were found at a home that caught fire this morning in San Francisco, according to San Francisco police officer Maria Oropeza. Police were called to the scene around 4:20 a.m. after firefighters put the one-alarm blaze out."

—San Francisco Chronicle,
February 5, 2006

"With at least tacit support from several local elected officials, operators of a San Francisco medical cannabis dispensary raided by U.S. drug agents last month thumbed their nose at federal authorities and handed out bags of pot-laced confections and marijuana cigarettes in Civic Center Plaza outside City Hall on Wednesday."

—San Francisco Chronicle,
January 10, 2006

"Braided rope made from 100% hemp is an item right out of antiquity. This incredibly strong natural rope is hand-made in Romania. The manufacturing of this hemp rope uses the same techniques practiced for hundreds of years. This is the same type of rope used in the old sailing ships."

—Ad from the Hemp Traders Weh site,
which sells products made from hemp

The Cannabis, or hemp, plant, also called marijuana, produces fibers, grows edible seeds (akenes), has an oil that is used as a fuel and a lubricant, contains a number of medicinal ingredients, produces psychedelic resin that can alter consciousness, and is illegal in most countries.

"A divided U.S. Supreme Court [6 to 3] on Monday said federal law enforcement can disregard state medical marijuana laws and seize plants and make arrests."

—Portland Oregonian, June 7, 2005

History Of Use

A relationship between Cannabis and Homo sapiens has existed for at least 10,000 years. From its probable origin in China or central Asia, hemp cultivation has spread to almost every country in the world. There is a variety of species; some Cannabis plants are better for fiber, some for food, some for medications, and some for inducing psychedelic effects.

The plant was probably first used for nutrition because primitive people were always searching for new sources of food. Our ancient ancestors undoubtedly experienced some psychedelic effects when the plant was eaten. Next Cannabis was most likely utilized as a fiber for rope and nets. After that various medicine men, especially the semi-legendary Chinese emperor Shen Nung (c. 2700 B.C.), experimented with Cannabis for its medicinal benefits. Finally, experimenters searched for different ways to extract and consume the plant's psychedelic components.

Around 1500 B.C. the Indian Vedas (which also praised Amanita mushrooms) described Cannabis as a divine nectar that could deter evil, bring luck, and cleanse man of sin. It was listed as one of the five sacred plants to bring about freedom from stress (Booth, 2004).

> "We speak to the five kingdoms of the plants with soma the most excellent among them. The darbha-grass, hemp, and mighty barley: they shall deliver us from calamity!"
>
> —Atharva Veda, VI 43

Indian writings also described Cannabis's medicinal use to relieve headaches, control mania, counteract insomnia, treat venereal disease, cure whooping cough, and even arrest tuberculosis (Touw, 1981). Over succeeding millennia

Cannabis continued to be used in all its forms. Galen, the "father of modern Western medicine," wrote in A.D. 200 that it was sometimes customary to give Cannabis to guests to induce enjoyment and mirth. In third-century Rome, ropes and sails for ships[5] riggings were made from hemp fiber (Brunner, 1977). Medieval physicians cultivated hemp for the treatment of jaundice or coughs and recommended weedy hemp to treat cancer.

Because Cannabis was not specifically banned in the Koran by the Prophet Mohammed, Islamic cultures spread its use to Africa and Europe. Hashish, the concentrated form of marijuana, was written about in certain ancient texts, some of them originating about A.D. 1000.

> "When he had earned his daily wage, he would spend a little of it on food and the rest on a sufficiency of that hilarious herb. He took his hashish three times a day: once in the morning on an empty stomach, once at noon, and once at sundown. Thus he was never lacking in extravagant gaiety."
>
> —"A Tale of Two Hashish Eaters" from *A Thousand and One Arabian Nights*

In later centuries the use of hashish and marijuana was discouraged then condemned in Islamic countries. In Africa beginning about 600 years ago, marijuana was used in social/religious rituals and in medicinal preparations to treat dysentery, fevers, asthma, and even the pain of childbirth (DuToit, 1980).

As the Age of Exploration increased the need for rope, sails, and paper, many newly established colonies were encouraged to grow the more fibrous variants of Cannabis and export the hemp to the mother country. Even George Washington had large fields of Cannabis growing on his plantation. Cannabis was widely cultivated in the Americas until the nineteenth century, when the end of slavery made it less profitable to harvest and process the plant. The importation of Cannabis into the Americas for the psychoactive effects of smoking are thought to have originated with African slaves kidnapped from Angola and brought to plantations in northeastern Brazil. From there it eventually spread north to the Caribbean Islands and Mexico (Courtwright, 2001).

After World War I, migrant laborers who worked in the United States introduced the habit of smoking marijuana for its psychoactive effects. Initially, its use was confined to poor and minority groups, but in the 1920s the use of Cannabis as a substitute for prohibited alcohol spread in popularity. Marijuana "tea pads," similar to opium dens, became popular. It is estimated that there were more than 500 "tea pads" in New York by the beginning of the 1930s. Many of the "tea pads" were simply apartments where tenants and their smoking friends would get together to smoke pot. Some of these gatherings soon evolved into "rent parties," where tenants charged daily admission fees to help make their rent payments (O'Brien, Cohen, Evans, et al., 1992; Booth, 2004).

This expanded use of marijuana alarmed prohibitionists, who were left without a cause when the Eighteenth Amendment was repealed. Added to this prohibitionist atmosphere was a series of crusading articles against the drug by the Hearst newspapers. They popularized the word marijuana in their campaign. As a result, the use of Cannabis (except for sterilized bird seed) was banned by the Marijuana Tax Act of 1937. Although medical use was still permitted, any prescribing of the substance was actively discouraged. Pharmaceutical manufacturers removed Cannabis from a list of 28 medications that were being widely prescribed at the time (Walton, 1938).

With the advent of World War II, the fear of an interruption in the importation of hemp fiber to America generated government support for locally grown hemp fields and plants that could turn it into ropes and fibers for the war effort. In addition, the Office of Strategic Services (OSS, later the Central Intelligence Agency) started a secret program to develop a speech-inducing drug to unseal the lips of spies during interrogations. One of the drugs they came up with was a potent extract of Cannabis that was odorless, tasteless, and colorless, code-named "TD," or truth drug. Remember that this was in the early 1940s, only a few years after marijuana had been banned as "the killer weed."

Since the end of World War II, the use of marijuana has been illegal in the United States and most other countries, although the level of enforcement varies widely from country to country. Currently, however, several countries are cultivating a fibrous variant of the Cannabis plant to supply pulp and fiber to make paper, textiles, and rope. France, Italy, Yugoslavia, and to a lesser extent England and Canada now permit the growing of hemp. The Netherlands permits personal use of marijuana in so-called coffee shops mainly in Amsterdam. In spite of restrictions, marijuana is still used in some form by 160 million people worldwide.

Epidemiology

"Before I tried marijuana myself I thought that it smelled like musk because everyone in the sixties and seventies used musk perfume to hide the real marijuana smell from the cops."

—30-year-old marijuana smoker

In 1960 only 2% of people in the United States (3.4 million) had tried any illegal drug. By the late 1960s, the growth of the counterculture, fueled by the Baby Boom, greatly increased the use of marijuana and other illicit drugs. By 1979, 68 million people in the United States had tried marijuana and 23 million were using it on a monthly basis. Its popularity led 10 states to decriminalize possession of small amounts of the drug for personal use, but by the 1990s the resurgence of the concept of complete prohibition had re-criminalized the use of "pot" in most states. It also greatly increased the number of people in prison for marijuana possession and use. By 1992 the monthly rate of use had dropped to one-third of its 1979 peak level, but recently those levels have begun to climb, particularly among teenagers.

By 2005 more than 14.6 million Americans (about 6% of the U.S. population 12 and older) were using marijuana on a monthly basis, an average of 18.7 joints, whereas 3.2 million used on a daily basis (SAMHSA, 2006).

- According to the Drug Abuse Warning Network, more than 80,000 visits to emergency rooms listed marijuana as a contributing factor.
- The National Institute of Justice's Arrestee Drug Abuse Monitoring Program found that 44% of adult male arrestees and 32% of adult female arrestees tested positive for marijuana, as did 57% of juvenile male arrestees and 32% of juvenile female arrestees. (DAWN, 2004 & 2005; Arrestee Drug Abuse Monitoring Program, 2005; United Nations Office on Drugs and Crime, 2005)

"You want to use it all the time. You want to be high, you want to hang out with the kids that are high so you get the same feeling or you're at the same level as them. You just want to hang out with them, just be cool."

—18-year-old marijuana smoker

Botany

"Most of the marijuana in the late sixties was 'brown Mexican,' but we also had access to 'Colombian gold,' 'Panama red,' 'Acapulco gold,' and 'Thai sticks,' so we had plenty of high-concentration THC. We also had connections for Vietnamese pot. They didnt check the QIs duffel bags. A lot of pot nowadays just makes you incapacitated or you munch and go to sleep or have just a 20-minute mystery trip or rush, then you munch, then crash out."

—48-year-old former marijuana smoker

There is much confusion over the various terms used to describe the Cannabis plant. Terms such as vulgaris, pedemontana, lupulus, Mexicana, and sinensis have been used in the past hundred years, but there is a growing consensus about some of the terminology. Cannabis is the botanical genus of all these plants. Hemp is generally used to describe Cannabis plants that are high in fiber content. Marijuana is used to describe Cannabis plants that are high in psychoactive resins (Booth, 2004).

Species

Over the years marijuana has had many street names: "pot," "muggles," "420," "Mary Jane," "grifa," "bud," "herb," "chronic," "dank," "da kind," "grass," "leaf," "ganja," "charas," "sens," "weed," and "dope." There are also hundreds of strains that sound like geographic brand names: "African black," "Panama red," "Acapulco gold," "Maui wowie," "Humboldt green," "BC [British Columbia] bud," and "Buddha Thai." Constant experimentation by growers has resulted in variations in the plant size, concentration of psychoactive resin, and even the shape of the leaf. Some botanists say that Cannabis sativa is the only true species; others think that there are three distinct species, but all agree that there are hundreds of unique variants of the plant (Emboden, 1981). Unfortunately, intensive hybridization and cultivation has made them hard to identify. In this book we designate three species: Cannabis sativa, Cannabis indica, and Cannabis ruderalis.

The most common species is Cannabis sativa, grown in tropical, subtropical, and temperate regions throughout the world. Variations of Cannabis sativa have sufficient quantities of active resins to cause psychedelic phenomena while other variations have a high concentration of fiber and are used for hemp. The average plant will grow from 5 to 12 ft. tall but can grow up to 20 ft. There are generally five thin serrated leaves on each stem plus two smaller vestigial leaves at the ends of the leaf clusters. Some variants have even more leaves. A typical plant will produce 1 to 5 lbs. of buds and smokable leaves, both of which contain high concentrations of the psychedelic resin called THC (tetrahydrocannabinol). It can grow in a variety of conditions.

The second species, Cannabis indicasometimes called "Indian hemp," is a shorter, bushier plant with fatter leaves and is generally not used for its fibers. It is especially plentiful in India, Afghanistan, Pakistan, and the Himalayas. It didn't make it to Europe until the mid-1800s, when its geographical area of cultivation expanded. Cannabis indica is the source of most of the world's hashish. Modifications of the plant

have resulted in a stronger, smellier variety, earning it the nickname "skunk weed" (Ratch, 2005). Many illegal growers have come to prefer Cannabis indica as the base plant on which to use the sinsemilla growing technique in the mistaken belief that Cannabis indica is legal because the law as written prohibits only Cannabis sativa. Legal challenges have resulted in the interpretation that it is marijuana that's illegal regardless of the specific species.

The third species, Cannabis ruderalis (weedy hemp), a small thin plant, has a small amount of THC and is especially plentiful in Siberia and western Asia. It is most likely the species that the historian Herodotus described the ancient Scythians using thousands of years ago in the Middle East.

Sinsemilla & Other Forms of Marijuana

The sinsemilla growing technique increases the potency of the marijuana plant and is used with both Cannabis indica and Cannabis sativa. The sinsemilla technique involves separating female plants from male plants before pollination. Female plants produce much more psychoactive resin than male plants especially when they are unpollinated and therefore bear no seeds. Sinsemilla means "without seeds" in Spanish. The term commercial grade refers to marijuana that is not grown by the sinsemilla technique.

Dried marijuana buds, leaves, and flowers can be crushed and rolled into "joints." They can also be smoked in pipes. In India and some other countries, marijuana in its various forms is smoked in chillums, which are cone-shaped pipes made out of clay, stone, or wood. Marijuana can also be taken in food and drinks, or the leaves can be chewed. In India and several other countries, marijuana is divided into three different strengths, each one coming from a different part of the plant.

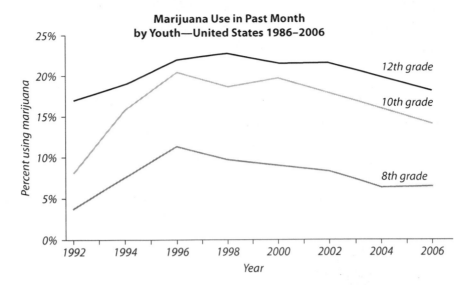

Marijuana Use in Past Month by Youth—United States 1986–2006

12th grade

10th grade

8th grade

Percent using marijuana

Year

FIGURE 1. In 1978, 37% of high school seniors used marijuana at least once a month. By 1992 that percentage had dropped to 12%; but after peaking in 1999, it was still 18.3% in 2006. Daily use for high school seniors rose from 1.9% in 1992 to 5% in 2006. This rise in monthly and daily use since 1992 is also apparent in the eighth and tenth grades (Monitoring the Future, 2006).

- Bhang is made from the stem and the leaves and has the lowest potency. In central Asia and India, it is often prepared as a drink, often with honey, sugar, molasses, and even yogurt.
- Ganja is made from the stronger leaves and the flowering tops. It is smoked alone or sometimes mixed with other herbs.
- Charas is the concentrated resin from the plant and is the most potent. It can be mixed with foods and eaten or smoked either alone or with other herbs (Ratch, 2005).

When the sticky resin is pressed into cakes, it is called "hashish"; the resin contains most of the psychoactive ingredients. This concentrated form of Cannabis is usually smoked in water pipes called "bongs" or "hookahs," or it can be added to a marijuana cigarette to enhance the potency of the weaker leaves. Bongs can also be used to smoke the less-concentrated parts of the marijuana plant. In India, Nepal, and other countries in the region, hashish use has been widespread. An early writer in the nineteenth century described five or six methods for collecting the resin and another dozen methods of preparing it for use, including pressed cakes, small pills, candies, or simply tiny balls of the dark brown resin (Bibra, 1855/1995).

Hash oil can be extracted from the plant (using solvents) and added to foods. Most often it is smeared onto rolling paper or dripped onto crushed marijuana leaves and smoked to enhance the psychoactive effects. The THC concentration of hash oil has been measured as high as 70%.

Growers

In 2006 federal agents discovered a 6-by-12-foot tunnel, 2,400 ft. long, under the U.S.-Mexico border in Tijuana. In the tunnel were 2 tons of marijuana, ready to be smuggled into the United States. Since 9/11, 20 tunnels (most of them smaller) have been found along this border. These discoveries emphasize the fact that the majority of the marijuana used in the United States comes from Mexico and Colombia. A disturbing recent change has been noted in California, where three-fourths of the marijuana seized in the state during the fall of 2002 was grown by Mexican cartels running growing operations in the richer soils of remote U.S. forests. The plantings contained anywhere from 2,000 to 10,000 plants (Meyers, 2006). The Campaign Against Marijuana Planting (CAMP) in California seized more than a million plants in 2005. A single bust in Oregon in 2006 netted 10,000 plants worth $50 million; another just north of San Francisco at Point Reyes National Seashore netted almost 23,000 plants. The federal Office of National Drug Control (ONDCP) policy estimates that growing 1 acre of marijuana damages 10 acres of land through runoff, excess fertilizer, deadly pesticides, and damage to trees and other foliage (Squatriglia, 2006). In the United States, 10% to 50% of the available marijuana is homegrown. Because of stiffer penalties and greater surveillance by law enforcement agencies, more growers have moved their operations indoors. The latest wrinkle is occurring in the suburbs, where drug traffickers buy ordinary-looking suburban homes and refit them with grow lights, plant beds, and bootlegged electricity as indoor growing operations. Thousands of plants were seized from a single four bedroom colonial home in New Hampshire (Ritter, 2007).

The indoor growing of marijuana has led to very high-potency plants grown all over the world. Some marijuana is even grown hydroponically (in water). Other major growing countries in the Western Hemisphere besides Canada, Colombia, Mexico, and the United States are Belize, Brazil, Guatemala, Jamaica, Trinidad, and Tobago. In the Far East,

Cambodia, Laos, Thailand, and the Philippines are big growers. The African and Middle Eastern countries Lebanon (greatly reduced in recent years), Morocco, Nigeria, and South Africa produce mostly Cannabis indica. In southwest and central Asia, Afghanistan and Pakistan are the big producers (DEA, 2006A).

The average street price of marijuana in the United States rose steadily from 1981 to a peak in 1991. Retail prices fell over the next decade but began to level off in the late 1990s to the present. Because the common unit of sale for marijuana is 1 oz. (called a "lid"), the average street price in the .United States ranges from $100 to $400 per "lid," although the high price has led to sales of smaller and smaller amounts. A gram (28.3 g equals 1 oz.) averages $10, while one-eighth of an ounce (about 3 to 4 g), the most common measure, goes for $50 to $60 (Marijuana Seeds, 2006; Office of National Drug Control Policy, 2006). The average marijuana joint uses 0.5 to 1 g of the substance. Prices for commercial-grade marijuana when bought in larger quantities have remained relatively stable (High Times, 2006). Prices for 1 lb. range widely:

- $50 to $100 in Mexico,
- $200 to $1,000 on the U.S.-Mexico border,
- $700 to $2,000 in the Midwest and the Northeast,
- $2,000 to $6,000 in northern California, and
- $900 to $6,000 in British Columbia.

The profits can be enormous: 500 lbs. of marijuana bought in Mexico for $50,000 can bring $400,000 in St. Louis.

Pharmacology

To date, researchers have discovered more than 420 chemicals in a single Cannabis plant.

Interestingly, some teenagers use the number 420 as their phone-beeper code to signal the availability of marijuana. At least 30 of these chemicals, called cannabinoids, have been studied for their psychoactive effects. The most potent psychoactive chemical by far is called A-9-tetrahydrocannabinol, or "THC" discovered in 1964 by two Israeli researchers. Cannabinol and cannabidiol are two other prominent cannabinoids, but they are not thought to have psychoactive properties. When smoked or ingested, these potent psychoactive chemicals are converted by the liver into more than 60 other metabolites, some of which are also psychoactive. When smoked, only about 20% of the THC in the joint is absorbed; however, the longer a lungful of smoke is held, the greater the amount of THC absorbed and the stronger the high.

The widespread use of the sin-semilla growing technique has increased the average concentration of THC from 1% to 3% in the 1960s to 4% to 15% and occasionally 25% since then (Ratch, 2005; DEA, 2006A). High-concentration THC marijuana has been around for many years—it just hasn't been so readily available. This means a user would have to smoke 3 to 5 of the weak joints from the 1960s and 1970s to equal just 1 of the stronger joints available today. Many of the early studies on marijuana—and many of the attitudes of the counterculture about the effects of the drug were based on the weaker plants. Today the greater strength of marijuana is an accepted fact by the using population. An accelerating level of research with higher percentages of THC has given some crucial insights into the psychoactive mechanisms of the drug.

Marijuana Receptors & Neurotransmitters

In 1988 and 1990, researchers detected receptor sites in the brain that were specifically reactive to THC (Hewlett, Evans & Houston, 1992). This discovery implied that the brain had its own natural neurotransmitters that fit into these receptor sites and that they affected the same areas of the brain as marijuana. These brain chemicals were called endogenous cannabinoid neurotransmitters or endocannabinoids.

Two years later researchers at the National Institute on Drug Abuse announced the discovery of anan-damide, an endocannabinoid that fits into the cannabinoid receptor sites (Devane, Hanus, Breuer, et al., 1992). A few years later, another endocannabinoid called 2-arachidonyl glycerol (2AG) was discovered. 2AG is more abundant but not as active as anandamide in the brain though it may be more active on other body receptors. There is evidence of other endocannabinoids that have yet to be discovered.

Receptors for anandamide were initially found in several areas of the limbic system, including the reward/reinforcement pathway. In succeeding years the two major receptors discovered were designated the CB_1 and CB_2 receptors. CB_2 receptors seem to be limited to the immune system and a few other sites in the lower body whereas CB' receptors are found mostly in the brain, in particular the hippocampus, amygdala, basal ganglia (including the nucleus accumbens), and cerebellum (Welch, 2005). These parts of the brain regulate the integration of sensory experiences with emotions as well as those controlling functions of learning, memory, a sense of novelty, motor coordination, and some automatic bodily functions. The presence of CB_1 anandamide receptors means that these areas of the brain are also quite affected by marijuana.

It is important to note that there are fewer anandamide receptors in the brainstem for marijuana, compared with endorphin receptors for opioids and norepinephrine receptors for cocaine, because this area of the brain controls heart rate, respiration, and other bodily functions. This is why dangerous overdoses can occur with cocaine and opioids, like respiratory depression or cardiac overstimulation, and why it is so difficult to physically overdose with marijuana (Smith, Comp-ton, Welch, et al., 1994; Huestis, Gorelick, Heish-man, et al., 2001). On the other hand, there are 10 times as many anandamides in the body as there are endorphins. They're involved in a vast range of physical and mental functions, most of which involve increasing or decreasing the sensitivity of our mind to certain sensory inputs.

Short-Term Effects

Physical Effects

The immediate physical effects of marijuana often include physical relaxation or sedation, some pain control, bloodshot eyes, coughing from lung irritation, an increase in appetite, and a small to moderate loss in muscular coordination. Other physical effects include a moderately increased heart rate, decreased blood pressure, decreased eye pressure (Marinol® capsules or marijuana joints are used as a treatment for glaucoma), increased blood flow through the mucous membranes of the eye resulting in conjunctivitis or red eye, and decreased nausea (capsules and joints are also used for cancer patients undergoing chemotherapy).

Marijuana impairs tracking ability (the ability to follow a moving object, such as a baseball) and causes a trailing phenomenon where one sees an afterimage of a moving object. Impaired tracking ability, the trailing phenomenon, and sedating effects make it more difficult to perform tasks that require depth perception and good hand/eye coordination, such as flying an airplane or catching a football.

Marijuana can act as a stimulant as well as a depressant, depending on the variety and the amount of chemical that is absorbed in the brain, the setting in which it is used, and the personality of the user.

> "Marijuana is not a downer for me, it's a speed thing. I have plenty of friends who smoke marijuana and become quiet. They can't speak. They become immobile. They're total veggies, you know, sitting around and cannot move whereas I become more active."
>
> —48-year-old marijuana smoker

Marijuana also causes a small, temporary disruption of the secretion of the male hormone testosterone. That might be important to a user with a hormonal imbalance or somebody in the throes of puberty and sexual maturation. The testosterone effect also results in a slight decrease in both sperm count and sperm motility in chronic "pot" users (Joy, Watson & Benson, 1999; Wilkins, Mellott, Markvitsa, et al., 2003; Marnell, 2005).

Marijuana increases hunger, often called "the munchies." Normally, the endocannabinoid system controls food intake through both central and peripheral mechanisms, particularly the CB_1 receptors in the hypothalamus. By flooding the receptors with THC, appetite is greatly increased. When marijuana is smoked, it doesn't seem to sharpen one's sense of taste; in fact, tests have shown that marijuana use does not change the perception of sourness, sweetness, saltiness, and bitterness nor does there appear to be an impairment of the satiation mechanisms. The enhancement of the sensory appeal of foods, especially in a friendly environment, does seem to increase, however. Once a person starts eating a food, the sense of novelty caused by marijuana (as described later in this section) makes the smoker pay attention to tastes and sensations.

"When I was I high, I got hungry and then I started eating and I couldn't stop and I'd keep going until I couldn't move. It tastes a lot better than normally. The taste seemed like it was more intense. Even stuff I hadn't really liked that much before ... it didn't make a difference. Before we smoked we made sure we had enough munchies on hand."

—18-year-old recovering marijuana user

Discovering the effects of cannabinoids on hunger has led to experiments with cannabinoid CBj antagonists (SR141716A and AM251) that block normal activity, thus leading to significant decreases in appetite (McLaughlin, Winston, Swezey, et al., 2003). SR141716A, marketed as Acomplia® (rimonabant), has been the subject of numerous clinical trials. It has been shown to reduce hunger by blocking the CB_1 receptors.

Mental Effects

Within a few minutes of smoking marijuana, the user becomes a bit confused and mentally separated from the environment. Marijuana produces a feeling of deja vu, where everything seems familiar but really isn't. Additional effects include drowsiness, an aloof feeling, and difficulty concentrating.

"It's kind of like life without a coherent thought. It's kind of like an escape. It's like when you go to sleep, you forget about things. It's like everything's dreamlike and there are no restraints on anything. You can have freedom to say what you want to say."

—16-year-old marijuana smoker

Stronger varieties of marijuana can produce giddiness, increased alertness, and major distortions of time, color, and sound. Very strong doses can even produce a sensation of movement under one's feet, visual illusions, and sometimes hallucinations.

"I have had illusions, not hallucinations, on marijuana but just where different colors stand out, things, different objects move, just little things that you never think twice about. It's just part of your high, I guess."

—11-year-old marijuana user

Two of the most frequently mentioned psychological problems with smoking marijuana are paranoia and a depersonification (detachment from one's sense of self).

"You can't be there for people when you're not inside yourself. And whenyou get loaded, you're not inside yourself. It's like you remove yourself from yourself and then you're another person."

—35-year-old marijuana user

Marijuana acts somewhat as a mild hypnotic. Charles Baudelaire, the nineteenth-century French poet, referred to it as "the mirror that magnifies." It exaggerates mood and personality and makes smokers more empathetic to others' feelings but also makes them more suggestible.

The effects of THC on the amygdala, the emotional center of the brain, are key to understanding many of the effects. The amygdala helps regulate appetite, pain, anxiety, fear, the suppression of painful memories, and, most important, the sense of novelty.

Novelty

Part of the amygdala's function is judging the emotional significance of objects and ideas that people encounter in their environment. For example, if a person encounters an unknown object, the amygdala is activated by the release of anandamides that alert his brain to beware of possible dangers or benefits, so the object is of greater interest. When a person uses marijuana, the THC artificially stimulates the amygdala, making even mundane objects interesting. Some users describe it as "virtual novelty" (drug-induced novelty). The senses themselves aren't sharpened, just the way the brain processes the information (Cermak, 2004).

> "When I smoked, I loved colors, shapes, smells, sounds, my spouse. I don't think I actually heard or saw or smelled better, I just paid more attention. Even the fifth rerun of Gilligan's Island episode #29 was interesting."
>
> —38-year-old recovering marijuana user

As the amygdala is continually bombarded with THC, the CBj receptors respond with delight. But soon, particularly with excess use, these cells react to the overstimulation by retracting into the cell membrane and becoming inactive (down regulation) (see Chapter 2). If marijuana is used chronically, these receptors are even dismantled and their numbers can be reduced by up to 70% (Breivogel, Scates, Beletskaya, et aL, 2003; Sim-Selley, 2003). This means that to a person who becomes down regulated and then stops smoking and has just a normal amount of anan-damide but way fewer receptor sites, even things that are truly novel may not have that freshness and everything becomes very boring. So to regain that sense, one has to continue to use (Cermak, 2004).

If a marijuana smoker isn't really interested in working, isn't really interested in studying, isn't really interested in a relationship, when he smokes his primitive brain takes over and says, "Forget it, let's not do this." Once CB_1 receptor sites are down regulated, it takes approximately two weeks for them to recover. But for really heavy smokers, it might take four to six weeks or longer.

Memory & Learning

The hippocampus is the part of the brain most involved in short-term memory. Normally, the hippocampus stores current input for immediate use. Eventually, the short-term information is shifted to long-term memory. The body's own anandamide determines how much of the hippocampus is available, depending on the complexity of the activity. For a straightforward sport like baseball, the hippocampus input is limited so only a small portion of it is made available. Cramming for an exam requires greater capacity, so more of the hippocampus is made available. When an external cannabinoid like THC is taken into the body, it severely limits the avail-able amount of hippocampal short-term memory.

> If you go home and have homework to do that night and you say 'Okay, I'm going to get stoned before I do my homework, you're never going to get your homework done."
>
> —High school student

Similar problems can occur on the job when there are a lot of details that have to be manipulated.

> "I d be doing the job and all of a sudden I'd look up and freeze and not know what to do. I would have a handful of

checks in my hand and just look at the machine for a while and think to myself, 'What is this? What do I do with it?' So I just stand there and think to myself, 'Okay; it's going to come. It's going to come.' And eventually it would."

—36-year-old male recovering marijuana smoker

As use is discontinued, the short-term memory is almost restored, but if previous experiences and facts were never processed through short-term memory, they will never be remembered. The more regular the use, the larger the chunks of one's life that are forgotten.

"I don't remember the years that I did smoke. I remember the most important things, but the little details I couldn't tell you. I don't remember what I ate a little bit ago."

—20-year old male marijuana smoker

Although marijuana slows learning and disrupts concentration by its influence on short-term memory, it has a much smaller effect on long-term memory. This explains why some students have been able to maintain good grades while using marijuana on a regular basis while others end up flunking out. A recent study of 150 heavy marijuana users in treatment found that not only memory but also attention span and cognitive functioning were impaired and, as expected, the heavier the use, the greater the impairment (Solowij, Stephens, Roffman, et al., 2002). Overall in one study, those who averaged a D in school were four times more likely to have used marijuana than those who got A's (SAMHSA, 2005).

"School was boring to a point before I started weed, but once I started smoking it more and more, it just got even more boring. I didn't want to go, I didn't want to interact at school. I went there and skipped a lot of classes. Actually I skipped more than half the year."

—18-year-old recovering marijuana abuser

With marijuana many thoughts and feelings are internalized. Long-term marijuana smokers feel that they're learning, thinking, feeling, and communicating better.

"When I got high I thought I was the smartest person in the world. I knew I had the answer to everything, and one day I sat down with the tape recorder and I started rattling off all this brilliance that I had; the next day when I woke up in the morning and I played it back, it was almost like I wasn't even speaking English."

—38-year-old recovering compulsive marijuana smoker

Marijuana affects the juvenile brain more severely than an adult brain. This is because in a juvenile's frontal lobes, around the age of 12, there is an explosion in the number of connections and synapses among the nerve cells. Over the succeeding 10 to 12 years, there is a gradual pruning process as these connections are strengthened or weakened. So when a person is experiencing a new idea or sensory input, the connections will be strengthened. Unused connections will be weakened and then break. Cannabinoid receptors are more dense here than in any other part of the cortex, so excess marijuana use can cause somewhat distorted thinking. For example, the ability to hone in on things that are important and ignore things that are not is reduced over time. This deficit can impair a person's ability to judge that which is dangerous and which situation has to be handled first.

The use of ecstasy and marijuana in combination is relatively popular among young people. Research has found that this combination has a synergistic negative effect on memory (Young, McGregor & Mallet, 2005).

Time

The distortion of a sense of time (temporal disintegration) is responsible for several of the perceived effects of marijuana. Dull repetitive jobs seem to go by faster. In Jamaica some cane field workers smoke "ganja" to make their hard, monotonous work pass by more quickly. On the other hand, students who smoke marijuana while studying (a more complex activity) get easily bored and often abandon their books.

The effects of distortion of the passage of time, impaired judgment, and short-term memory loss result in a user's inability to perform multiple and interactive tasks, like installing a computer program, while under the influence (Stafford, 1992; Joy, Watson & Benson, 1999; Wilkins, Mellott, Markvitsa, et al., 2003; Marnell, 2005). A study of current and former marijuana users tested the smokers at 1, 7, and 28 days after stopping various levels of use. Significant impairment was found at days 1 and 7 for heavy users, but by day 28 the difference in impairment had mostly disappeared (Pope, Gruber, Hudson, et al., 2001).

Long-Term Effects

Respiratory Problems

Although the main psychoactive substances are different (THC vs. nicotine), the smoke of both marijuana and nicotine contains a mixture of toxic gases and particulate matter. As smoking becomes chronic, so does irritation to the breathing passages. Because marijuana is grown under a wide variety of conditions and is unrefined, the joints made from the buds and/or leaves are harsh, unfiltered, irregular in quality, and composed of many different chemicals. Therefore, when it is inhaled and held in the lungs, smoking four to five joints gives the same exposure to the lungs and mucous membranes as smoking a full pack of cigarettes, according to studies by Dr. Donald Tashkin at UCLA (Tashkin, Simmons & Clark, 1988; Joy, Watson & Benson, 1999; Tashkin, 2005). For these and other reasons, a major concern of health professionals is the damaging effect that marijuana smoking has on the respiratory system. Marijuana smoking on a regular basis leads to symptoms of increased coughing with acute and chronic bronchitis. In microscopic studies of these mucous membranes, Dr. Tashkin has found that most damage occurs in the lungs of those who smoke both cigarettes and marijuana. This is significant because approximately 75% of marijuana smokers also smoke cigarettes (Richter, Kaur, Rezni-cow, et al, 2005).

In the series of slides (Figure 6-2), the normal ciliated surface epithelial cells in the mucous membranes of a nonsmoker of either cigarettes or marijuana (6-2a) show healthy, densely packed cilia that clear the breathing passages of mucous, dust, and debris. The breathing passage of a chronic marijuana smoker (6-2b) shows increased numbers of mucous-secreting surface epithelial cells that do not have cilia, so phlegm production is increased but is not cleared as readily from the breathing passages.

Finally, the breathing passage of a chronic smoker of both marijuana and cigarettes (6-2c) shows that the normal surface cells have been completely replaced by nonciliated cells resembling skin, so the smoker has to cough to clear any mucous from the lungs because the ciliated cells are gone.

> "I'm sure I've done some damage to my lungs. I mean, you can't put that kind of tar down in your system, heated tar going into your system constantly for 23 years, and sit here and say there's nothing wrong and nothing has happened. Surely something has happened."
>
> —48-year-old marijuana smoker

Although marijuana smoking damages lung tissue, whether it causes cancer is unclear. Some of the changes involving the cell nucleus suggested to researchers that malignancy may be a consequence of regular marijuana smoking because the changes observed are precursors of cancer. In 2006, however, Dr. Tashkin and other researchers at UCLA released a study funded by the National Institute on Drug Abuse of 1,200 people with lung, neck, or head cancer and another 1,000 controls and found no link between marijuana smoking and lung cancer, even, among heavy marijuana smokers. Cigarette smokers were found to have a 20-fold increased risk for cancer if they smoked two packs or more per day. As an explanation for this lowered cancer risk in marijuana smokers, some researchers postulate

that the THC in marijuana might kill aging cells that could become cancerous (Tashkin, 2006).

Immune System

Epidemiologic studies have identified marijuana as a cofactor in the progression of HIV infection. Animal studies at UCLA found that the administration of marijuana increased the replication of the immunodeficiency virus and measurably suppressed immune function (Roth, Tashkin, Whittaker, et al., 2005). Another animal study found that THC can lead to enhanced growth of tumors due to suppression of the anti-tumor immune response, including breast cancer (McKallip, Nagarkatti & Nagarkatti, 2005).

Some evidence suggests that heavy marijuana use can also make users more susceptible to a cold, the flu, and other viral infections. If such were the case, it could be somewhat counterproductive for people who are already immune depressed to smoke marijuana for therapeutic purposes. In addition, the user is further exposing the lungs to pathogens, such as fungi and bacteria, found in marijuana smoke. The total health impact of marijuana on the immune system remains unclear.

Acute Mental Effects.

There is still much debate about whether marijuana will cause a psychosis or serious mental illness rather than just increasing paranoia, acute anxiety, or depression. One reason is because it is hard to separate other factors, especially pre-existing mental problems, from the precipitating influence of marijuana. Often the use of marijuana (particularly that with high levels of THC) will tip the mental balance of someone just holding on. In a number of studies of patients in treatment, thorough investigation found the vast preponderance of psychoses and mental problems to be pre-existing (Os, Bak, Hanssen, et al., 2002; Grinspoon, Bakalar & Russo, 2005).

Some users believe that they have lost control of their mental state. Besides paranoia there is often a belief that they have severely damaged themselves or that their underlying insecurities are insurmountable. These acute problems are usually treatable, but it is problematic when the symptoms persist. Recovery counselors have seen a number of cases of people who, after experiencing a bad trip, don't come all the way back and may have problems going on with their lives. They experience continued confusion, difficulty concentrating, and memory problems and feel as though their mind is in a fog ...

> "I once worked with a 13-year-old client who had no premorbid symptoms that could be identified prior to his thirteenth birthday, when his friends turned him on to a honey blunt, which is a cigar packed with marijuana soaked in honey and dried. It happened to be very strong sinsemilla, and he experienced an acute anxiety reaction followed by a hallucinogen persisting perceptual disorder, including a profound depression and an inability to concentrate. We don't know how long these problems will last."
>
> —Counselor, Genesis Recovery Center

Even veteran smokers who've been smoking some low-grade "pot" and then get some strong "BC bud" sinsemilla may feel that somebody has slipped them a psychedelic like PCP or LSD. They experience anxiety and paranoia that then creates even more anxiety.

There is also an increase in the practice of mixing marijuana with other drugs like cocaine,

amphetamine, and PCP that can cause exaggerated reactions. Some users even smoke joints that have been soaked in formaldehyde and embalming fluid ("clickems" or "fry") for a bigger kick. "Clickems" give a PCP-like effect when smoked.

Tolerance, Withdrawal & Addiction

Tolerance

Tolerance to marijuana occurs fairly rapidly, even though initially smokers become more sensitive, not less, to desired effects (inverse tolerance). Although high-dose chronic users can recognize the effects of low levels of THC in their systems, they are able to tolerate much higher levels without some of the more severe emotional and psychic effects experienced by first-time users. Current research suggests that pharmacodynamic tolerance (reduction of nerve ceil sensitivity to marijuana) is the mechanism rather than reduced bioavailability (speeding up the breakdown of the drug known as drug dispositional tolerance).

> "Originally, when we first got it, we could smoke, say two bong loads and be just totally stoned whereas now we have to keep continuously smoking just to keep the high going, even with the higher-potency stuff."
>
> —24-year-old recovering marijuana user

One great concern is that marijuana persists in the body of a chronic user for up to three months, though the major effects last only four to six hours after smoking. These residual amounts in the body can disrupt some physiological, mental, and emotional functions.

Withdrawal

Because there is not the rapid onset of withdrawal from marijuana as with alcohol or heroin, many people deny that withdrawal occurs. The withdrawal from marijuana is more drawn out because much of the THC has been retained in the brain and only after a relatively long period of abstinence will the withdrawal effects appear.

> "Sometimes people who've been smoking for five years decide to quit They stop 1, 2, 3 days, even a week, and they (especially those who think marijuana is benign), say, 'Wow, I feel great marijuana's no problem. I have no withdrawal. It's nothing at all.' Then they start up again. They never experience withdrawal. We see that withdrawal symptoms to marijuana are delayed sometimes for several weeks to a month after a person stops."

—Counselor, Genesis Recovery Center

The discovery by French scientists in 1994 of an antagonist that instantly blocks the effects of marijuana enabled researchers to search for true signs of tolerance, tissue dependence, and withdrawal symptoms in long-term users. Experiments demonstrated that cessation of marijuana use could cause true physical withdrawal symptoms. Dr. Billy Martin of the Medical College of Virginia gave the THC antagonist SR14176A to rats that had been exposed to marijuana four days in a row. The antagonist negated the influence of the marijuana. Within 10 minutes the rats exhibited immediate physical withdrawal behaviors that included "wet dog shakes" and facial rubbing, which is the rat equivalent of withdrawal. These experiments indicated that marijuana dependence occurs more rapidly than previously suspected (Rinaldi-Carmona, Barth,

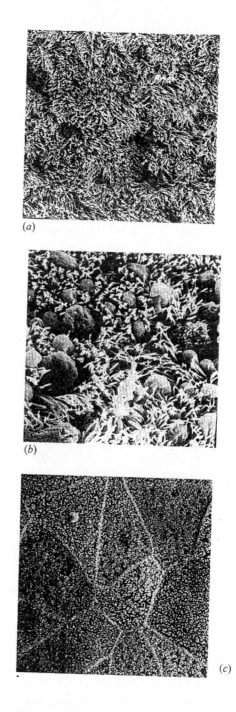

FIGURE 2. (a) Healthy mucous membrane of non-smoker. (b) Mucous membrane of a marijuana smoker. (c) Mucous membrane of a marijuana and cigarette smoker.

Courtesy of Dr. Donald Tashkin, Pulmonary Research Department, UCLA Medical Center, Los Angeles, CA

Heau-line, et al,, 1994; Tsou, Patrick & Walker, 1995; Aceto, Scates & Martin, 2001).

Withdrawal effects of marijuana include:

- anger, irritability, anxiety, and/or aggression;
- aches, pains, chills;
- depression;
- inability to concentrate;
- slight tremors;
- sleep disturbances;
- decreased appetite and stomach pain;
- sweating; and
- craving.

Not everyone will experience all of these effects, but everyone will experience some of them, especially craving. Recent human research demonstrated that irritability, anxiety, aggression, and even stomach pain caused by marijuana withdrawal occurred within three to seven days of abstinence (Haney, Ward, Comer, et al., 1999; Kouri, Pope & Lukas, 1999; Budney, Hughes, Moore, et al., 2001; Zickler, 2002).

> "I would break into a sweat in the shower. I could not maintain my concentration for the first month or two. To really treasure my sobriety, it took me about three or four months before I really came out of the fog and really started getting a grasp of what was going on around me."
>
> —38-year-old recovering marijuana addict

Addiction

Just as the refinement of coca leaves into cocaine and opium into heroin led to greater abuse of those drugs, so have better sinsemilla cultivation techniques leading to higher THC concentrations increased the compulsive liability of marijuana use.

Unlike opiates, sedative-hypnotics, alcohol, and some stimulants, psychological addiction is more of a factor than physical addiction.

> "I thought I could control it because when I woke up in the morning, I didn't get high for the first hour and a half. I figured an hour and a half that proves that I'm not hooked on this stuff because I don't really need it."
>
> —Recovering user in Marijuana Anonymous, a 12-step program

The research of the 1990s and 2000s has provided a different view of the addiction potential of this substance. Today many people smoke the drug in a chronic, compulsive way and have difficulty discontinuing their use. Like cocaine, heroin, alcohol, nicotine, and other addictive drugs, marijuana does have the ability to induce compulsive use in spite of the negative consequences it may be causing in the user's life.

> "Today's potent form of marijuana is causing a lot more problems than we saw in the 1960s. I never treated a single marijuana self-admitted addict in the clinic throughout the sixties nor the seventies and pretty much through the eighties. But by the late eighties, we started seeing people coming in. Every one of them came in on their own volition, saying, 'Help me. I want to stop smoking pot. It is causing me these problems, causing me to have memory problems, causing me to be too spaced out. I have withdrawal symptoms. I want to stop and I can't.' At our program in San Francisco, we have about 100

patients who are in treatment at any-given time specifically for marijuana addiction."

—Darryl Inaba, Pharm.D., former CEO and president, Haight Ashbury Free Clinic Foundation

Although the dependence liability of marijuana is supposedly lower than with other drugs, the bottom line, as with any addiction, is the consequences.

"What are the consequences? Is something costing you more money than you should be spending? Is it jeopardizing your job? Is it jeopardizing your relationship with your spouse or your lover or your children? Are you alienated because of that? Those are the consequences."

—36-year-old recovering marijuana abuser

"Why am I doing this? What's wrong with me? Why do I have to keep doing this? And I did this for a good eight to 10 years. I started buying dime bags, figuring it would cost a lot more and then eventually I'd get the point. It didn't work. I just kept on buying."

—38-year-old recovering marijuana abuser

Is Marijuana a Gateway Drug?

In antidrug movies from the 1930s like Reefer Madness and Marijuana, Assassin of Youth, the claim was that marijuana physically and mentally changed users, so they started using heroin and

cocaine and became helpless addicts. The exaggeration of this idea undermined drug education because people who smoked marijuana didn't become raving lunatics or depraved dope fiends. The experimenters who had tried marijuana said, "I tried marijuana and that didn't happen, so I guess they're lying about all the drugs."

This exaggeration and resultant ridicule of propagandistic or scare films and books probably caused more drug abuse than it prevented. It also obscured an important idea: the real role that marijuana use plays in future drug use and abuse.

"I've been in a 12-step program [Narcotics Anonymous] for a little over six years, and I'm not going to say, like, one and one equal two, but just about everybody I meet in the 12-step program started out with either marijuana or alcohol."

—Recovering marijuana addict

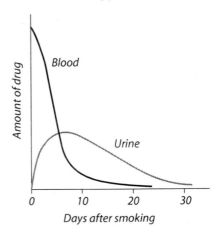

Marijuana Blood Level vs. Urine Level (approximations)

FIGURE 3. This chart shows the blood and urine levels of marijuana over time. The marijuana persists in the urine longer. The majority of drug testing measures only marijuana in the urine.

Marijuana is a gateway drug in the sense that if people smoke it, they will probably hang around others who smoke it or use other drugs, so the opportunities to experiment with other drugs are greater. Viewed from this perspective, it is not surprising that most users of other illicit drugs have used marijuana first but only after they began using alcohol and/or nicotine (Kandel, Yamaguchi & Chen, 1992; Kandel & Yamaguchi, 1993; Joy, Watson & Benson, 1999).

No two people will have the exact same reaction to marijuana, but what has been observed is that those who continue to use it regularly establish a pattern of use and begin to find opportunities where drugs other than marijuana are available. There is also growing evidence that the use of any addictive drug at an early age changes vulnerable young brain functions that makes a person more likely to develop addiction.

> "The majority of people that I know, that I hang around with, if they ain't smoking weed, they're smoking crack or drinking. I'm not saying that they are bad people, but that's just how it is."
>
> —30-year-old poly drug user who started smoking marijuana at the age of 13

A study of 311 young adults in Australia who were identical or fraternal twins found that those who smoked Cannabis by age 17 had a 2.1 to 5.2 times higher chance of other drug use, alcohol dependence, and drug abuse/dependence than those who didn't smoke it. There was no significant difference in drug/alcohol use or dependence between fraternal or identical twins, emphasizing the direct effect of marijuana and of environmental influences (Lynskey, Heath, Bucholz, et al., 2003). A Dutch study of twins found that early Cannabis use in one twin increased that individual's later illicit drug use but did not increase future drug use in the twin who did not use marijuana while young (Lynskey, Vink & Boomsma, 2006).

Marijuana (Cannabis) & The Law

Marijuana has never been out of favor over the past 40 years in the United States and is still popular at the start of the twenty-first century. Internationally, marijuana is the most widely used illicit drug in countries such as Australia, Canada, Costa Rica, El Salvador, Mexico, Panama, and South Africa (DEA, 2006B). Penalties vary widely from country to country.

In the United States, the penalties for marijuana use or possession vary from federal laws to state laws and from state to state. Federal laws focus more on heavy trafficking, although there are penalties for simple possession and personal use. For example, sale of 200 to 2,000 pounds will result in federal penalties of 5 to 40 years and up to a $2 million fine. State penalties are for possession or sale. Possession of up to 1 lb. will bring sentences of 180 days to 2 years in Texas and up to 4 years in New York (National Organization for the Reform of Marijuana Laws, 2006). In 2004, 44.2% of the 1,745,712 arrests for drug abuse violations were for marijuana, more than 90% for possession alone (Drug War Facts, 2006). Marijuana arrests went from 401,982 in 1980 to 771,605 in 2004.

- Austria, Belgium, Germany, Greece, Ireland, Italy, and Spain don't prosecute for possession of small amounts for personal use.
- In England Cannabis is designated as a "class B" drug by the Misuse of Drugs Act of 1971. Possession could lead to a five-year prison term, though most sentences handed down are minimal.

- In the Netherlands use is kept within the so-called coffee shop system, and sales outside of this system are illegal.
- In Japan people can go to jail for possessing less than 1 g of marijuana. Smugglers with a few hundred grams, up to a few kilograms, are routinely sent to prison for three to four years. Foreigners caught with marijuana are deported after serving their sentence, often with up to a lifetime ban (e.g., Paul McCartney).
- Countries with a death penalty for drug dealing (usually hard drugs) and in some cases possession are Algeria, Indonesia, Iran, Malaysia, Singapore, Thailand, and Turkey.
- In India you can get up to 10 years for smoking Cannabis.
- In Venezuela drug carriers face minimum 10-year prison sentences. (TheSite.org, 2006)

Worldwide the push for the medical use of marijuana has caused a reassessment of many of the legal penalties for use and even sale (e.g., medical marijuana clubs). In the United States, approval by a number of states of the medical use of marijuana has come in conflict with the 2005 Supreme Court ruling that allowed federal law to supercede state-enacted marijuana laws. (There is more on medical marijuana later in this chapter.)

Marijuana, Driving & Drug Testing

In more and more arrests for reckless driving or in investigations at the scene of an accident, the driver is tested for marijuana and other drugs. There are four problems associated with marijuana testing:

- the drug persists for a number of days in the body and can sometimes still be detected weeks after use;

- the elimination rate varies radically compared with alcohol, which has a defined rate of metabolism;
- there is a scarcity of good data about the level of marijuana in the blood vs. the level of impairment;
- and, most important, usually there is another drug besides marijuana in the system, especially alcohol.

So even if marijuana has a relatively small effect, it is magnified by polydrug use and abuse. Added to the fact that 65% of heavy drinkers also use marijuana, it's no wonder that positive polydrug test results are the rule and not the exception in drivers arrested for driving while under the influence (Gieringer, 1988; SAMHSA, 2005).

When it comes to driving a car, tests showed lower levels of impairment after smoking a small amount of marijuana compared with drinking a small amount of alcohol. As the dosages increased, impairment for the marijuana smokers increased but not as fast as it did for drinkers. Interestingly, the smokers thought they did worse than they actually did while the drinkers thought they did better. Drinking boosts overconfidence whereas marijuana makes the drivers overly wary and even paranoid (Mathias, 1996).

"At first I wouldn't drive when I was stoned, but after it became more of a habit and it didn't do as much to me. I was more conscientious of my driving. I would drive the speed limit. I didn't want to get pulled over."

—11-year-old male marijuana user

One study found that 60% of marijuana smokers failed a field sobriety test 2.5 hours after smoking moderate amounts; other tests have shown some impairment 3 to 7 hours after smoking. Some tests even showed minimal impairment up to 8 hours later (Reeve, Robertson, Grant, et al., 1983; Hollister, 1986; Smiley, 1986).

The problem is that repetitive tasks such as normal, uneventful driving are not huge problems when smoking marijuana, but if a complicated driving situation arises that requires decision-making and swift reaction time, the chances of error when marijuana is in the system are significantly increased. In a number of U.S. studies, 4% to 14% of drivers who were injured or killed in accidents tested positive for marijuana or marijuana and another drug (Ramaekers, Berghaus, van Laar, et al., 2004). On the other hand, though 2.5% of fatal crashes in a French study involved marijuana, 11 times that amount (28.6%) involved alcohol. As a side note, a further survey of 6,766 French drivers considered at fault in accidents found that 681 were positive for marijuana (Laumon, Gadegbeku, Martin, et al., 2005).

Testing machines can measure minute amounts of the THC metabolite but are generally calibrated to start registering at 50 nanograms per milliliter (ng/mL) in urine samples. The 50 ng level doesn't necessarily measure impairment but only the fact that marijuana was used. Generally, for long-term smokers it would take about 3 weeks before they wouldn't register on a test with a 50 ng/mL cutoff and another 3 weeks to be completely negative. In a few instances, it has taken 10 weeks for the drug to clear completely. Someone who smoked a joint at a party but is not a longtime user usually tests negative 24 to 48 hours after use. The Olympic Committee uses just 15 ng as its cutoff level.

Medical Use of Marijuana

After the Ninth U.S. Circuit Court of Appeals in San Francisco ruled that Congress did not have the constitutional authority to regulate the non-commercial cultivation and use of marijuana that does not cross state lines, the U.S. Supreme Court, in a 6-to-3 decision, ruled that the federal government had the right to supercede state laws that permitted the medical use of marijuana and that Congress had acted within its mandate to control interstate trade (Egelko, 2005). This was but the latest skirmish in the battle to legalize marijuana at the very least for medical purposes and at the most for unrestricted use.

Over the past 150 years or so, the medical profession has attempted to clinically and scientifically examine the use of Cannabis and its extracts for medicinal purposes. Because there were a limited number of all-purpose medications available over the millennia (e.g., opium, theriac, willow bark), substances that had real therapeutic effects were prized. Dr. William O'Shaughnesy spurred curiosity about the drug in Europe in the 1830s. In 1860 in a report to the Ohio State Medical Society, Cannabis researcher and physician Dr. R. R. McMeens said he was convinced of its immense value because of the immediate action of the drug in appeasing the appetite for chloral hydrate or opium and restoring the ability to appreciate food. He also recommended it as a treatment for disordered bowels, as a diuretic, and as a sleeping tonic (McMeens, 1860).

As in the present day, there were also warnings about the drug's dangers. For example, in 1890, in writing about his 30 years of experience using Cannabis medicinally, Dr. J. Russel Reynolds said that the problems included a wide variation in the strength of any Cannabis indica preparation, that people vary widely in their reaction to the same dose, and that if high concentrations are taken, severe reactions are quite possible (Reynolds, 1890). By 1900 a number of prominent drug companies marketed Cannabis extracts and patent medicines as cures for a variety of illnesses.

Historically marijuana has been used:

- as a muscle relaxant;
- as a painkiller (analgesic);
- as an appetite stimulant;
- to control spasms and convulsions;
- to calm anxiety;
- to treat asthma;
- to treat jaundice, beriberi, and ague;
- to stimulate childbirth;
- to relieve coughs (anti-tussive);
- to treat withdrawal from opiates and alcohol; and
- as an antibiotic.

Passage of the Marijuana Tax Act of 1937 discouraged research for many years until the 1980s. By 1996 a number of states had passed laws permitting medicinal use of the drug. The resumption of research has explored and in some cases recommended Cannabis for some types of glaucoma, nausea and pain control, to subdue uncontrolled movements (e.g., multiple sclerosis), and to stimulate weight gain for wasting illnesses such as cancer and AIDS (Mikuriya, 1973; Aldrich, 1997; Gurley, Aranow & Katz, 1998; Earlywirie, 2002; Booth, 2004; Grinspoon, Bakalar & Russo, 2005; Ratsch, 2005; Pertwee, 2006). A recent study of AIDS patients at San Francisco General Hospital found substantial pain relief from smoking marijuana. The most pain relief occurred on the first day of use (Russel, 2007).

There is evidence that marijuana does reduce intraocular pressure in glaucoma patients, does calm nausea, does reduce some pain, and does encourage people to eat, though there are other drugs that are also effective or in some cases better. The fact that there are other medications as or more effective than those under examination, however, has never been a bar to the development and prescribing of less effective ones (e.g., pain killers, sedative-hypnotics, and antidepressants). The medicinal use of psychoactive substances that have therapeutic value has always created conflict between those who minimize or simply accept the dependency and collateral health liabilities and those who don't. The over-and under-prescription of opiates is a prime example of this kind of conflict.

A recent report by the U.S. General Accounting Office found that in Alaska, Hawaii, and Oregon and where prescribing Cannabis is legal, the average medical marijuana user is male (70%) and in his 40s (70%) (Medical Marijuana, 2002). In the states where it is legal to prescribe, there are marijuana buyers' clubs and growers who supply marijuana for those who have a medical marijuana card, prescription, or license. There has been abuse of the system in several states due to over-prescription of the medical marijuana cards, sometimes to people who just don't want to be hassled by law-enforcement for their recreational use of the drug. A somewhat similar problem has existed for years with opiates, sedative-hypnotics, and even ADHD stimulant medications such as Ritalin® in the United States and abroad. Some states allow growing by authorized users of medical marijuana or by their registered suppliers. In almost all states, however, growing by unauthorized users is illegal even if they are supplying their drug to medical marijuana buyers' clubs (Egelko, 2002).

Synthetic THC called dronabinol (Marinol®) is theoretically available for treatment of these health problems but in practice is rarely prescribed. People say they prefer marijuana in its smokable form because it works faster than Marinol.® If they smoke, they can smoke as much or as little as they need to relieve symptoms, whereas if they take a premeasured Marinol® capsule, it may be too much or not enough for their condition. In 2006 a second synthetic marijuana drug was reintroduced into the United States—Cesamet®— which has been used in Canada since 1981. Cesamet® or Marinol® can cost $30 per day. In 2004 a third product— Sativex®—was developed and conditionally approved to be used in spray form in an inhaler. Sativex® was approved in 2005 in Canada to treat multiple sclerosis. It is being directed at many of the 110,000 multiple sclerosis sufferers in the United Kingdom. Worldwide an estimated 2.5 million people have MS; 400,000 in the United . States (Willing, 2004).

A major obstacle with smoking or ingesting marijuana for medical purposes is the great variation in the amount of active ingredients in any given marijuana plant. Variations in A-9-THC potency, the relative concentration of other active cannabinoids, and the inconsistency of botanical factors make it difficult to rely on this substance to treat medical problems. For example, some forms of marijuana have been shown to increase intraocular pressure, making someone's glaucoma worse, although normally most forms of marijuana will lower intraocular pressure.

Beyond the physiological effects, there are the mental effects of marijuana. Like opium cure-alls, such as theriac and laudanum, and even prescription opiates or sedative-hypnotics, it is often the mental effects of calming, anxiety relief, or mild euphoria that make people feel good and think they are getting better even if the drug isn't helping the illness as much as it's supposed to.

There is, however, reluctance in the medical community to prescribe or even approve of marijuana for medical use for several reasons, including those already stated.

- Marijuana smoke contains a number of irritants, carcinogens, pathogens, fungi, insecticides, and other chemicals, most of which have not been studied. If marijuana is baked in brownies or otherwise eaten, the respiratory problems are avoided but the 420 or more compounds contained in marijuana remain, along with all their side effects.

- Marijuana is a psychoactive drug with dependency potential, which is particularly problematic for those who are recovering from abuse or addiction. It can cause its own dependency or relapse to other dependencies.

Medical research about marijuana continues in many countries. Since the 1970s more than 14,000 scientific studies have been conducted, yet results remain conflicting, making it difficult to substantiate appropriate medical use of marijuana.

1999 Report From The Institute Of Medicine To The ONDCP

In 1996 the federal Office of National Drug Control Policy commissioned a study by the Institute of Medicine of the National Academy of Sciences to review the scientific evidence and do field research concerning the health benefits and risks of marijuana. When the ensuing report, entitled Marijuana and Medicine: Assessing the Science Base, was released in 1999, both sides of the argument (pro-and anti-marijuana forces) went in front of the media and translated the report, colored by what they thought it said. The result was that unless one read the original report, it was extremely difficult to know what was actually written.

Some Conclusions of the Report

- Cannabinoids likely have a natural role in pain modulation, control of movement, and memory.
- Scientific data indicate the potential therapeutic value of cannabi-noid drugs, primarily THC, for pain relief, for control of nausea and vomiting, and as an appetite

stimulation; smoked marijuana, however, is a crude THC delivery system that also delivers harmful substances.

- The psychological effects of cannabinoids, such as anxiety reduction, sedation, and euphoria, can influence the potential therapeutic value.
- Numerous studies suggest that marijuana smoke is an important risk factor in the development of respiratory disease.

Some Recommendations of the Report

- Research should continue into the physiological effects of synthetic and plant-derived cannabinoids and the natural function of cannabinoids in the body.
- Clinical trials of cannabinoid drugs for symptom management should be conducted with the goal of developing safe, reliable, and rapid-onset delivery systems.

- Psychological effects of cannabinoids such as anxiety reduction and sedation, which can influence medical benefits, should be evaluated in clinical trials.

(Joy, Watson & Benson, 1999; the full report is available online at http://newton.nap.edu/catalog/6376.html)

In April 2006 the Food and Drug Administration declared that "no sound scientific studies" support the medical use of smoked marijuana. The statement seems to ignore two of the main conclusions of the report, which emphasize the importance of finding a less damaging delivery system but does accept studies about the efficacy of marijuana for pain, nausea, and wasting diseases. As with so many pronouncements about marijuana, political considerations are in a constant battle with scientific information as well as with those who would simply like marijuana to be legalized (Harris, 2006).

Hallucinogens (Psychedelics)

By Glen Hanson, Peter J. Venturelli, and Annette E. Fleckenstein

Introduction

A person on LSD who becomes depressed, agitated, or confused may experience these feelings in an overwhelming manner that grows on itself. The best solution is to remove disturbing influences, get to a safe, comforting environment, and reassure the "tripper" that things are alright. It may comfort those who fear that they are losing their minds to be reminded that it will end in several hours. (from Erowid 2007)

This quote from an experienced user illustrates the sensory and emotional distortions that can be caused by using hallucinogens or psychedelics. The word psychedelic comes from the Greek root meaning "mind-revealing" (Harvard Mental Health Letter 2006). In this chapter, we begin with a brief historical review of the use of hallucinogens, tracing the trend in the United States from the 1960s to today. Next, the nature of hallucinogens and the effects they produce are examined.

The rest of the chapter addresses the various types of psychedelic agents — LSD types, phenylethylamines (including Ecstasy), anticholinergics, and other miscellaneous substances.

The History of Hallucinogen Use

People have known and written about drug-related hallucinations for centuries. Throughout the ages, individuals who saw visions or experienced hallucinations were perceived as being holy or sacred, as receiving divine messages, or possibly as being bewitched and controlled by the devil. There are many indications that medicine men, shamans, witches, oracles, and perhaps mystics and priests of various groups were familiar with drugs and herbs that caused such experiences and today are known as hallucinogens (National Institute on Drug Abuse [NIDA] 2001).

Before the 1960s, several psychedelic substances, such as mescaline from the peyote cactus, could be obtained from chemical supply houses with no restriction in the United States.

Abuse of hallucinogens did not become a major social problem in this country until this decade of racial struggles, the Vietnam War, and violent demonstrations. Many individuals frustrated with the hypocrisy of "the establishment" tried to "turn on and tune in" by using hallucinogens as pharmacological crutches.

Psychedelic drugs became especially popular when some medical professionals such as then-Harvard psychology professor, Timothy Leary, reported that these drugs allowed users to get in touch with themselves and achieve a peaceful inner serenity (Associated Press 1999). At the same time, it became well publicized that the natural psychedelics (such as mescaline and peyote) were and had been for many years used routinely by some religious organizations of Native Americans for enhancing spiritual experiences. This factor contributed to the mystical, supernatural aura associated with hallucinogenic agents and added to their enticement for the so-called dropout generation.

With widespread use of LSD, it was observed that this and similar drugs may induce a form of psychosis-like schizophrenia (American Psychiatric Association [APA] 2000). The term psychotomimetic was coined to describe these compounds; this term means "psychosis mimicking" and is still used in medicine today. The basis for the designation is the effects of these drugs that induce mental states that impair an individual's ability to recognize and respond appropriately to reality.

By the mid-1960s, federal regulatory agencies had become concerned with the misuse of hallucinogens and the potential emotional damage caused by these drugs. Access to hallucinogenic agents was restricted, and laws against their distribution were passed. Despite the problems associated with these psychedelics, some groups demanded that responsible use was possible and that they be allowed legal access to these substances.

The Native American Church

The hallucinogen peyote plays a central role in the ceremonies of Native Americans who follow a religion that is a combination of Christian doctrine and Native American religious rituals. Members of this church are found as far north as Canada. They believe that God made a special gift of this sacramental plant to them so that they might commune more directly with Him. The first organized peyote church was the First-Born Church of Christ, incorporated in 1914 in Oklahoma. The Native American Church of the United States was chartered in 1918 and is the largest such group at present (approximately 100,000-200,000 members).

Because of the religious beliefs of the members of the Native American Church concerning the powers of peyote, when Congress legislated against its use in 1965, it allowed room for religious use of this psychedelic plant. The American Indian Religious Freedom Act of 1978 was an attempt by Congress to allow the members of the Native American

---

Key Terms

hallucinogens
   substances that alter sensory processing in the brain, causing perceptual disturbances, changes in thought processing, and depersonalization

psychedelics
   substances that expand or heighten perception and consciousness

psychotomimetic
   substances that cause psychosis-like symptoms

Church access to peyote due to constitutional guarantees of religious freedom. Due to controversy inspired by the original piece of legislation, an amendment to the 1978 act was signed in 1994, which specifically protected the use of peyote in Native American Church ceremonies. This amendment also prohibits use of peyote for nonreligious purposes (Native American Church 2007). However, despite these efforts by Congress to resolve this issue, controversies continue to arise (see "Case in Point," Peyote and the Rights of Native Americans: How Far Should It Go?).

Timothy Leary and the League of Spiritual Discovery

In 1966, 3 years after being fired by Harvard because of his controversial involvement with hallucinogens (Associated Press 1999), Timothy Leary undertook a constitutional strategy intended to retain legitimate access to another hallucinogen, LSD. He began a religion called the League of Spiritual Discovery; LSD was the sacrament. This unorthodox religious orientation to the LSD experience was presented in a manual called The Psychedelic Experience (Leary et al. 1964), which was based on the Tibetan Book of the Dead. It became the "bible" of the psychedelic drug movement.

The movement grew, but most members used street LSD and did not follow Leary's directions. Leary believed that the hallucinogenic experience was only beneficial under proper control and guidance. But most members of this so-called religion merely used the organization as a front to gain access to an illegal drug. Federal authorities did not agree with Leary's freedom of religion interpretation and in 1969 convicted him for possession of marijuana and LSD and sentenced him to 20 years imprisonment (Stone 1991). Before being incarcerated, Leary escaped to Algeria and wandered for a couple of years before being extradited to the United States. He served several years in jail and was released in 1976.

Even in his later years, Leary continued to believe that U.S. citizens should be able to use hallucinogens without government regulation. He died in 1996 at the age of 75 years, revered by some but despised by others (Associated Press 1999; "Many Were Lost" 1996).

Hallucinogen Use Today

Today, the use of hallucinogens (excluding marijuana) is primarily a young-adult phenomenon (Johnston 2007). Although the use rate has not returned to that of the late 1960s and early 1970s (approximately 16%), in high school seniors lifetime use in 2006 was 8.3% (Johnston 2007). (See Table 12.1.) It has been speculated that this popularity reflects the ignorance of a new generation about the potential problems of the hallucinogens.

The Nature of hallucinogens

Agreement has not been reached on what constitutes a hallucinogenic agent (O'Brien 2006), for several reasons. First, a variety of seemingly unrelated drug groups can produce hallucinations, delusions, or sensory disturbances under certain conditions. For example, besides the traditional hallucinogens (such as LSD), high doses of anticholinergics, cocaine, amphetamines, and steroids can cause hallucinations.

In addition, responses to even the traditional hallucinogens can vary tremendously from person to person and from experience to experience. Multiple mechanisms are involved in the actions of these drugs, which contribute to the array of responses that they can cause. These drugs most certainly influence the complex inner workings of the human mind and have been described as

Peyote and the Rights of Mative Americans: How Far Should it Go?

Jonathan Fowler, a member of the Grand Traverse Band of Ottawa and Chippewa Indians, requested a judge allow his 4-year-old son to ingest peyote with him, as part of a religious ritual at the Native American Church of the Morning Star. The boy's mother opposed the request, fearing potential neurological damage to the boy. Although the use of peyote in Native American rituals is legal in all 50 states, the judge ruled against Fowler, stating that the boy could use peyote when he becomes old enough to comprehend its effects and with permission from both parents. Several Native American congregations who use peyote already have age limitations indicating who can take the substance during religious rites.

Source: Center for Cognitive Liberty and Ethics. "Court Says No Peyote for Native American Boy" (22 April 2003). Available www.cognitiveliberty.org/dil/peyote_boy.html.

psychedelic, psychoiogenic, or psychotomimetic. The features of hallucinogens that distinguish them from other drug groups are their ability to alter perception, thought, and feeling in such a manner that does not normally occur except in dreams or during experiences of extreme religious exaltation (NIDA 2001). We examine these characteristics throughout this chapter.

Sensory and Psychological Effects

In general, LSD is considered the prototype agent against which other hallucinogens are measured (NIDA 2001). Typical users experience several stages of sensory experiences; they can go through all stages during a single "trip" or, more likely, will pass through only some. These stages are as follows:

1. Heightened, exaggerated senses
2. Loss of control
3. Self-reflection
4. Loss of identity and a sense of cosmic merging

The following illustrations of the stages of the LSD experience are based primarily on an account by Solomon Snyder (1974), a highly regarded neuroscientist (one of the principal discoverers of endorphins; see Chapter 4), who personally experienced the effects of LSD as a young resident in psychiatry.

Altered Senses

In his encounter with LSD, Snyder used a moderate dose of 100 to 200 micrograms and observed few discernible effects for the first 30 minutes except some mild nausea. After this time had elapsed, objects took on a purplish tinge and appeared to be vaguely outlined. Colors, textures, and lines achieved an unexpected richness. Perception was so exaggerated that individual skin pores "stood out and clamored for recognition" (Snyder 1974, p. 42). Objects became distorted; when Snyder focused on his thumb, it began to swell, undulate, and then moved forward in a menacing fashion. Visions filled with distorted imagery occurred when his eyes were closed. The sense of time and distance changed dramatically; "a minute was like an hour, a week was like an eternity, a foot became a mile" (Snyder 1974, p. 43). The present seemed to drag on forever, and the concept of future lost its meaning. The exaggeration of perceptions and feelings gave the sense of more events occurring in a time period, giving the impression of time slowing.

An associated sensation described by Snyder is called synesthesia, a crossover phenomenon between senses. For example, sound develops visual dimensions, and vice versa, enabling the user to see sounds and hear colors. These altered sensory experiences are described as a heightened sensory awareness and relate to the first component of the psychedelic state (NIDA 2001).

Loss of Control

The second feature of LSD also relates to altered sensory experiences and a loss of control (O'Brien 2006). The user cannot determine whether the psychedelic trip will be a pleasant, relaxing experience or a "bad trip," with recollections of hidden fears and suppressed anxieties that can precipitate neurotic or psychotic responses. The frightening reactions may persist for a few minutes or several hours and be mildly agitating or extremely disturbing. Some bad trips can include feelings of panic, confusion, suspicion, helplessness, and a total lack of control. The following example illustrates how terrifying a bad trip can be:

> I was having problems breathing [and] my throat was all screwed up. The things that entered my mind were that I was dead and people were saying good-bye, because they really meant it. I was witnessing my own funeral. I was thinking that I was going to wake either in the

back seat of a cop car or in the hospital. (From Venturelli's files, interview with a 19-year-old male, 1995.)

Replays of these frightening experiences can occur at a later time, even though the drug has not been taken again; such recurrences are referred to as flashbacks (NIDA 2001) or hallucinogen persisting perception disorder (Halpern and Pope 2003).

It is not clear what determines the nature of the sensory response. Perhaps it relates to the state of anxiety and personality of the user or the nature of his or her surroundings. It is interesting that Timothy Leary tried to teach his "drug disciples" that "turning on correctly means to understand the many levels that are brought into focus; it takes years of discipline, training and disciple-ship" ("Celebration #1" 1966). He apparently felt that, with experience and training, you could control the sensory effects of the hallucinogens. This is an interesting possibility but has never been well demonstrated.

Self-Reflection

Snyder (1974) made reference to the third component of the psychedelic response in his LSD experience. During the period when sensory effects predominate, self-reflection also occurs. While in this state, Snyder explained, the user "becomes aware of thoughts and feelings long hidden beneath the surface, forgotten and/or repressed" (p. 44). As a psychiatrist, Snyder claimed that this

---

Key Terms

psychotogenic
  substances that initiate psychotic behavior

Key Terms

synesthesia
  a subjective sensation or image of a sense other than the one being stimulated, such as an auditory sensation caused by a visual stimulus

TABLE 1. Trends (Shown in Percentages) in the Use of LSD and All Hallucinogens by 8th Graders Through Young Adults, 1994-2006

	Used during lifetime					Used during year					Used during month				
	1994	1996	1999	2004	2006	1994	1996	1999	2004	2006	1994	1996	1999	2004	2006
8th graders															
LSD	3.7	5.1	4.1	1.8	2.8	2.4	3.5	2.4	1.1	0.9	1.1	1.5	1.1	0.5	0.4
All hallucinogens	4.3	5.9	4.8	3.5	3.4	2.7	4.1	2.9	2.2	2.1	1.3	1.9	1.3	1.0	0.9
10th graders															
LSD	7.2	9.4	8.5	2.8	2.7	5.2	6.9	6.0	1.6	1.7	2.0	2.4	2.3	0.6	0.7
All hallucinogens	8.1	10.5	9.7	6.4	6.1	5.8	7.8	6.9	4.1	4.1	2.4	2.8	2.9	1.6	1.3
12th graders															
LSD	10.5	12.6	12.2	4.6	3.3	6.9	8.8	8.1	2.2	1.7	2.6	2.5	2.7	0.7	0.6
All hallucinogens	11.4	14.0	13.7	9.7	8.3	7.6	10.1	9.4	6.2	4.9	3.1	3.5	3.5	1.9	1.5

	Used during lifetime				Used during year				Used during month			
	1994	1996	2001	2006	1994	1996	2001	2006	1994	1996	2001	2006
Young Adults												
LSD	13.8	15.0	16.0	6.8	4.0	4.5	3.4	2.5	1.1	0.7	0.7	—
All hallucinogens	15.9	15.4	18.3	14.9	5.1	4.9	5.4	5.7	1.6	1.4	1.2	—
Ecstasy	3.8	5.2	13.0	12.3	0.7	1.7	7.5	5.2	0.2	0.3	1.8	—

*For this survey, inhalants and marijuana were not considered as hallucinogens.

Sources: Johnston, L, P. O'Malley, and J. Bachman. "Monitoring the Future National Results on Adolescents Drug Use. Overview of Key Findings, 2002." Lansing, MI: University of Michigan, 2003.

Johnston, L. "Monitoring the Future 2006." Available www.monitoringthefuture.orgj/new.html.

new perspective can lead to valid insights that are useful psychotherapeutic exercises.

Some psychotherapists have used or advocated the use of psychedelics for this purpose since the 1950s, as described by Sigmund Freud, to "make conscious the unconscious" (Snyder 1974, p. 44). Although a case can be made for the psychotherapeutic use of this group of drugs, the Food and Drug Administration (FDA) has not approved any of these agents for psychiatric use. The psychedelics currently available are considered to be too unpredictable in their effects and possess substantial risks (Abraham et al. 1996). Not only is their administration not considered to be significantly therapeutic, but their use is also deemed a great enough risk that the principal hallucinogenic agents are classified (i.e., scheduled) as controlled substances (see Chapter 3 and Appendix B).

Loss of Identity and Cosmic Merging

The final features that set the psychedelics apart as unique drugs were described by Snyder (1974) as the "mystical-spiritual aspect of the drug experience." He claimed, "It is indescribable. For how can anyone verbalize a merging of his being with the totality of the universe? How do you put into words the feeling that 'all is one,' 'I am of the all,' 'I am no longer.' One's skin ceases to be a boundary between self and others" (p. 45). Because consumption of hallucinogen-containing plants has often been part of religious ceremonies, it is likely that this sense of cosmic merging and union with all humankind correlates to the exhilaratingly spiritual experiences described by many religious mystics.

The loss of identity and personal boundaries caused by hallucinogens is not viewed as being so spiritually enticing by all. In particular, for individuals who have rigid, highly ordered personalities, the dissolution of a well-organized and well-structured world is terrifying because the drug destroys the individual's emotional support. Such an individual finds that the loss of a separate identity can cause extreme panic and anxiety. During these drug-induced panic states, which in some ways are schizophrenic-like, people have committed suicide and homicide. These tragic reactions are part of the risk of using hallucinogenics and explain some of the FDA's hesitancy to legalize or authorize them for psychotherapeutic use.

Key Terms

flashbacks
recurrences of earlier drug-induced sensory experiences in the absence of the drug

Mechanisms of Action

As with most drugs, hallucinogens represent the proverbial "double-edged sword." These drugs may cause potentially useful psychiatric effects for many people. However, the variability in positive versus negative responses, coupled with lack of understanding as to what factors are responsible for the variables, have made these drugs dangerous and difficult to manage.

Some researchers have suggested that all hallucinogens act at a common central nervous system (CNS) site to exert their psychedelic effects. Although this hypothesis has not been totally dis-proven, there is little evidence to support it. The fact that so many different types of drugs can cause hallucinogenic effects suggests that multiple mechanisms are likely responsible for their actions.

The most predictable and typical psychedelic experiences are caused by LSD or similar agents. Consequently, these agents have been the primary focus of studies intended to elucidate the nature of hallucinogenic mechanisms. Although LSD has effects at several CNS sites, ranging from the spinal cord to the cortex of the brain, its effects on the neurotransmitter serotonin most likely account for its psychedelic properties (Nichols 2004). That LSD and similar drugs alter serotonin activity has been proven; how they affect this transmitter is not so readily apparent.

Although many experts believe changes in serotonin activity are the basis for the psychedelic properties of most hallucinogens, a case can be made for the involvement of norepinephrine, dopamine, acetylcholine, and perhaps other transmitter systems as well (see Chapter 4). Only

additional research will be able to sort out this complex but important issue.

Types of Hallucinogenic Agents

Due to recent technological developments, understanding of hallucinogens has advanced; even so, the classification of these drugs remains somewhat arbitrary. Many agents produce some of the pharmacological effects of the traditional psychedelics, such as LSD and mescaline.

A second type of hallucinogen includes those agents that have amphetamine-like molecular structures (referred to as phenylethylamines) and possess some stimulant action; this group includes drugs such as DOM (dimethoxymethylamphetamine), MDA (methylenedioxyamphetamine), and MDMA (methylenedioxymethamphetamine or Ecstasy). These agents vary in their hallucinogen or stimulant properties. MDA is more like an amphetamine (stimulant), whereas MDMA is more like LSD (hallucinogen). In large doses, however, each of the phenylethylamines causes substantial CNS stimulation.

The third major group of hallucinogens comprises the anticholinergic drugs, which block some of the receptors for the neurotransmitter acetylcholine (see Chapter 4). Almost all drugs that antagonize these receptors cause hallucinations in high doses. Many of these potent anticholinergic hallucinogens are naturally occurring and have been known, used, and abused for millennia.

Traditional Hallucinogens: LSD Types

The LSD-like drugs are considered to be the prototypical hallucinogens and are used as the basis of comparison for other types of agents with psychedelic properties. Included in this group are LSD itself and some hallucinogens derived from plants, such as mescaline from the peyote cactus,

---

Key Terms

ergotism
    poisoning by toxic substances from the ergot fungus Claviceps purpurea

---

psilocybin from mushrooms, dimethyltryptamine (DMT) from seeds, and myristicin from nutmeg. Because LSD is the principal hallucinogen, its origin, history, and properties are discussed in detail, providing a basis for understanding the other psychedelic drugs.

Lysergic Acid Diethylamide (LSD)

LSD is a relatively new drug, but similar compounds have existed for a long time. For example, accounts from the Middle Ages tell about a strange affliction that caused pregnant women to abort and others to develop strange burning sensations in their extremities. Today, we call this condition ergotism and know that it is caused by eating grain contaminated by the ergot fungus. This fungus produces compounds related to LSD called the ergot alkaloids (Goldstein 1994; NIDA 2007b). Besides the sensory effects, the ergot substances can cause hallucinations, delirium, and psychosis.

In 1938, Albert Hofmann, a scientist for Sandoz Pharmaceutical Laboratories of Basel, Switzerland, worked on a series of ergot compounds in a search for active chemicals that might be of medical value. Lysergic acid was similar in structure to a compound called nikethamide, a stimulant, and Hofmann tried to create slight chemical modifications that might merit further testing. The result of this effort was the production of lysergic acid diethylamide, or LSD. Hofmann's experience with this new compound gave insight into the effects of this drug (NIDA 2001).

Soon after LSD was discovered, the similarity of experiences with this agent to the symptoms of schizophrenia were noted, which prompted researchers to investigate correlations between the two (Weber 2006). The hope was to use LSD as a tool for producing an artificial psychosis to aid in understanding the biochemistry of psychosis (NIDA 2001). Interest in this use of LSD has declined because it is generally accepted that LSD effects differ from natural psychoses.

The use of LSD in psychotherapy has also been tried in connection with the treatment of alcoholism, autism, paranoia, schizophrenia, and various other mental and emotional disorders (Weber 2006). Therapeutic use of LSD has not increased to any great extent over the years because of its limited success, legal aspects, difficulty in obtaining the pure drug, adverse reactions to the drug ("bad trips" can occur under controlled as well as uncontrolled conditions), and rapid tolerance buildup in some patients.

Nonmedical interest in LSD and related drugs began to grow during the 1950s and peaked in the 1960s, when LSD was used by millions of young Americans for chemical escape. On rare occasions, a "bad trip" would cause a user to feel terror and panic; these experiences resulted in well-publicized accidental deaths due to jumping from building tops or running into the pathway of oncoming vehicles (U.S. Department of Justice 1991).

As with other hallucinogens, the use of LSD by teenagers declined somewhat over the 1970s and 1980s but began to rise again in the early 1990s. The reason for this rise was thought to relate to a decline in the perceived dangers of using LSD and an increase in peer approval (Johnston 1999). However, surveys have demonstrated a dramatic drop in LSD use in 2006 that has not been explained (Johnston 2007; Table 12.1). Of high school seniors sampled in 1975, 11.3% had used LSD sometime during their life; that number declined to 8.6% in 1992, rebounded to 12.2% in 1999, and tumbled to 4.6% in 2004 and further to 3.3% in 2006. LSD users are typically college or high school students, white, middle-class, and risk-takers (Johnston et al. 1996; Johnston 2007).

Synthesis and Administration LSD is a complex molecule that requires about 1 week to be synthesized. Because of the sophisticated chemistry necessary for its production, LSD is not manufactured by local illicit laboratories but requires the skills of a trained chemist (U.S. Department of Justice 2002, 2003). Because of LSD's potency, it has been difficult to locate illicit LSD labs; small quantities of LSD are sufficient to satisfy the demand and can be easily transported without detection. However, in 2000 a large lab was raided in Kansas resulting in a 95% decrease in LSD supplies in the United States by 2004, perhaps contributing to its decreased use in this country (Philadelphia Inquirer 2006).

The physical properties of LSD are not distinctive. In its purified form, LSD is colorless, odorless, and tasteless. It can be purchased in several forms, including tiny tablets (about one tenth the size of aspirins, called microdots), capsules, thin squares of gelatin called "window panes," or more commonly dissolved and applied to paper as "blotter acid" and cut up into 0.25-inch squares for individual dosing (Publishers Group 2002). Each square is swallowed or chewed and represents a single dose. One gram of LSD can provide 10,000 individual doses and be sold on the streets for $50,000. Although LSD usually is taken by mouth, it is sometimes injected. It costs about $1-10/dose (Schaffer Library 2007).

Physiological Effects Like many hallucinogens, LSD is remarkably potent. The typical dose today is 20 to 30 micrograms, compared with a typical dose of 150 to 300 micrograms in the 1960s. This difference in dose likely explains why today fewer users of LSD are experiencing severe side effects (NIDA 2007b). In monkeys, the lethal dose has been determined to be about 5 milligrams per kilogram of body weight.

When taken orally, LSD is readily absorbed and diffused into all tissues. It passes through the placenta into the fetus and through the blood-brain barrier. The brain receives about 1% of the total dose.

Within the brain, LSD is particularly concentrated in the hypothalamus, the limbic system, and the auditory and visual reflex areas. Electrodes placed in the limbic system show an "electrical storm," or a massive increase in neural activity, which might correlate with the overwhelming flood of sensations and the phenomenon of synesthesia reported by the user (NIDA 2001). LSD also activates the sympathetic nervous system; shortly after the drug is taken, body temperature, heart . rate, and blood pressure rise, the person sweats, and the pupils of the eyes dilate. Its effects on the parasympathetic nervous system increase salivation and nausea (NIDA 2007b). These systemic effects do not appear to be related to the hallucinogenic properties of the drug.

The effect of LSD begins within 30 to 90 minutes after ingestion and can last up to 12 hours. Tolerance to the effects of LSD develops more rapidly and lasts longer than tolerance to other hallucinogens (NIDA 2001). Tolerance develops very quickly to repeated doses, probably because of a change in sensitivity of the target cells in the brain rather than a change in its metabolism. Tolerance wears off within a few days after the drug is discontinued. Because there are no withdrawal symptoms, a person does not become physically dependent, but some psychological dependency on LSD can occur (NIDA 2007b).

Behavioral Effects Because LSD alters a number of systems in the brain, its behavioral effects are many and variable among individuals (Goldstein 1995). The following sections address common CNS responses to this drug.

Creativity and Insight. A question often raised by researchers interested in experimenting with LSD is this: Does LSD help expand the mind, increasing insight and creativity? This question is extremely difficult to answer because no one has ever determined the origin of insight and creativity. Moreover, each of us views these qualities differently.

Subjects under the influence of LSD often express the feeling of being more creative, but creative acts such as drawing and painting are hindered by the motor impairment caused by LSD. The products of artists under the influence of the drug usually prove to be inferior to those produced before the drug experience. Paintings done in LSD creativity studies have been described as reminiscent of "schizophrenic art."

In an often-cited study, creativity, attitude, and anxiety tests on 24 college students found that LSD had no objective effect on creativity, although many of the subjects said they felt they were more creative (McGlothin et al. 1967). This paradox is noted in several studies of LSD use. The subjects believe they have more insight and provide better answers to life's problems, but they do not or cannot demonstrate this increase objectively. Overt behavior is not modified, and these new insights are short-lived unless they are reinforced by modified behavior.

In spite of these results, some researchers still contend that LSD can enhance the creative process. For example, Oscar Janigar, a psychiatrist at the University of California, Los Angeles, claimed to have determined that LSD does not produce a tangible alteration in the way a painter paints; thus, it does not turn a poor painter into a good one. However, Janigar claimed that LSD does alter the way the painter appraises the world and allows the artist to "plunge into areas where access was restricted by confines of perceptions" and consequently becomes more creative (Tucker 1987, p. 16).

Adverse Psychedelic Effects. It is important to remember that there is no typical pattern of response to LSD. The experience varies for each user as a function of the person's set, or expectations, and setting, or environment, during the experience (Publishers Group 2002). Two of the major negative responses are described as follows (NIDA 2007b; Pahnke et al. 1970):

1. The psychotic adverse reaction, or "Breakout," is an intense, nightmarish experience. The subject may have complete loss of emotional control and experience paranoid delusions, hallucinations, panic attacks, psychosis, and catatonic seizures. In rare instances, some of these reactions are prolonged, lasting days.

2. The nonpsychotic adverse reaction may involve varying degrees of tension, anxiety, fear, depression, and despair but not as intense a response as the "freakout."

A person with deep psychological problems or a strong need to be in conscious control or one who take's the drug in an unfavorable setting is more likely to have an adverse reaction than a person with a well-integrated personality.

Severe LSD behavioral toxicity can be treated with tranquilizers or a sedative like a benzodiazepine.

Perceptual Effects. Because the brain's sensory processing is altered by a hallucinogenic dose of LSD, many kinds of unusual illusions can occur. Some users report seeing shifting geometrical patterns mixed with intense color perception; others observe the movement of stationary objects, such that a speck on the wall appears as a large blinking eye or an unfolding flower. Interpretation of sounds can also be scrambled; a dropped ashtray may become a gun fired at the user, for instance. In some cases, LSD alters perceptions to the extent that people feel they can walk on water or fly through the air. The sensation that the body is distorted and even coming apart is another common effect, especially for novice users. Thoughts of suicide and sometimes actual attempts can be caused by use of LSD as well (NIDA 2007b; U.S. Department of Justice 1991).

Many LSD users find their sense of time distorted, such that hours may be perceived as years or an eternity. As discussed earlier, users may also have a distorted perception of their own knowledge or creativity; for instance, they may feel their ideas or work are especially unique, brilliant, or artistic. When analyzed by a person not on LSD or explained after the "trip" is over, however, these ideas or creations are almost always quite ordinary.

In sum, LSD alters perception such that any sensation can be perceived in the extreme. An experience can be incredibly beautiful and uplifting. However, sometimes the experience can be very unpleasant.

The flashback is an interesting but poorly understood phenomenon of LSD use. Although usually thought of as being adverse, sometimes flashbacks are pleasant and even referred to as "free trips." During a flashback, sensations caused by previous LSD use return, although the subject is not using the drug at the time.

This head was sculpted by a university student while under the influence of LSD.

There are three broad categories of negative LSD-related flashbacks:

1. "Body trip recurrence of an unpleasant physical sensation
2. "Bad mind trip": recurrence of a distressing thought or emotion
3. Altered visual perception: the most frequent type of recurrence, consisting of seeing dots, flashes, trails of light, halos, false motion in the peripheral field, and other sensations

Flashbacks are most disturbing because they come on unexpectedly. Some have been reported years after use of LSD; for most people, however, flashbacks usually subside within weeks or months after taking LSD (NIDA 1999b). The duration of a flashback is variable, lasting from a few minutes to several hours (Fleckenstein 2000).

Although the precise mechanism of flashbacks is unknown, physical or psychological stresses and some drugs such as marijuana may trigger these experiences (Goldstein 1995). It has been proposed that flashbacks are an especially vivid form of memory that becomes seared into the subconscious mind due to the effects of LSD on the brain's transmitters.

Treatment consists of reassurance that the condition will go away and use of a sedative such as diazepam (Valium), if necessary, to treat the anxiety or panic that can accompany the flashback experience.

Genetic Damage and Birth Defects
Experiments conducted in the mid-1960s suggested that LSD could cause birth defects, based on the observation that, when LSD was added to a suspension of human white blood cells in a test tube, the chromosomes of these cells were damaged. From this finding, it was proposed that when LSD was consumed by human beings, it could damage the chromosomes of the male sperm, female egg, or cells of the developing infant. Such damage theoretically could result in congenital defects in offspring (Dishotsky etal. 1971).

Carefully controlled studies conducted after news of LSD's chromosomal effects were made, public have not supported this hypothesis. Experiments have revealed that, in contrast to the test tube findings, there is no chromosomal damage to white blood cells or any other cells when LSD is given to a human being (Dishotsky et al. 1971).

Studies have also shown that there are no carcinogenic or mutagenic effects from using LSD in experimental animals or human beings, with the exception of the fruit fly. (LSD is a mutagen in fruit flies if given in doses that are equivalent to 100,000 times the hallucinogenic dose for people.) Teratogenic effects occur in mice if LSD is given early in pregnancy. LSD may be teratogenic in rhesus monkeys if it is injected in doses (based on body weight) exceeding at least 100 times the usual hallucinogenic dose for humans. In other studies, women who took street LSD but not those given pure LSD had a higher rate of spontaneous abortions and births of malformed infants; this finding suggests that contaminants in adulterated LSD were responsible for the fetal effects and not the hallucinogen itself (Dishotsky et al. 1971).

Early Human Research In the 1950s, the U.S. government— specifically, the Central Intelligence Agency (CIA) and the army — became interested in reports of the effects of mind-altering drugs, including LSD. Unknown to the public at the time, these agencies conducted tests on human beings to learn more about such compounds and determine their usefulness in conducting military and clandestine missions. These activities became public when a biochemist, Frank Olson, killed himself in 1953 after being given a drink laced with LSD. Olson had a severe psychotic reaction and was being treated for the condition when he jumped out of a 10th-story window. His family was told only that he had committed suicide. The connection to LSD was not uncovered until 1975. The court awarded Olson's family $750,000 in damages in 1976.

In 1976, the extent of these studies was revealed; nearly 585 soldiers and 900 civilians had been given LSD in poorly organized experiments in which participants were coerced into taking this drug or not told that they were receiving it. Powerful hallucinogens such as LSD can cause serious psychological damage in some subjects, especially when they are unaware of what is happening.

The legal consequences of these LSD studies continued for years. As recently as 1987, a New York judge awarded $700,000 to the family of a mental patient who killed himself after having been given LSD without an explanation of the drug's nature. The judge said that there was a "conspiracy of silence" among the army, the Department of Justice, and the New York State Attorney General to conceal events surrounding the death of the subject, Harold Blauer.

Mescaline (Peyote)

Mescaline is one of approximately 30 psychoactive chemicals that have been isolated from the peyote cactus and used for centuries in the Americas (see "Here and Now," Peyote: An Ancient Indian Way). One of the first reports on the peyote plant was made by Francisco Hernandez to the court of King Philip II of Spain. King Philip was interested in reports from the earlier Cortes expedition about strange medicines the natives used and sent Hernandez to collect information about herbs and medicines. Hernandez worked on this project from 1570 to 1575 and reported on the use of more than 1200 plant remedies as well as the existence of many hallucinogenic plants. He was one of the first to record the eating of parts of the peyote cactus and the resulting visions and mental changes.

In the 17th century, Spanish Catholic priests asked their Indian converts to confess to the use of peyote, which they believed was used to conjure up demons. However, nothing stopped its use. By 1760, use of peyote had spread into what is now the United States.

Peyote has been confused with another plant, the mescal shrub, which produces dark red beans that contain an extremely toxic alkaloid called cytisine. This alkaloid may cause hallucinations, convulsions, and even death. In addition, a mescal liquor is made from the agave cactus. Partly because of misidentification with the toxic mescal beans, the U.S. government outlawed the use of both peyote and mescaline for everyone except members of the Native American Church (Mims 2000). Mescaline has been used for decades by this group as part of their religious sacrament. A recent study suggested that long-term religious use of peyote does not have significant psychological effects or cause problems with cognitive performance in Native Americans (Halpern et al. 2005).

Mescaline is the most active drug in peyote; it induces intensified perception of colors and euphoria in the user. However, as Aldous Huxley said in The Doors of Perception (1954), his book about his experimentation with mescaline, "Along with the happily transfigured majority of mescaline takers there is a minority that finds in the drug only hell and purgatory." After Huxley related his experiences with mescaline, it was used by an increasing number of people.

Physiological Effects The average dose of mescaline that will cause hallucinations and other physiological effects is from 300 to 600 milligrams. It may take up to 20 peyote (mescal) buttons (ingested orally) to get 600 milligrams of mescaline.

Based on animal studies, scientists estimate that a lethal dosage is 10 to 30 times greater than that which causes behavioral effects in human beings. (About 200 milligrams is the lowest mind-altering dose.) Death in animals results from convulsions and respiratory arrest. Mescaline is perhaps 1000 to 3000 times less potent than LSD and 30 times less potent than another common hallucinogen, psilocybin (Mathias 1993). Psilocybin is discussed later in this chapter.

Mescaline's effects include dilation of the pupils (mydriasis), increase in body temperature, anxiety, visual hallucinations, and alteration of body image. The last effect is a type of hallucination in which parts of the body may seem to disappear or to become grossly distorted. Mescaline induces vomiting in many people and some muscular relaxation (sedation). Apparently, there are few aftereffects or drug hangover feelings at low doses. Higher doses of mescaline slow the heart and respiratory rhythm, contract the intestines and the uterus, and cause headache, difficulty in coordination, dry skin with itching, and hypertension (high blood pressure).

Mescaline users report that they lose all awareness of time. As with LSD, the setting for the "trip" influences the user's reactions. Most mescaline users prefer natural settings, most likely due to the historical association of this drug with Native Americans and their nature-related spiritual experiences (often under the influence of this drug). The visual hallucinations achieved depend on the individual. Colors are at first intensified and may be followed by hallucinations of shades, movements, forms, and events. The senses of smell and taste are enhanced. Some people claim (as with LSD) that they can "hear" colors and "see" sounds, such as the wind. Synesthesia occurs naturally in a small percentage of cases.

At low to medium doses, a state of euphoria is reported, often followed by a feeling of anxiety and less frequently by depression. Occasionally, users observe themselves as two people and experience the sensation that the mind and the body are separate entities. A number of people have had cosmic experiences that are profound — almost religious — and in which they discover a sense of unity with all creation. People who have this sensation often believe they have discovered the meaning of existence.

Mechanism of Action Within 30 to 120 minutes after ingestion, mescaline reaches a maximum concentration in the brain. The effects may persist for as long as 9 or 10 hours. Hallucinations may last up to 2 hours and are usually affected by the dose level. About half the dose is excreted unchanged after 6 hours and can be recovered in the urine for reuse (if peyote is in short supply). A slow tolerance builds up after repeated use, and there is cross-tolerance to LSD. As with LSD, mescaline intoxication can be alleviated or stopped by taking a dose of chlorpromazine (Thorazine), a tranquilizer, and to a lesser extent by taking diazepam (Valium). Like LSD, mescaline probably exerts much of its hallucinogenic effects by altering serotonin systems (Aghajanian and Marck 2000).

Analysis of street samples of mescaline obtained in a number of U.S. cities over the past decade shows that the chemical sold rarely is authentic. Regardless of color or appearance, these street drugs are usually other hallucinogens, such as LSD, 2,6-dimethoxy-4-methylamphetamine (DOM), or PCP. If a person decides to take hallucinogenic street drugs, "let the buyer beware." Not only is the actual content often different and potentially much more toxic than bargained for (they are frequently contaminated), but the dosage is usually unknown even if the drug is genuine.

Psilocybin

The drug psilocybin has a long and colorful history. Its principal source is the Psilocybe mexicana mushroom of the "magic" variety (Goldstein 1994; U.S. Department of Justice 2002). It was first used by some of the early natives of Central America more than 2000 years ago. In Guatemala, statues of mushrooms that date back to 100 B.C. have been found. The Aztecs later used the mushrooms for ceremonial rites. When the Spaniards came into Mexico in the 1500s, the natives were calling the Psilocybe mexicana mushroom "God's flesh" (Harvard Mental Health Letter 2006). Because of this seeming sacrilege, the natives were harshly treated by the Spanish priests.

Gordon Wasson identified the Psilocybe mexicana mushroom in 1955. The active ingredient was extracted in 1958 by .Albert Hofmann, who also synthesized LSD. Doing research, Hofmann wanted to make certain he would feel the effects of the mushroom, so he ate 32 of them, weighing 2.4 grams (a medium dose by Native American standards) and then recorded his hallucinogenic reactions (Burger 1968).

Timothy Leary also tried some psilocybin mushrooms in Mexico in 1960; apparently, the experience influenced him greatly. On his return to Harvard, he carried out a series of experiments using psilocybin with student groups. Leary was careless in experimental procedures and did some work in uncontrolled situations. His actions

---

Here and Now

Peyote: An Ancient Indian Way

Members of the Native American Church use the buttons of the hallucinogenic peyote cactus to brew a sacramental tea as sacred to them as the bread and wine of the Christian Eucharist. As described by one member, "Peyote is a gift given to the Indians, but its ways cannot be obtained overnight; It has to be done with sincerity. It becomes part of your way of life. One has to walk that walk" Those who accept this form of worship believe that respectful use of peyote can be a gateway to the realm of the spirit, visions, and guidance. The use of peyote as part of the latest New Age craze is very disturbing to members of this church and is viewed almost as a form of sacrilege.

Source: Mtms, B. "Peyote: When the Ancient Indian Way Collides with a New Age Craze." Salt Lake Tribune 258 (I July 1999); A-10. Native American Church. (2008). Availabfewww.nativeamericanchurch.com/.

caused a major administrative upheaval, ending in his departure from Harvard.

One of Leary's questionable studies was the "Good Friday" experiment in which 20 theological students were given either a placebo or psilocybin in a double-blind study (that is, neither the researcher nor the subjects know who gets the placebo or the drug), after which all attended the same 2.5-hour Good Friday service. The experimental group reported mystical experiences whereas the control group did not (Pahnke and Richards 1966). Leary believed that the experience was of value and that, under proper control and guidance, the hallucinatory experience could be beneficial.

Psilocybin is not very common on the street. Generally, it is administered orally and is eaten either fresh or dried. Accidental poisonings are common for those who mistakenly consume poisonous mushrooms rather than the hallucinogenic variety.

The dried form of these mushrooms contains from 0.2% to 0.5% psilocybin. The hallucinogenic effects produced are quite similar to those of LSD, and there is a cross-tolerance among psilocybin, LSD, and mescaline. The effects caused by psilocybin vary with the dosage taken. Up to 4 milligrams cause a pleasant experience, relaxation, and some body sensation. In some subjects, higher doses cause considerable perceptual and body image changes, accompanied by hallucinations, as illustrated in the following quote:

> The first time I 'shroomed, everything looked like it was made of plastic, like everything could be folded up or something. Whatever somebody told me, I would believe it to be true. Like if I was drinking a beer and someone told

me it was tequila, I would taste tequila. (From Venturelli's files, interview with a 20-year-old male, 1995.)

In extreme cases, psilocybin can even induce the first stages of schizophrenia-like psychosis (Vollenwelder et al. 1998). Psilocybin stimulates the autonomic nervous system, dilates the pupils, and increases the body temperature. There is some evidence that psilocybin is metabolized into psilocin, which is more potent and may be the principal active ingredient. Psilocin is found in mushrooms, albeit in small amounts. Like the other hallucinogens, psilocybin apparently causes no physical dependence.

Trypiamines Some compounds related to the tryptamine class of drugs (molecules that resemble the neurotransmitter serotonin) have hallucinogenic properties and can exist naturally in herbs, fungi, and animals or can be synthesized in the laboratory. Most of these compounds are Schedule I drugs and illegal (Drug Enforcement Agency [DEA] 2002b). Two examples are discussed in this section.

Dimelhylttyptamine (DMT). DMT is a short-acting hallucinogen found in the seeds of certain leguminous trees native to the West Indies and parts of South America (Schultes 1978). It is also prepared synthetically in illicit laboratories. For centuries, the powdered seeds have been used as a snuff called cohoba in pipes and snuffing tubes. The Haitian natives claim that, under the influence of the drug, they can communicate with their gods. Its effects may last less than 1 hour, which has earned it the nickname "the businessman's lunch break" drug.

DMT has no effect when taken orally; it is inhaled either as smoke from the burning plant or in vaporized form. DMT is sometimes added to parsley leaves or flakes, tobacco, or marijuana to induce its hallucinogenic effect. The usual dose is 60 to 150 milligrams. In structure and action, it is similar to psilocybin although not as powerful. Like the other hallucinogens discussed, DMT does not cause physical dependence.

Foxy. The synthetic substance chemically named S-methoxy-A^A^-diisopropyltryptamine (Foxy) is a relatively new hallucinogen. This drug has been used at raves and clubs in Arizona, California, New York, and Florida. It was added to the DEA Schedule I category in 2004 (Wikipedia 2007). At lower doses, Foxy can cause euphoria; at higher doses, its effects are similar to LSD (DEA 2002b).

Nutmeg High doses of nutmeg can be quite intoxicating, causing symptoms such as drowsiness, stupor, delirium, and sleep. Prison inmates have known about this drug for years, so in most prisons use of spices such as nutmeg is restricted.

Nutmeg contains 5% to 15% myristica oil, which is responsible for the physical effects. Myristicin (about 4%), which is structurally similar to mescaline, and elemicin are probably the most potent psychoactive ingredients in nutmeg. Myristicin blocks release of serotonin from brain neurons. Some scientists believe that it can be converted in the body to MDMA (a close relative of MDA, discussed later), which also affects the CNS. Mace, the exterior covering of the nutmeg seed, also contains the hallucinogenic compound myristicin.

Two tablespoons of nutmeg (about 14 grams) taken orally cause a rather unpleasant "trip" with a dreamlike stage; rapid heartbeat, dry mouth, and thirst are experienced as well. Agitation, apprehension, and a sense of impending doom may last about 12 hours, with a sense of unreality persisting for several days (Claus et al. 1970).

Phenyiethylaniine Hallucinogens

The phenylethylamine drugs are chemically related to amphetamines. Phenylethylamines have varying degrees of hallucinogenic and CNS stimulant effects, which are likely related to their ability to release serotonin and dopamine, respectively. Consequently, the phenylethylamines that predominantly release serotonin are dominated by their hallucinogenic action and are LSD-like, whereas those more inclined to release dopamine are dominated by their stimulant effects and are amphetamine-like.

Dimethoxymethylamphetamine

The basic structure of dimethoxymethylamphetamine (DOM or STP) is amphetamine. Nonetheless, it is a fairly powerful hallucinogen that seems to work through mechanisms similar to those found with mescaline and LSD. In fact, the effects of DOM are similar to those caused by a combination of amphetamine and LSD, with the hallucinogenic effects of the drug overpowering the amphetamine-like physiological effects.

"Designer" Amphetamines

"Designer" amphetamines were discussed in Chapter 10 but are presented again here owing to their hallucinogenic effects. Their hybrid actions as psychedelic stimulants not only make them a particularly fascinating topic for research, but also provide a unique experience described by drug abusers as a "smooth amphetamine" or entactogens (implying that the pleasurable sensation of touch is enhanced) . This characterization likely accounts for the popularity of the designer amphetamines (de la Torre et al. 2004) .

3,H-Methylenedioxyamphetamine (MDA) MDA, first synthesized in 1910, is structurally related to both mescaline and amphetamine. Early research found that MDA is an anorexiant (causing loss of appetite) as well as a mood elevator in some persons. Further research has shown that the mode of action of MDA is similar to that of amphetamines. It causes additional release of the neurotransmitters serotonin, dopamine, and norepinephrine.

MDA has been used as an adjunct to psychotherapy. In one study, eight volunteers who had previously experienced the effects of LSD under clinical conditions were given 150 milligrams of MDA. Effects of the drug were noted between 40 and 60 minutes following ingestion by all eight subjects. The subjective effects following administration peaked at the end of 90 minutes and persisted for approximately 8 hours. None of the subjects experienced hallucinations, perceptual distortion, or closed-eye imagery, but they reported that the feelings the drug induced had some relationship to those previously experienced with LSD. The subjects found that both drugs induced an intensification of feelings, increased perceptions of self-insight, and heightened empathy with others during the experience. Most of the subjects also felt an increased sense of aesthetic enjoyment at some point during the intoxication. Seven of the eight subjects said they perceived music as "three-dimensional" (Naranjo et al. 1967).

On the street, MDA has been called the love drug because of its effects on the sense of touch and the attitudes of the users. Users often report experiencing a sense of well-being (likely a stimulant effect) and heightened tactile sensations (like a hallucinogenic effect) and thus increased pleasure through sex and expressions of affection. Those under the influence of MDA frequendy focus on interpersonal relationships and demonstrate an overwhelming desire or need to be with or talk to people. Some users say they have a very pleasant "body high" — more sensual than cerebral, and more emphatic than introverted. For these reasons, MDA is sometimes used by persons attending raves, much like MDMA or Ecstasy (Kalant 2001).

The unpleasant side effects most often reported are nausea, periodic tensing of muscles in the neck, tightening of the jaw and grinding of the teeth, and dilation of the pupils. Street doses of MDA range from 100 to 150 milligrams. Serious convulsions and death have resulted from larger doses, but in these cases the quantity of MDA was not accurately measured. Ingestion of 500 milligrams of pure MDA has been shown to cause death. The only adverse reaction to moderate doses reported is a marked physical exhaustion, lasting as long as 2 days (Marquardt et al. 1978).

An unpleasant MDA experience should be treated the same as a bad trip with any hallucinogen. The person should be "talked down" (reassured) in a friendly and supportive manner. The use of other drugs is rarely needed, although medical attention may be necessary. Under the Comprehensive Drug Abuse Prevention and Control Act of 1970, MDA is classified as a Schedule I substance; illegal possession is a serious offense.

Methylenedioxymethamphetamine (MDMA) MDMA is a modification of MDA but is thought to have more psychedelic and less stimulant activity (for example, euphoria) than its predecessor. MDMA is also structurally similar to mescaline. This drug has become known as Ecstasy, XTC, and Adam (Zickler 2000). (Ecstasy was also discussed in Chapter 10.)

MDMA was synthesized in 1912 to suppress appetite, but due to bizarre side effects it was withdrawn from development until it became widely used in the 1980s (Adam 2006). This designer amphetamine can be produced easily (DEA 2002a). Although the synthesis can be done by local illicit laboratories (Hyslop 2000), most of the MDMA supplies in this country are smuggled in from outlaw drug laboratories in European countries such as the Netherlands (Cool Nurse 2007). The unusual psychological effects it produces are part of the reason for its popularity. The drug causes euphoria, increased energy, increased sensitivity to touch, and lowered inhibitions. Many users claim it intensifies emotional feelings without sensory distortion and that it increases empathy and awareness both of the user's body and of the aesthetics of the surroundings (Farley 2000). Some consider MDMA to be an aphrodisiac. Because MDMA lowers defense mechanisms and reduces inhibitions, it has even been used during psychoanalysis (Cloud 2000). In fact, recently MDMA was approved by the FDA to be tested as a psychotherapeutic drug with the ultimate objective of determining its value in the treatment of patients suffering from posttraumatic stress disorder (PTSD) (Multidisciplinary Association for Psychedelic Studies [MAPS] 2007).

MDMA — popularized in the 1980s by articles in Newsweek (Adler 1985), Time (Toufexis 1985), and other magazines — recently was again touted on the national newsstands as a drug with euphoric effects, potential therapeutic value, and lack of serious side effects. MDMA is popular with college-age students and young adults (Office of National Drug Control Policy [ONDCP] 2008). Because of its effect of enhancing sensations, MDMA has been used as part of a countercultural rave scene, including high-tech music and laser light shows. Observers report that MDMA-linked rave parties are reminiscent of the acid parties of the 1960s and 1970s. The latest cycle of MDMA popularity peaked in 2001 and was being used by 10% of high school seniors (Johnston 2007). However, due to reports of MDMA neurotoxicity and persistent negative side effects, use of this drug has decreased dramatically and by 2006 was being used by only 4.1% of high school seniors (Johnston 2007).

Because of the widespread abuse of MDMA, the DEA prohibited its use by formally placing it on the Schedule I list in 1988 (Office of National Drug Control Policy [ONDCP] 2008). At the time of the ban, it was estimated that as many as 200 physicians were using the drug in psychotherapy (Greer and Tolbert 1990) and an estimated 30,000 doses per month were being taken for recreational purposes. Currently, MDMA is referred to as a "club drug" because of its frequent use at rave dances, clubs, and bars (Office of National Drug Control Policy [ONDCP] 2008). A dose of this drug is readily affordable at $10 to $20 (Hegadoran et al. 1999).

MDMA is usually taken orally, but it is sometimes snorted or even occasionally smoked. After the high starts, it may persist for minutes or even an hour, depending on the person, the purity of the drug, and the environment in which it is taken. When coming down from an MDMA-induced high, people often take small oral doses known as "boosters" to get high again. If they take too many boosters, they become very fatigued the next day. The average dose is about 75 to 150 milligrams; toxic effects have been reported at higher doses (Cami et al. 2000). Some statistics suggest that almost 50% of the tablets sold as MDMA actually contain other drugs such as aspirin, caffeine, cocaine, methamphetamine, or pseudoephedrine (Tanner-Smith 2006).

There is disagreement as to the possible harmful side effects of MDMA. Use of high doses can cause psychosis and paranoia (Parrott 2000a). Some negative physiological responses caused by recreational doses include dilated pupils, dry mouth and throat, clenching and grinding of teeth (resulting in the use of baby pacifiers), muscle aches and stiffness (in 28% of users), fatigue (in 80% of users), insomnia (in 38% of users), agitation, and anxiety. Some of these reactions can be intense and unpredictable. Under some conditions, death can be caused by hyperthermia (elevated body temperature), instability of the autonomic nervous system, and kidney failure (Burke 2001).

Several studies have demonstrated long-term damage to serotonin neurons in the brain following a single high dose of either MDMA or MDA, which may result in impaired memory, diminished ability to process information, and heightened im-pulsivity (Parrott 2000b; Williams 2002). Although the behavioral significance of this damage in people is not clear, at the present time caution using this drug is warranted (see "Here and Now," MDMA's Casual User).

There has been considerable debate as to the addictive properties of MDMA. Some claim this drug is like LSD with little likelihood of causing physical dependence, whereas others claim its properties are likely to be more amphetamine-like. Part of the difficulty in sorting out this controversy is that most moderate MDMA users also use other drugs, making it difficult to determine which effects are specifically attributable to the MDMA. The potential to cause addiction and dependence by MDMA is likely somewhere between that of amphetamine and LSD. Because of its ability to cause euphoria and release dopamine in the brain, it is very probable that use by smoking or injection can cause significant dependence.

Anticholinergic Hallucinogens

The anticholinergic hallucinogens include naturally occurring alkaloid (bitter organic base) substances that are present in plants and herbs found around the world. These drugs are often mentioned in folklore and in early literature as being added to potions. They are thought to have killed the Roman Emperor Claudius and to have poisoned Hamlet's father. Historically, they have been the favorite drugs used to eliminate inconvenient people (Marken et al. 1996). Hallucinogens affecting the cholinergic neurons also have been used by South American Indians for religious ceremonies (Schultes and Hofmann 1980) and were probably used in witchcraft to give the illusion of flying, to prepare sacrificial victims, and

even to give some types of marijuana ("superpot") its kick.

The potato family of plants (Solanaceae) contain most of these mind-altering drugs. The following three potent anticholinergic compounds are commonly found in these plants: (1) scopolamine, or hyoscine; (2) hyoscyamine; and (3) atropine. Scopolamine may produce excitement, hallucinations, and delirium even at therapeutic doses. With atropine, doses bordering on toxic levels are usually required to obtain these effects (Schultes and Hofmann 1973). All of these active alkaloid drugs block some acetylcholine receptors (see Chapter 4).

These alkaloid drugs can be used as ingredients in cold symptom remedies because they have a drying effect and block production of mucus in the nose and throat. They also prevent salivation; therefore, the mouth becomes uncommonly dry and perspiration may stop. Atropine may increase the heart rate by 100% and dilate the pupils markedly, causing inability to focus on nearby objects. Other annoying side effects of these anticholinergic drugs include constipation and difficulty in urinating. These inconveniences tend to discourage excessive abuse of these drugs for their hallucinogenic properties. Usually, people who abuse these anticholinergic compounds are receiving the drugs by prescription (Marken et al. 1996).

Anticholinergics can cause drowsiness by affecting the sleep centers of the brain. At large doses, a condition occurs that is similar to a psychosis, characterized by delirium, loss of attention, mental confusion, and sleepiness (Carlini 1993). Hallucinations may also occur at higher doses. At very high doses, paralysis of the respiratory system may cause death.

Although hundreds of plant species naturally contain anticholinergic substances and consequently can cause psychedelic experiences, only a few of the principal plants are mentioned here.

Atropa Belladonna: The Deadly Nightshade Plant

Knowledge of Atropa belladonna is very old, and its use as a drug is reported in early folklore. The name of the genus, Atropa, is the origin for the drug name atropine and indicates the reverence the Greeks had for the plant. Atropos was one of the three Fates in Greek mythology, whose duty it was to cut the thread of life when the time came. This plant has been used for thousands of years by assassins and murderers. In Tales of the Arabian Nights, unsuspecting potentates were poisoned with atropine from the deadly nightshade or one of its relatives. Fourteen berries of the deadly nightshade contain enough drug to cause death.

The species name, belladonna, means "beautiful woman." In early Rome and Egypt, girls with large pupils were considered attractive and friendly. To create this condition, they would put a few drops of an extract of this plant into their eyes, causing the pupils to dilate (Marken et al. 1996). Belladonna has also enjoyed a reputation as a love potion.

Mandragora Officinarum: The Mandrake

The mandrake contains several active psychedelic alkaloids: hyoscyamine, scopolamine, atropine, and mandragorine. Mandrake has been used as a love potion for centuries but has also been known for its toxic properties. In ancient folk medicine, mandrake was used to treat many ailments in spite of its side effects. It was recommended as a sedative, to relieve nervous conditions, and to relieve pain (Schultes and Hofmann 1980), as portrayed in the 2007 movie, Pan's Labyrinth.

The root of the mandrake is forked and, viewed with a little imagination, may resemble the human body (as portrayed in the Harry Potter and the Chamber of Secrets movie in 2002). Because of this resemblance, it has been credited with human attributes, which gave rise to many superstitions in the Middle Ages about its magical powers. Shakespeare referred to this plant in Romeo and Juliet. In her farewell speech, Juliet says, "And shrieks like mandrakes torn out of the earth, that living mortals hearing them run mad."

Here and Now

MDMA's Casual User

A study examined fifteen regular Ecstasy users, fifteen novice (first-time) Ecstasy users, and fifteen control subjects who attended a Saturday night rave. The regular users consumed, on average, L8 MDMA tablets, the novice users took 1.4 MDMA tablets, and the control subjects had no drug except alcohol. All groups reported positive moods during the dance; However, 2 days later, the Ecstasy users felt significantly more depressed, unsociable, unpleasant, and less good-tempered than the control subjects. Verbal recall was also diminished in MDMA users, who remembered only 60% to 70% of the words remembered by the control subjects. Those who used Ecstasy regularly had the most difficulty remembering.

Source: Parrott, A., and J. Lasky, "Ecstasy (MDMA) Effects Upon Mood and Cognition: Before, During and After a Saturday Night Dance." Psychophar-macology 139 (1998): 261-268.

Hyoscyamus Niger: Henbane

Henbane is a plant that contains both hyoscyamine and scopolamine. In a.d. 60, Pliny the Elder spoke of henbane: "For this is certainly known, that if one takes it in drink more than four leaves, it will put him beside himself" (Jones 1956). Henbane was also used in the orgies, or bacchanalias, of the ancient world.

Although rarely used today, henbane has been given medicinally since early times. It was frequently used to cause sleep, although hallucinations often occurred if given in excess. It was likely included in witches' brews and deadly concoctions during the Dark Ages (Schultes and Hofmann 1980).

Datura Stramonium: Jimsonweed

The Datura genus of the Solanaceae family includes a large number of related plants found worldwide. The principal active drug in this group is scopolamine; there are also several less active alkaloids.

Throughout history, these plants have been used as hallucinogens by many societies. They are mentioned in early Sanskrit and Chinese writings and were revered by the Buddhists. There is also some indication that the priestess (oracle) at the ancient Greek Temple of Apollo at Delphi was under the influence of this type of plant when she made prophecies (Schultes 1970). Before the supposed divine possession, she appeared to have chewed leaves of the sacred laurel. A mystic vapor was also reported to have risen from a fissure in the ground. The sacred laurel may have been one of the Datura species, and the vapors may have come from burning these plants.

Jimsonweed gets its name from an incident that took place in 17th-century Jamestown. British soldiers ate this weed while trying to capture Nathaniel Bacon, who had made seditious remarks about the king. Although still abused occasionally by adventuresome young people, the anticholinergic side effects of jimsonweed are so unpleasant that it rarely becomes a long-term problem (Lein-wand 2006; Tiongson and Salen 1998).

Other Hallucinogens

Technically, any drug that alters perceptions, thoughts, and feelings in a manner that is not normally experienced except in dreams can be classified as a hallucinogen. Because the brain's sensory input is complex and involves several neurotransmitter systems, drugs with many diverse effects can cause hallucinations (NIDA 2001).

Four agents that do not conveniendy fit into the principal categories of hallucinogens are discussed in the following sections.

Phencyclidine

Phencyclidine (PCP) is considered by many experts as the most dangerous of the hallucinogens (APA 2000; Maier 2003). PCP was developed in the late 1950s as an intravenous anesthetic. Although it was found to be effective, it had serious side effects that caused it to be discontinued for human use (NIDA 2001). Sometimes when people were recovering from PCP anesthesia, they experienced delirium and manic states of excitation lasting 18 hours (APA 2000). PCP is currently a Schedule II drug, legitimately available only as an anesthetic for animals but has even been banned from veterinary practice since 1985 because of its high theft rate. Most, if not all, PCP used in the United States today is produced illegally (National Drug Intelligence Center 2004).

Street PCP is mainly synthesized from readily available chemical precursors in clandestine laboratories. Within 24 hours, cooks (the makers of street PCP) can set up a lab, make several gallons of the drug, and destroy the lab before the police can locate them. Liquid PCP is then poured into containers and ready for shipment (Maier 2003).

PCP first appeared on the street drug scene in 1967 as the PeaCe Pill In 1968, it reappeared in New York as a substance called hog. By 1969, PCP was found under a variety of guises. It was sold as angel dust and sprinkled on parsley for smoking. Today, it is sold on the streets under many different slang names, including angel dust, supergrass, killerweed, embalming fluid, bobbies, dippies, hydro a, and purple haze, to mention a few (Dewan 2003; Maier 2003).

In the late 1960s, PCP began to find its way into a variety of street drugs sold as psychedelics. By 1970, authorities observed that phencyclidine was used widely as a main ingredient in psychedelic preparations. It has been frequently substituted for and sold as LSD, mescaline, marijuana, and cocaine (Maier 2003; National Drug Intelligence Center 2004).

One difficulty in estimating the effects or use patterns of PCP is caused by variance in drug purity. Also, there are about 30 analogs of PCP, some of which have appeared on the street. PCP has so many other street names that people may not know they are using it or they may have been deceived when buying what they thought was LSD or mescaline (Dewan 2003). Users may not question the identity of the substances unless they have a bad reaction.

PCP is available as a pure, white crystalline powder, as tablets, or as capsules. However, because it is usually manufactured in makeshift laboratories, it is frequently discolored by contaminants from a tan to brown with a consistency ranging from powder to a gummy mass (U.S. Department of Justice 1991). PCP can be taken orally, smoked, sniffed, or injected (NIDA 2007c). In the late 1960s through the early 1970s, PCP was mostly taken orally, but it is now commonly snorted or applied to dark brown cigarettes, leafy materials such as parsley, mint, oregano, marijuana, or tobacco, and smoked (U.S. Department of Justice 2003). By smoking PCP, the experienced user is better able to limit his or her dosage to a desired level. After smoking, the subjective effects appear within 1 to 5 minutes and peak within the next 5 to 30 minutes. The high lasts about 4 to 6 hours, followed by a 6-to 24-hour "comedown" (APA 2000).

In the 1979 national drug survey performed by the National Institute on Drug Abuse, about 7% of U.S. high school seniors had used PCP in a 12-month period; however, in 2004, that rate had declined to 0.7% (Johnston 2007).

Physiological Effects Although PCP may have hallucinogenic effects, it can cause a host of other physiological actions, including stimulation, depression, anesthesia, and analgesia. The effects of PCP on the CNS vary greatly. At low doses, the most prominent effect is similar to that of alcohol intoxication, with generalized numbness. As the dose of PCP increases, the person becomes even more insensitive and may become fully anesthetized. Large doses can cause coma, convulsions, and death (APA 2000).

The majority of peripheral effects are apparently related to activation of the sympathetic nervous system (see Chapter 5). Flushing, excess sweating, and a blank stare are common, although the size of the pupils is unaffected. The cardiovascular system reacts by increasing blood pressure and heart rate. Other effects include side-to-side eye movements (called nystagmus), muscular incoordination, . double vision, dizziness, nausea, and vomiting (National Drug Intelligence Center 2004). These symptoms occur in many people taking medium to high doses.

Psychological Effects PCP has unpleasant effects most of the time it is used. Why, then, do people use it repeatedly as their drug of choice?

PCP has the ability to markedly alter the person's subjective feelings; this effect may be

Jimsonweed Abuse in Idaho

Jimsonweed is a natural herb whose medicinal purposes include treatment for asthma, muscle spasms, and whooping cough. Its dangerous side effects include hallucinogenic actions and induction of a rapid heartbeat. Because of the effects jimsonweed has on the body, and because it is a legal, uncontrolled substance, adolescents have been known to take this herb for its psychedelic properties. For example, a new wave of jimsonweed abuse in eastern Idaho recently resulted in several teenagers entering the emergency room in drug-induced comas. Jimsonweed is a fairly accessible and somewhat inexpensive herb that is dangerous not only because of its biological effects, but also because of the variability of its side effects' intensity from batch to batch.

Source: "Jimson Weed Abuse in Idaho" (2003). Available www.drug-rehabs.org/content.php?cid=1097&state=Idaho.

reinforcing, even though the alteration is not always positive. Some say use of PCP makes them feel godlike and powerful (Maier 2003). There is an element of risk, not knowing how the trip will turn out. PCP may give the user feelings of strength, power, and invulnerability (NIDA 2007c). Other positive effects include heightened sensitivity to outside stimuli, a sense of stimulation and mood elevation, and dissociation from surroundings. Also, PCP is a social drug; virtually all users report taking it in groups rather than during a solitary experience. PCP also causes serious perceptual distortions. Users cannot accurately interpret the environment and as a result may do what appear to be absurd things such as jump out of a window thinking they can fly (APA 2000).

Chronic users may take PCP in "runs" extending over 2 to 3 days, during which time they do not sleep or eat. In later stages of chronic administration, users may develop outright paranoia, unpredictable violent behavior, and auditory hallucinations (APA 2000). Law enforcement officers claim to be more fearful of suspects on PCP than of suspects on other drugs of abuse. Often such people seem to have superhuman strength and are totally irrational and very difficult — even dangerous — to manage (NIDA 2007a; 2007c).

PCP has no equal in its ability to produce brief psychoses similar to schizophrenia (Jentsch and Roth 1999). The psychoses — induced with moderate doses given to normal, healthy volunteers — last about 2 hours and are characterized by changes in body image, thought disorders, estrangement, autism, and occasionally rigid inability to move (catatonia, or catalepsy). Subjects report feeling numb, have great difficulty differentiating between themselves and their surroundings, and complain afterward of feeling extremely isolated and apathetic. They are often violently paranoid during the psychosis (APA 2000; Medical Letter 1996). When PCP was given experimentally to hospitalized chronic schizophrenics, it made them much worse not for a few hours but for 6 weeks. PCP is not just another hallucinogen — many authorities view it as much more dangerous than other drugs of abuse (Dewan 2003; Maier 2003).

Medical Management The diagnosis of a PCP overdose is frequently missed because the

Key Terms

jimsonweed
a potent hallucinogenic plant

A Legal High, Least for Now

One user described smoking Salvia divinorum he purchased legally at a local health shop near his home. He related an experience unlike any other that gave him a consciousness-expanding journey. His body felt disconnected, resulting in people and objects taking on a car-toonish, surreal, and marvelous appearance. Abruptly the visions ended and the user found himself back in his room with his "sitter" (a person designated to watch the drug user to prevent accidents or harm — this was recommended on the product's package). The user felt awkward and clumsy when talking or trying to stand. Within a couple of minutes his mind felt clear although his body was damp from sweating. The whole experience lasted approximately 5 minutes. The user admits little is known about the adverse effects of Salvia and acknowledges the need for additional study. But in the interim, products containing legal hallucinogenic herbs such as Sahia are available in shops throughout the United States and around the world without regulation.

Source: Vince, G. "Legally High." New Scientist (30 September 2006): 40-45

symptoms often closely resemble those of an acute schizophrenic episode.

Simple, uncomplicated PCP intoxication can be managed with the same techniques used in other psychedelic drug cases. It is important to have a quiet environment, limited contact with an em-pathic person capable of determining any deterioration in the patient's physical state, protection from self-harm, and the availability of hospital facilities. Talking down is not helpful; the patient is better off isolated from external stimuli as much as possible.

Valium is often used for its sedating effect to prevent injury to self and to staff and also to reduce the chance for severe convulsions. An antipsychotic agent (for example, haloperidol [Haldol]) is frequently administered to make the patient manageable (Jaffe 1990).

The medical management of a comatose or convulsing patient is more difficult. The patient may need external respiratory assistance and external cooling to reduce fever. Blood pressure may have to be reduced to safe levels and convulsions controlled. Restraints and four to five strong hospital aides are often needed to prevent the patient from injuring himself or herself or the medical staff. After the coma lightens, the patient typically becomes delirious, paranoid, and violently assaultive.

Effects of Chronic Use Chronic PCP users may develop a tolerance to the drug; thus, a decrease in behavioral effects and toxicity can occur with frequent administration. Different forms of dependence may occur when tolerance develops. Users may complain of vague cravings after cessation of the drug. In addition, long-term difficulties in memory, speech, and thinking persist for 6 to 12 months in the chronic user (NIDA 2007c). These functional changes are accompanied by personality deficits such as social isolation and states of anxiety, nervousness, and extreme agitation (APA 2000).

Key Terms

analogs
  drugs with similar structures

Ketamine

Ketamine has received attention lately as a club drug. Its annual use in 2006 by high school seniors was 1.4% (Johnston 2007). Almost all persons who abuse ketamine have abused at least three other illicit drugs (Center for Substance Abuse Research [CESAR] 2006). Ketamine, like PCP, was originally developed for its general anesthetic properties (NIDA 2001). Its effects resemble those of PCP except they are more rapid and less potent (NIDA 2001). Depending on the dose, ketamine can have many effects, ranging from feelings of weightlessness to out-of-body or near-death experiences. Ketamine, often referred to as "Special K," has been abused as a "date rape" drug like other CNS depressants, such as Rohypnol or gamma-hydroxybutyrate (GHB) (see Chapter 6; NIDA 2001). Abuse of ketamine has been reported in many cities throughout the United States, and the drug is sometimes snorted as a substitute for cocaine. Several deaths have been linked to ketamine overdoses (NIDA 2007a).

Dextromethorphan

Dextromethorphan is the active ingredient used in many OTC cough medicines because of its ability to suppress the cough reflex (CESAR 2005). However, when consumed in high quantities (approximately ten times the recommended dose), it can cause some hallucinogenic effects much like PCP and ketamine do. These effects can vary and have been described as ranging from a mild stimulant effect to a complete dissociation from one's body. The effects can last for several hours. Abuse of dextromethorphan is typically done by teenagers and is sometimes referred to as "roboing" (CESAR 2005).

Marijuana

In high doses, marijuana use can result in image distortions and hallucinations (Nunez and Gurpegui 2002). Some users claim that marijuana can enhance hearing, vision, and skin sensitivity, although these claims have not been confirmed in controlled laboratory studies.

Although typical marijuana use does not appear to cause severe emotional disorders like the other hallucinogens, some experts suggest it can aggravate underlying mental illness such as depression. Each month, thousands of people seek professional treatment due to marijuana-related problems (Narconon 2007). In contrast to other hallucinogens that have a combination of stimulant and psychedelic effects, high doses of marijuana cause a combination of depression and hallucinations and enhance the appetite (Fleckenstein 2000). Marijuana is discussed thoroughly in Chapter 13.

Natural Substances

Naturally Occurring Hallucinogens

Many plants contain naturally occurring hallucmo gens. As already discussed, examples of such substances include mescaline from the peyote cactus, psilocybin from psilocybe mushrooms, and anticholinergic drugs such as atropine from the deadly nightshade plant, mandrake, or jimsonweed. Although some of these plants have been used for medicinal purposes for centuries, typically the therapeutic benefit has not been a consequence of the hallucinogenic effects of the substance. For example, anticholinergic drugs usually cause CNS depression and induce sleep; therefore, herbs that contain these drugs have been used as sleep potions. The hallucinogenic properties of some natural products, such as peyote, are viewed as positive by some cultures. As already mentioned, peyote is employed in a religious context as a sacrament for the Native American Church. In the United States today, the hallucinogen-containing natural substances are generally not viewed as therapeutic and are more likely to be used for their mind-altering properties as recreational drugs by adolescents (see "Case in Point," Jimsonweed Abuse in Idaho). In 2006 there were almost 1,000 reported incidents of poisonings with these hallucinogenic plants, most frequently by kids trying to get high (Leinwand 2006). Some users claim because these are natural rather than synthetic sources of a hallucinogenic episode, that somehow it makes the experience more rewarding and desirable. There is no evidence that the natural-versus-synthetic features of a hallucinogen areresponsible for the quality of a drug-induced hallucination. Frequently, consumption of these seeds and weeds causes severe hallucinations, dry mouth, hyperthermia, seizures, and occasionally death (Leinwand 2006).

Salvia Divinorum

Occasionally, obscure hallucinogenic herbs make their way into the culture of hallucinogenic substance users.. This migration has become easier because of the Internet and specialized web sites that provide information (some accurate and much available in shops throughout the United States and around the world without regulation.

anecdotal) and the means to acquire these typically natural substances. For example, a relatively recent hallucinogenic fad has been the use of the Mexican herb Salvia divinorum, a drug that did not reach the United States until the late 1980s (Allday 2007). This bright, leafy green plant can be smoked or chewed (Allday 2007). This relatively unknown plant is referred to as "diviner's mint" and is legal in most of the United States despite its ability to cause intense hallucinations, "out-of-body" experiences, and short-term memory loss (Jones 2001; Pienciak 2003). Promotions for these products include advertising claims such as "The Mazatec people have preserved Salvia divinorum and the knowledge surrounding its use for hundreds of years. We are privileged to have them share their sacred herb with us" (Jones 2001, p. A14). The dried herb can sell for as much as $15 to $50 a hit (Allday 2007). The drug typically makes the user introverted while "altering the conscious in unusual ways" (Vince 2006; see "Here and Now," A Legal High, At Least for Now). Although national drug information sources and law enforcement officers are not well informed about this hallucinogenic herb, the DEA has started to take notice and it has been outlawed in four states (Allday 2007). Law enforcement agencies claim to be watching carefully to see whether its use will cause significant health or social problems. This herb can have dramatic effects on perception similar to LSD (Allday 2007), causing hallucinations when chewed or smoked (Lein-wand 2003). It typically is not used in social settings and often is used only once because the effects can be quite unpleasant, often triggering a lack of coordination and frightening perceptions (Simmie 2003). Because of its frequent negative consequences, this herb is not viewed as particularly addicting (Pienciak 2003).

Over-the-Counter Medication and Herbal or Dietary Supplement Use in College

Dose Frequency and Relationship to Self-Reported Distress

By Michael Stasio and Kim Curry

Objective: *A growing number of researchers have examined the use of over-the-counter (OTC) medications and herbal or dietary supplements among college students. There is concern about the efficacy and safety of these products, particularly because students appear to use them at a higher rate than does the general public. Participants and Methods: The authors administered surveys to college students (N = 201) to assess the frequency of use in the past week. Results: A substantial percentage reported using OTC medications (74.1%), herbal or dietary supplements (70.6%), or both concurrently (61.2%). Dose frequency of OTC medications was the best predictor of self-reported emotional distress in the past week. Higher doses of products containing pseudoephedrine or valerian were associated with self-reported anxiety. Conclusions: These data further reflect an increasing trend toward self-medication among college students. Investigators must conduct reliability and validity studies to evaluate the clinical utility of the measurement tool developed in this study.*

Keywords: *college students, distress, herbs, over-the-counter, supplements*

The trend toward self-medication in the United States is clearly reflected in the increasing use of over- the-counter (OTC) medicines and herbal or dietary supplements. Kennedy[1] analyzed data from 31,044 adults who participated in the 2002 National Health Interview Survey and estimated that approximately 19% of adults in the United States had used an herbal or dietary supplement in the past 12 months, nearly double the percentage

Michael J. Stasio, Kim Curry, Kelly M. Sutton-Skinner, & Destinee M. Glassman, "Over-the-Counter Medication and Herbal or Dietary Supplement Use in College: Dose Frequency and Relationship to Self-Reported Distress," *Journal of American College Health*, vol. 56, no. 5, pp. 535-547. Copyright © 2008 by Heldref Publications. Reprinted with permission.

reported in 1999. Researchers have been studying this trend closely,

because despite widespread use of these products, their efficacy and safety have not been well studied, and some products with known health risks remain on the market. For example, although the US Food and Drug Administration (FDA) in 2004 prohibited the sale of the stimulant ephedra (ma huang) because of reports citing risks to cardiovascular and central nervous system functions, the product remains available while legal appeals are pending.[2] Furthermore, there is strong evidence that common OTC sedative antihistamines cause deficits in attention, concentration, psycho- motor functioning, and verbal learning.[2-4]

Given the research findings and known risks, college health professionals must obtain reliable and accurate information about students' OTC medication and herbal or dietary supplement use. Underscoring this point is evidence that college students use these products more frequently than do members of the general public. For example, Newberry et al[5] surveyed 272 college students to assess the use frequency of nonvitamin, non-mineral dietary supplements (daily, weekly, or monthly) and found that 48% of participants reported using at least 1 product in the past month. Although that survey yielded information about participants' patterns of use, few currently available instruments focus on individual dose frequency of a particular substance used in the past week. Such a measurement tool would increase the reliability of participants' responses more so than instruments that require participants to estimate frequency of product use over the past month or year. One of our goals in the present study—and one that sits well under the umbrella of the Healthy Campus 2010 initiative[6]—was to pilot test the format of an easy-to-use tool assessing dose frequency of OTC medications and herbal or dietary supplements that students could

complete as part of the assessment procedures conducted at university health and counseling centers.

Many college students experience considerable emotional distress, particularly related to anxiety and depression. For example, in the 2005 American College Health Association National College Health Assessment survey (N = 54,111) students commonly reported anxiety (13.4%), depression (19.6%), and serious thoughts of suicide (10.2%) in the past year, and many more reported feelings of hopelessness (63.8%), sadness (80.7%), and a sense of being overwhelmed (93.8%).[7] Results from the National Epidemiologic Survey on Alcohol and Related Conditions showed notable co-occurrences of anxiety and substance-use disorders (17.75%) as well as depression and substance-abuse disorders (20.13%).[8] It is therefore reasonable to ask whether students' self-reported emotional distress is associated with use of OTC and herbal or dietary supplements. Kava (Piper methysticum), for instance, is a ceremonial herb originating from the Polynesian Islands that has known sedative and anxiolytic effects and is used as an alternative to medications commonly prescribed for anxiety.[9,10] Few researchers have examined the relationship between the use of kava—or other herbal sedatives such as valerian—and college students' reported experiences of emotional distress.

OTC Medications and General Safety

The FDA defines OTC medications as drugs characterized by low potential for misuse, usefulness by consumers in self- diagnosed conditions, and ability to be safely used without the involvement of a medical provider.[11] OTC medications, also known as nonprescription medications, give patients the ability to manage the treatment of many common medical conditions while freeing the healthcare system to expend resources on more serious diseases and conditions. The FDA increasingly converts prescribed drugs to OTC status. Rizzo[12] noted that this practice is consistent with the national move toward consumerism in health care and the preference of many healthcare consumers to self-medicate.

A few investigators have attempted to illustrate safety issues surrounding the use of OTC medications. Although these medications have demonstrated benefits outweighing their risks, they are not without side effects. For example, loratadine, a popular antihistamine, has been shown to increase the likelihood of some cardiac dysrrhythmias.[13] Another safety issue is intentional overdose. Lo[14] reviewed the medical records of 95 Canadian patients who engaged in intentional overdose of medication. Although 71% of overdose attempts were limited to prescription drugs, younger patients and patients with a diagnosis of substance abuse were most likely to attempt overdose with OTC medications. The most common OTC medication used for overdose was acetaminophen.

College Student Use of OTC Medication

General Use

Findings from college student samples generally show that a high percentage of participants used OTC medications. Burak and Damico[15] surveyed 471 students and found that almost 89% reported using at least 1 of 24 commonly advertised medications (M = 2.3). The authors found that the 3 most commonly used medications were Advil—which 83.86% of the sample used—Midol, and Excedrin, which were used by 32.91% and 32.48%, respectively. In fact, the majority of students used analgesics without consulting their physician, suggesting a familiarity and comfort with this type of medication. Regarding sex, most researchers have found that women purchase and use OTC medications more than do men.[16,17] The products most often purchased are cold and flu relievers (53%), ibuprofen (49.9%), aspirin (49.2%), cough medications (44.8%), and vitamins (36.5%). In addition, women reportedly are more likely to abuse laxatives, whereas men tend to abuse a combination of OTC medications and alcohol.[17]

Howland et al[18] studied OTC medication use in college seniors suffering from allergy symptoms and found that 63.0% of the sample reported moderate to severe symptoms in the past year. The investigators found that 91.1% of students reporting allergy symptoms used OTC medications to treat them; 55.5% also used prescription medications. This finding is important to note in this age group because evidence suggests that certain types of allergy medications—notably sedative antihistamines—can impair a range of cognitive functions.

Age and participation in some extracurricular groups also have been linked to OTC medication use. In general, people younger than 60 purchase OTC medications more regularly and favor drug deregulation more than do older individuals.[17] Younger and older adults do not differ in their use of some types of medications: both are equally likely to have purchased and used pain relievers, cold remedies, and antacids. Regarding extracurricular participation, Simons et al[19] surveyed 317 undergraduate college students and found that those who participated in drinking games, collegiate sports, and Greek organizations had a higher rate of both OTC and prescription drug use than did those who did not participate. A majority of freshmen used OTC and prescription medication, but less than one-third reported illicit drug use. In addition, past substance abuse was the best predictor of OTC and prescription medication use, whereas past 30-day alcohol use (to which 96% of the sample admitted) was the next best predictor of OTC drug use.

Use of OTC Pain Medications and Sleep Aids

Researchers have shown that the use of OTC medications to relieve pain begins at an early age. Reid[20] surveyed 651 junior high school students in Canada, and 75% reported self-administering OTC pain medication. The students experienced pain symptoms including headache, ear and throat pain, stomach pain, menstrual pain, and musculoskeletal pain. The most common medication selected was acetaminophen. The author noted that 6% to 20% of students were taking medication that may not have been appropriate, given their reported symptoms. More than half of the students had taken pain medication within the past 3 months without consulting an adult.

Pillitteri et al[21] studied insomnia in a sample of 278 undergraduate and graduate students and found that more than 80% had difficulty falling asleep 1 to 4 nights per month. Among women, 11.4% used OTC sleep medications, and 10.9% used alcohol to induce sleep. Among men, 6.4% used OTC sleep medications, and 23.4% used alcohol to induce sleep. The authors also noted that 1 OTC nighttime cold medication listed 10% alcohol as one of the active ingredients.

OTC Medications with Neuropsychological Effects

Stein and Strickland[3] reviewed the neuropsychological effects of commonly used prescription and nonprescription medications. Two widely used drugs—sedative antihistamines and pseudoephedrine—have direct central nervous system effects and are often combined in cold remedies. Thirty million Americans, for instance, report using anti- histamines (H_1 antagonists) each year to treat allergy symptoms. First-generation antihistamines, such as diphenhydramine or chlorpheniramine, have known sedative effects. Deficits in psychomotor function, attention, concentration, memory, and driving skills have been associated with use of such sedative antihistamines. In an imaging study using positron emission tomography, Mochizuki et al[4] found that the use of d-chlorpheniramine alternately increased and decreased activity in the areas of the brain responsible for attention and visual spatial processing. Although Stein and Strickland[3] noted that the effects of regular sedative antihistamine use have not been well studied in clinical trials, Charlton[22] recently recommended that individuals who are self-managing anxiety disorders should consider diphenhydramine and chlorpheniramine. Pseudoephedrine, which is used primarily as a decongestant, is a stimulant that mimics the actions of norepinephrine and epinephrine. Unfortunately, few investigators have examined the effect of pseudoephedrine on cognitive functioning.

Use of Herbs and Dietary Supplements

Herbs

A considerable number of adults and adolescents report using herbs and dietary supplements. Kennedy[1] analyzed the use of complementary and alternative medicines in a sample of more than 30,000 adults who participated in the 2002 National Health Interview Survey. The findings yielded a weighted estimate of 38.2 million Americans (18.9%) who had used an herb or supplement product in the past 12 months. The prevalence of use was higher for women (21.0%) than for men (16.7%) and higher for college graduates (25.3%) than for people who did not complete high school (10.4%). The percentage of 18- to 24-year-olds who used at least 1 of these products in the past 12 months was 16.1%. Participants used several herbal products frequently, among them Echinacea (38.4%), ginseng (23.0%), and garlic supplements (18.6%). Interestingly, only 34% of respondents indicated they routinely informed medical professionals of their use of herbs and dietary supplements.

Wilson et al[23] surveyed about 1,300 adolescents aged 14 to 19 years and found a relatively higher lifetime rate of herb and supplement use (46.2%), although the inclusion of vitamins in this category likely accounted for the difference.

Vitamins and Minerals

Fennell[24] examined the past-year use of vitamins and minerals of about 24,800 adults who participated in the 2000 National Health Interview Survey. The results revealed an effect of sex: women reported higher use of vitamins or minerals than did men (57.9% vs. 46.0%, respectively). In addition, non-Latino whites, older participants, and those who had completed college reported higher use of vitamins and minerals. A slight majority of participants had used vitamins or minerals (52.7%) in the past year, and a notable number of respondents reported using multiple vitamins (40.1%), vitamin C (20.5%), and vitamin E (17.1%.) Wilson et al[23] found similar results regarding the use of vitamins among adolescents: lifetime use was 66.9%, and current use was 54.2%.

Weight Loss Supplements and Performance Enhancers

Products marketed to promote weight loss and improve athletic performance often contain stimulants. Haller et al[25] noted that bitter orange (Citrus aurantium) contains the active ingredient synephrine and has quickly replaced the recently banned drug ephedra in some weight loss supplements. Researchers are beginning to conduct laboratory studies in which they examine the use and physiological effects of products containing synephrine. Haller and colleagues[25] used a double-blind, placebo-controlled study to test the effects of synephrine on 10 individuals; results showed that Xenadrine EFX, a multi-ingredient formulation, increased systolic and diastolic blood pressure, as well as heart rate, over synephrine alone or placebo. They concluded that these ephedra-free weight loss products were cardiovascular stimulants similar to ephedra, although the observed effects were unlikely caused by synephrine alone.

Although college athletes may be reluctant to report their use of drugs to enhance performance, there is evidence that some use stimulants toward this end. In one recent study, Bents et al[26] administered questionnaires to 122 National Collegiate Athletic Association Division 1 hockey players to assess their use of performance-enhancing drugs. A majority of players (58%) reported past or present use of at least 1 performance-enhancing drug, and participants reported use of pseudoephedrine (48% lifetime; 24% current use) and ephedrine (38% lifetime; 11% current use).

Use of Herbs with Neuropsychological Effects

Several herbal preparations also have general psychotropic effects. The most commonly used products of this type are ginkgo biloba, kava, St. John's wort, and valerian. Ken- nedy[1] extrapolated the following use-percentage estimates from a large sample of US adults: ginkgo biloba (20.1%), St. John's wort (11.5%), kava (6.4%), and valerian (5.6%). Beaubrum and Gray[27] reviewed the psychotropic properties

of these preparations. US adults use ginkgo biloba, made from parts of the gingko (maidenhair, kew) tree, primarily to prevent or treat memory problems, including those related to dementia. St. John's wort, made from the hypericum plant, is commonly used as an antidepressant, and evidence suggests that it blocks the reuptake of both norepinephrine and serotonin. Kava (also known as kava kava) is prepared from a shrub native to Polynesia and the Pacific Islands and acts primarily as an anxiolytic. Kava is one of the few herbal psychotropics with a known active ingredient—kavapyrones—although its mechanism of action remains unclear. Valerian has been shown to have primarily sedative and anticonvulsive effects by both increasing production and blocking reuptake of gamma-aminobutyric acid.

The cognitive effects and risks associated with the use of these preparations have either not been well studied or are just beginning to emerge. For instance, St. John's wort is commonly used to treat mild to moderate depression, yet its potential health risks are not fully understood. Hypericin, which is believed (but not yet proven) to be the active ingredient in St. John's wort, may interact with medications such as digoxin or warfarin and lessen the effects of antiretroviral regimens used in HIV treatment.[27,28] St. John's wort also reportedly decreases the efficacy of certain oral contraceptives.[1] Last, Van Rijswijk et al[29] studied the characteristics of those who use OTC psychotropic medication and found that users experienced more psychological symptoms or distress—but not somatic problems—than did nonusers.

Emotional Distress and Self-Medication

College students experience a variety of medical problems and emotional distress. According to the American College Health Association,[7] the most common symptoms include allergies (52.2%), back pain (51.2%), sinus infection (33.4%), depression (19.6%), and anxiety (13.4%). Such findings are likely related to the numerous demands (eg, academic, social, financial) that college environments place on students at a key developmental time when many are also struggling with independence and choices related to relationships, lifestyles, and careers. Healthy Campus 2010,[6] the national healthcare agenda for students aged 18 to 25, features several objectives that are affected by self-medication among college students. These include preventive health care, healthcare access, and alcohol and drug use. Steinman[16] found a positive relationship between high school students' OTC medication use and the presence of depressive affect, violent behavior, and the use of alcohol and illicit drugs. The author suggested that students' experience of stress and the tendency toward maladaptive coping strategies interact to influence the use (and misuse) of OTC medications and other drugs. In addition, higher levels of prosocial behavior were associated with less misuse of OTC medications and other substances.

Hart and Hill[30] studied the influence of premenstrual distress on the generalized use of OTC analgesics. The authors hypothesized that women who experienced higher levels of premenstrual distress were more likely to use analgesics beyond the premenstrual phase in a typical week than were women experiencing lower levels of premenstrual distress. Women who experienced premenstrual symptoms used analgesics more frequently and in higher doses than did women who did not experience such distress. The authors also observed that the frequency of analgesic use correlated positively with symptoms such as pain, water retention, autonomic reactions, and negative affect, whereas the average quantity of analgesic use correlated positively with pain and negative affect. The authors argue that the relationship between analgesic use and premenstrual distress may generalize beyond the premenstrual phase to the use of analgesics for somatic (ie, stress) and negative mood symptoms.

Summary and Rationale for Current Study

Use of OTC medications and herbal or dietary supplements allows consumers a role in self-management of health. Such use is consistent with the ongoing trend toward self-medication in the United States. Evidence shows that adolescents and young adults are active users of OTC medications and other nonprescription products, and this use increases with the presence of health symptoms. Few researchers have examined the use of both OTC and herbal or dietary supplements in the college population. We are unaware of assessment tools that measure recent volume of use in this population. OTC medications and herbal or dietary supplements may be misused or abused. Several such preparations are known to have psychotropic effects. There is a need for further study to document quantity of specific products and the relationship between self-medication and the presence of health symptoms.

METHODS

Participants

Students (N = 201) enrolled at a private southeastern university participated in this study (125 women and 76 men, M age = 22.3 years, SD = 4.85). The sample consisted of 126 students from the College of Liberal Arts and Sciences, 70 students from the College of Business, and 5 students who classified themselves as undeclared. The majority of participants were upper-division students (15 freshmen, 37 sophomores, 62 juniors, 79 seniors, and 4 graduate students). Participants volunteered for this study, and we did not compensate them for participation. (We did offer extra course credit at the instructors' discretion.) The university's institutional review board approved the study.

Materials

Reliably measuring the frequency of OTC medication and herbal and dietary supplement use is important, particularly as it relates to the delivery of clinical services at college health centers. Researchers in most studies cited in the literature reduced respondents' estimated use frequency data to a yes-no dichotomy to indicate use of one of these types of products during at least one time period (eg, 12- month, lifetime). A limitation to this approach is the tempered reliability of the resulting data. For example, although it is helpful to know that use of an herbal product at least once in the past 12 months may be linked to the use other substances, data reflecting current use (eg, weekly) would lessen respondents' recall bias, increase the reliability of the data, and improve the quality of the clinical assessment.

Survey Construction

The survey developed for this study was a paper-and-pen- cil measure of past-week dose frequency for various OTC medications and herbs or dietary supplements. A small group of professionals that consisted of a practicing pharmacist and 2 university faculty members (a nurse practitioner and a clinical psychologist) developed the survey. The instrument consisted of a general list of commonly available OTC medications and herbs or dietary supplements, with extra space provided for participants to write in any products they used that were not listed. Categories of OTC medications included allergy, cough and cold, indigestion /constipation, pain relievers, and sleep aids. Categories of herbs and dietary supplements included herbs, performance enhancers, vitamins and minerals, and weight loss supplements. We constructed all categories to reflect those that consumers would likely see when purchasing these products at drug and other retail stores, with the rationale that such continuity would increase the instrument's ease of use (see Appendix A).

The survey design allowed participants to estimate the number of product doses used on each day of the previous week in blank boxes arranged in rows. The survey resembled a typical behavioral self-monitoring tool designed to measure frequency of any selected target behavior. The following directions appeared at the top of the survey: "Write the number of adult recommended doses taken per day (1, 2, 3, or 4) in each box that corresponds to days DURING THE PAST WEEK. If zero (0) doses taken, leave box blank." We asked participants to estimate their use of various products over the past week (versus taking the survey home and making daily entries for the next week, as is the case in most self-monitoring procedures) to maximize the number of completed surveys returned. Appendix B presents a portion of the survey as an example of its design and appearance.

In addition to the survey, we gave participants a handout with brief descriptions of each of the products listed. We did so to provide them with extra information as needed about the products and to minimize the length of the administration sessions. We compiled product descriptions directly from the manufacturers (either from the packaging materials or product Web site). An example of a typical product description is: "Benadryl. Diphenhydramine is used to treat cold and allergy symptoms, suppress cough, treat motion sickness, and induce sleep."

Design and Procedure

We recruited survey participants in a quasi-random fashion. We e-mailed instructors from each department to ask whether they would be willing to yield 10-15 minutes of

a regular class period for students to complete the survey. We administered the survey to students in 20 classes in the College of Liberal Arts and Sciences and to 13 classes in the College of Business. We followed a standard protocol for each administration session. We first distributed, reviewed, and collected the anonymous informed consent. (As a way to increase the accuracy of responses, we did not require students to sign their names.) We gave participants the handout that contained brief product descriptions and then distributed the survey. We waited until participants had finished the survey before collecting it. Students generally completed the survey in 10 minutes.

RESULTS

We first analyzed the data to ascertain the percentage of students, across several demographic groups, who reported using OTC medications, herbal and dietary supplements, and both concurrently. We coded all use percentages dichotomously (yes or no). We also compiled the reported number of adult recommended doses used per week for each product. We chose the median as the best measure of central tendency for all dose-frequency data because these distributions were nonsymmetrical. We compared use percentages between demographic groups (eg, spring vs summer term) with a chi-square test for goodness of fit. We compared dose frequencies with the median test, a nonparametric procedure that tests whether 2 samples come from a population with the same median; it also yields a chi-square statistic. We estimated effect sizes for significant chi-square test results by computing the phi coefficient ($) as recommended by Gravetter and Wallnau.[31] We did not test for changes in use percentage and dose frequency within each demographic group because the assumption of independence was not met (ie, the same student may have contributed to the use percentage and dose frequency of both OTC medications and

TABLE 1. Doses of Over-the-Counter Medications and Herbs and Supplements Used in the Past Week, by Demographic Group and Product Type

Demographic	n	Over-the-counter medication		Herbs and supplements		Both used concurrently	
		%	Median dose frequency	%	Median dose frequency	%	Median dose frequency
All participants	201	74.1	5.0	70.6	10.0	61.2	14.0
Academic term							
Spring	101	80.2*	10.0**	79.2*	17.5**	67.3	32.0**
Summer	100	68.8	5.0	62.0	12.0	55.0	20.0
Sex							
Male	76	64.5*	9.0	71.1	15.0	56.6	27.0
Female	125	80.0	8.0	70.4	14.0	64.0	27.0
Age (y)							
17–20	100	72.0	8.0	71.0	14.0	64.0	28.0
> 21	99	75.8	9.0	69.6	14.5	57.6	28.0
College							
CLAS	126	80.2*	8.0	74.6	15.0	64.3	25.0
COB	70	64.3	8.0	64.3	14.0	54.4	24.0
Class							
Freshman	15	80.0	10.5	73.3	13.0	66.7	25.0
Sophomore	38	81.1	7.5	75.7	14.0	73.0	27.0
Junior	62	71.0	7.5	74.2	14.0	66.1	26.0
Senior	79	70.9	8.5	63.3	16.5	49.4	27.0
Extracurricular activity[a]							
Exercise 3 times/wk	118	75.2	7.0	72.6	16.5	65.0	27.0
Greek	53	66.0	10.0	77.4	14.0	67.9	31.5
Intramural	40	75.0	8.5	72.5	14.0	62.5	28.5
ROTC	21	71.4	9.0	85.7	16.0	66.7	32.0
Varsity sport	13	69.2	4.0	61.5	15.5	61.5	36.0

Note. CLAS = College of Liberal Arts and Sciences; COB = College of Business; ROTC = Reserve Officers' Training Corps.
[a]Nonexclusive groups; tests done between yes–no group membership.
*Significant χ² test difference (*p* < .05) between groups for use percentage.** Significant χ² difference (*p* < .05) between groups for median dose frequency.

herbs and dietary supplements). Table 1 presents these data.

Initial analyses using the entire sample showed that most students (74.1%) reported using OTC medication in the past week ($x^2[1, N = 201] = 46.81$, p < .001, $ = .48). A similarly large proportion of students (70.6%) reported using an herb or dietary supplement in the past week ($\%^2[1, N = 201] = 34.27$, p < .001, $ = .41). Fewer students— although still a majority (61.2%)—reported concurrent use of both product types in the past week compared with those who used either 1 product or neither ($x^2[1, N = 201] = 10.08$, p = .002, $ = .22). Median weekly dose frequencies for students

who reported using OTC medications, herbs and dietary supplements, and both product types concurrently were 5.0, 10.0, and 14.0, respectively.

Analysis of Product Use by Demographic Groups

The analysis of demographic variables began with academic term (spring, summer). We found that academic term had a consistent effect on both the use percentage and median dose frequency reported for each product type. A marginally greater percentage of students reported using OTC medications in the spring term (80.2%) than

TABLE 2. Doses of Over-the-Counter (OTC) Medications and Herbs and Supplements Used in the Past Week by Product Type and Academic Term

				Academic term		
	Total (N = 201)		Spring (n = 101)		Summer (n = 100)	
Product type	%	Median dose frequency	%	Median dose frequency	%	Median dose frequency
OTC medication						
Allergy	30.8	4.5	30.7	6.0	31.0	3.0
Cough and cold**	11.4	4.0	12.9	7.0	10.0	2.5
Indigestion/constipation	9.0	2.5	10.9	3.0	7.0	2.0
Pain reliever**	59.7	5.0	62.4	6.0	57.0	3.0
Sleep aid***	23.9	5.0	30.7	6.0	17.0	3.0
Herbs and supplements						
Herbal*	31.3	7.0	37.6	7.0	23.0	7.0
Performance enhancer	16.4	7.0	17.8	9.5	15.0	5.0
Vitamins and minerals*	59.7	12.0	66.3	13.0	51.0	10.0
Weight loss*	14.4	7.0	19.8	7.0	9.0	3.0

*Significant χ^2 difference (p < .05) between spring and summer use percentage.** Significant χ^2 difference (p < .05) between spring and summer median dose frequency.*** Significant χ^2 difference (p < .05) between spring and summer median dose frequency and use percentage.

in the summer term (68.8%; X^2[1, N = 201] = 3.90, p = .048, $ = .13). The median dose frequency for OTC medications was also greater in the spring term (10.0) than in the summer (5.0; x^2[1, N = 153] = 11.12, p < .001, $ = .27). We found similar results for herbs and supplements; a greater percentage of students reported using them in the spring (79.2%) versus the summer term (62.0%; X^2[1, N = 201] = 7.17, p = .007, $ = .19). We found the median dose frequency of herbs and dietary supplements to be greater in the spring term (17.5) than in the summer (12.0; X^2[1, N = 145] = 5.90, p = .015, $ = .20). Last, the median dose frequency of concurrent use of OTC medications and herbs and supplements was notably greater in spring (32.0) than in summer (20.0; X^2[1, N = 123] = 16.72, p < .001, $ = .36). The difference between concurrent use percentages in the spring term (67.3%) versus the summer (55.0%) was not statistically significant (x^2[1, N = 201] = 3.11, p = .073, ns).

Next, we analyzed the influence of several other demographic groups on students' use of the products under investigation. From among the

variables sex, age, college, class, and extracurricular participation, only sex and college influenced the percentage of students who reported OTC medication use. A significantly greater proportion of women (80.0%) than men (64.5%) reported using OTC medications in the past week (x^2[1, N = 201] = 5.94, p = .015, $ = .17). We observed no effect of sex on the use percentage of herbs and supplements, concurrent use of both product types, or median dose frequency for any product type. We also found that students enrolled in the College of Liberal Arts and Sciences were more likely to report using OTC medications in the past week (80.2%) than were their College of Business counterparts (64.3%; x^2[1, N = 201] = 6.44, p = .040, $ = .18). Just as in the results for the sex variable, no other effect of college was statistically meaningful. The extracurricular groups included exercise > 3 times per week, Greek participant, intramural athlete, Reserve Officer Training Corps participant, and varsity athlete. Membership in any of these groups had little influence on either the percentage of students who used OTC medicines or herbal products or the number of times per week they used them.

Analysis of Product Use by Academic Term

With the next series of analyses, we explored changes in use patterns between the spring and summer terms for specific types of nonprescription products. As in the previous analyses, we used chi-square tests of goodness of fit to compare differences in use percentage and median tests to compare differences in median dose frequency. First, we calculated total use percentages and median dose frequencies for each product type. The products reportedly used most in the past week were pain relievers (59.7%) and vitamins and minerals (59.7%). About one-third of participants reported using allergy medication (30.8%) and herbs (31.3%) in the past week, and about one-fourth (23.9%) reported using sleep aids. Next, we calculated the use percentages and median dose frequencies and analyzed them by academic term (see Table 2).

Considering categories of OTC medications, we found that the percentage of students who reported using sleep aids in the spring term (30.7%) was greater than the percentage of summer users (17.0%; $\%^2$[1, n = 201] = 5.18, p = .023, $ = .16). Among the remaining variables tested— allergy, cough and cold, indigestion/constipation, and pain relievers—we found no difference in the percentage of student use between the spring and summer terms. Regarding median dose frequency, however, we observed several differences. The median dose frequency for those using pain relievers was significantly greater in the spring term (6.0) than it was in summer (3.0; X^2[1, N = 120] = 17.85, p < .001, $ = .29). For students who reported using sleep aids, the median dose frequency was also greater in the spring term (6.0) than it was in summer (3.0; $\%^2$[1, N = 48] = 6.00, p = .021, $ = .35). This same pattern held

for the median dose frequency of cough and cold medication in the spring (7.0) compared with the summer term (2.5; $\%^2$[1, N = 23] = 10.14, p = .001, $ = .66).

An analysis of use patterns for categories of herbs and supplements revealed that the percentage of students who reported using herbal products in the spring term (37.6%) was significantly greater than those reporting use in the summer term (23.0%; X^2[1, N = 201] = 5.08, p = .023, $ = .16). The percentage of those using weight loss products in the spring term (19.8%) also was greater than the percentage of those of used these products in the summer (9.0%; X^2[1, N = 201] = 4.74, p = .029, $ = .15). The use percentage reported for vitamins and minerals was also greater in the spring (66.3%) than it was in the summer term (51.0%; X^2[1, N = 201] = 4.87, p = .027, $ = .15). Last, median tests revealed no effect of academic term on the median dose frequency for herbal products, performance enhancers, vitamins and minerals, or weight loss supplements.

Analysis of Product Use and Physical and Emotional Distress

With the next series of analyses, we examined the relationship between the use of nonprescription products and the reported presence of physical illness or personal distress in the past week. We computed both the percentage of students reporting each type of problem and the number of problems reported. Given the large number of significance tests required to investigate these relationships, we adopted the more conservative alpha level of p = .01. We dichotomously coded (yes-no) whether a participant reported physical or adjustment problems, to indicate the presence or absence of problems related to anxiety, eating, mood, physical health, sexuality, and sleeping. Group membership by problem type was nonexclusive (ie, students could endorse more than one

TABLE 3. Students Reporting Physical Illness or Personal Distress in the Past Week and the Number of Problems Reported

Problems in past week	n	%
Type		
Anxiety	54	26.9
Eating	32	15.9
Mood	50	24.9
Physically ill	54	29.9
Sexual	10	5.0
Sleeping	67	33.3
Any type	137	68.2
Number reported		
0	64	31.8
1	61	30.3
2	38	18.9
3	24	11.9
4	8	4.0
5	5	2.5

problem). Regarding the total sample, a significant majority of students (n = 137) reported that they had experienced at least 1 problem in the past week ($X^2[1, N = 201] = 26.51$, p < .001, $ = .36). The number of past-week problems ranged from 0 to 5 (M = 1.32, SD = 1.28). Roughly one-third of the participants reported no problems in the past week (31.8%), whereas another third reported 1 problem (30.3%; see Table 3).

In subsequent analyses, we tested whether academic term influenced either the percentage of students reporting particular types of problems or the average number of problems reported. We submitted the percentage data to a series of chi-square analyses that revealed no effect of academic term on any problem type. We found no differences between spring and summer term in the proportion of students who reported distress related to anxiety ($x^2[1, N = 201] = 0.35$, p = .553, ns), eating ($x^2[1, N = 201] = 2.28$, p = .131, ns), mood ($x^2[1, N = 201] = 0.38$, p = .540, ns), physical illness ($X^2[1, N = 201] = 2.39$, p = .121, ns), sexuality ($x^2[1, N = 201] = 1.64$, p = .200, ns), sleeping ($x^2[1, N = 201] = 0.40$, p = .842, ns), or any problem ($x^2[1, N = 201] = 1.23$ p = .776, ns).

The average number of problems reported by students in the spring term (M = 1.47, SD = 1.39) was not significantly different from the average reported in summer (M = 1.18, SD = 1.16; F[1, 199] = 2.49, p = .116, ns).

We next analyzed the relationships among product use, median dose frequency, and number of past-week physical and adjustment problems. We screened the data prior to the application of linear regression analysis. Predictor variables included OTC medication use (yes or no), OTC medication dose frequency, herb and supplement use (yes or no), and herb and supplement dose frequency. The total number of past-week physical and adjustment problems served as the dependent variable. The predictor variables, as expected, were intercorrelated (range: r = .10-.48), but we ruled out colinearity after examining the colinearity diagnostics in SPSS (SPSS, Inc, Chicago, IL; Condition Index = 4.09), as recommended by Keith.[32] Results of this analysis showed that only 1 predictor—OTC medication dose frequency—explained a significant portion of the variance in the number of problems reported in the past week (B[N = 195] = .28, SE = .01, p = .001, $R^2 = .061$).

The previous finding prompted a series of logistic regression analyses in which we examined how well the dose frequencies of OTC medications predicted the presence of each category of physical illness and personal distress reported. Predictor variables (entered simultaneously) were the dose frequencies of classes of OTC medications (allergy, cough and cold, indigestion, pain relievers, and sleep aids), and the dependent measures were the presence or absence of each reported problem. Dose frequency of cough and cold medication was positively related to past-week physical illness (r = .48) and explained a significant portion of variance in category membership ($AR^2 = .28$). The dose frequency of sleep aids also was positively related to sleep problems (r = .36) and explained a significant amount of variance in student endorsement of this problem ($AR^2 = .28$). Interestingly, dose frequencies of both pain relievers and sleep aids were positively correlated with past-week anxiety ($r = .26$ and .19, respectively), and both variables predicted endorsement of this type of distress ($AR^2 = .08$ and .05, respectively). Table 4 presents the data for this analysis.

Analysis of Selected Pain Relievers and Psychotropic Agents

Last, we examined the relationship between selected pain relievers and drugs with known neuropsychological effects and students' endorsement of anxiety. The dose frequencies of 2 pain relievers—acetaminophen and ibuprofen—were each composites of 3 OTC medications containing that drug. Two of the drugs (typically used as sleep aids) with central nervous system effects—diphenhydramine and valerian—were also composites of different products. We conducted a series of point-biseral correlations between the various drugs and past-week anxiety. The dose frequency of psuedoephedrine was positively related to endorsement of anxiety ($r = .23$, $N = 201$, $p = .001$). Similarly, increased doses of valerian were positively related to endorsement of anxiety distress ($r = .22$, $N = 201$, $p = .002$), as was increased doses of ibuprofen ($r = .20$, $N = 201$, $p = .002$). Table 5 presents results from this analysis.

COMMENT

These data support the assertion that a considerable percentage of college students use OTC medication (74.1%) and herbal or dietary supplements, including vitamins and minerals (70.4%). The high frequency of OTC medication use was actually lower than previously reported in one college sample,[15] although those data were limited to lifetime use of popularly advertised medications and did not examine a range of medications used in the past week. Regarding use of herbal or dietary supplements, the high frequency of use we found was greater than expected, given that 19% of respondents in the 2002 National Health Interview Survey[1] and 48% of a recent college sample[5] reported use of a non- vitamin, nonmineral supplement in the past year.

One explanation for these discrepancies is that we included the use of vitamins and minerals in the total percentage calculations, whereas other investigators did not. However, when we removed vitamins and minerals from the herbal or dietary supplement total, the use percentage remained substantial at 50.2%. Another possibility for the high use rates we found is that the study was truly anonymous: participants did not have to sign their names to the consent form to participate (and thus may have provided more accurate data.) Another factor may have been the format of the survey, which assessed use frequency over the past week rather than in the past month or year. We assert that these data reflect larger trends toward self-medication and pharmacotherapy among US college students and thus indicate that students' use of these products is considerable.

Regarding previously well-studied demographic variables such as sex and age, our data partially support previous findings. Similar to most work, a greater percentage of women than men in our study reported past-week OTC medication use, although the effect was modest ($\$ = .17$). Sex influenced neither the percentage of students who used herbal or dietary supplements in the past week nor the dose frequency with which they used them. These findings suggest that sex differences are less pronounced among college students and generally replicate findings by Newberry et al.[5] Although previous study findings hold that use of OTC and herbal or dietary

TABLE 4. Logistic Regression Model Summary Predicting Reported Problem Types From Dose Frequencies of Over-the-Counter Medications Used in Past Week

Problem type	Significant predictor	B	SE	R^2	χ^2	p
Anxiety	Pain reliever	.10	0.03	.08	10.57	< .001
	Sleep aid	.14	0.06	.05	6.36	.001
Eating	—					
Mood	Allergy	.11	0.05	.03	4.10	.047
Physically ill	Cough and cold	1.00	0.31	.28	42.72	< .001
Sexual	—					
Sleeping	Sleep aid	.30	0.68	.16	25.19	< .001

Note. The following predictors were entered simultaneously: allergy, cough and cold, indigestion/constipation, pain reliever, and sleep aid. Each predictor represents the dose frequencies of that medication. $N = 201$. For each chi-square test, $N = 201$ and $df = 1$.

supplements tends to increase with age, we found no effect of age on reported use patterns. This finding was not surprising, given that only 12% of participants in this sample were aged older than 24 years.

An important aspect of the current study was that we assessed both use percentage and dose frequency of various OTC medications and herbal or dietary supplements.

Differences between the 2 were particularly evident when we compared spring and summer academic terms. Not only did a greater percentage of students use OTC medications and herbal or dietary supplements in the spring term than in summer term, but they also self-administered them more often. One explanation may be simply that students are more likely to experience allergy symptoms in the springtime than in the summertime, so the difference may be due to an increase in the use of allergy medication. Further inspection did not support this claim: we observed no difference in either the use percentage or dose frequency for allergy medications between the spring and summer terms.

Another possible reason for this term effect may be related to the increased academic demands related to the final exam period. In spring, we administered the surveys 3 weeks before the final exam period when students' stress levels were likely to be higher than at other times during the term. In summer, when campus activity is usually lower, we handed out surveys during the second week of the term and on average 5 weeks before final exams. Higher levels of academic demand may have led to more students experiencing stress and ultimately using more OTC medication and herbal or dietary supplements as a method of coping. However, the data do not seem to support this claim either. Analyses revealed no differences between spring and summer academic terms in either the percentage of students reporting physical illness, anxiety, depression, sleep problems, or in the total number of problems reported. Increased self-medication in the spring term is apparently unrelated to the length of time prior to final exams. Instead, these data suggest that the relationship between self-reported distress and self-medication exists independently of academic term. Thus, a strong explanation for differences in use percentage and frequency of these products between spring and summer terms is lacking.

A considerable percentage (68.2%) of the sample reported past-week physical illness or emotional distress. Students self-reported problems related to anxiety (26.9%), mood (24.9), and sleep (33.3%) more frequently than in previous studies. For example, Dusselier et al[33] found that most college students experienced "depression/anxiety/seasonal affective disorder" either never

Drug	n	%	Median dose frequency	r_{pb} (Anxiety)	p
Pain reliever					
Aspirin	6	3.0	2.0	−.04	.578
Acetaminophen[a]	57	28.4	4.0	−.01	.847
Ibuprofen[b]	77	38.3	4.0	.20	.002
Psychotropic agent					
Diphenhydramine[c]	49	24.4	4.0	.16	.018
Ginkgo biloba	9	4.5	7.0	−.02	.766
Kava	3	1.5	7.0	.11	.118
Pseudoephedrine	29	14.4	4.0	.23	.001
St. John's wort	10	5.0	6.0	.12	.095
Valerian[d]	19	9.5	4.0	.22	.002

[a]Includes Midol, Tylenol, and generic.
[b]Includes Advil, Motrin, and generic.
[c]Includes Benydrl, Sominex, and Tylenol PM.
[d]Includes Alluna, Melatrol, and generic.

or rarely (M = 1.56, SD = 0.87). Participants in that sample also reported experiencing sleep difficulties either rarely or sometimes (M = 2.17, SD = 0.95). Data from the National Epidemiologic Survey on Alcohol and Related Conditions reveal that (independent of substance use) 9.2% of participants experienced a mood disorder and 11.1% experienced an anxiety disorder.[8] One confound in comparing those findings to ours is that the national survey used the clinical diagnostic criteria set forth in the Diagnostic and Statistical Manual of Mental Disorders, 4th edition.[34]

Another main finding here was that dose frequency (not use percentage) was most strongly associated with students' self-reported distress. In particular, regression analyses demonstrated that the dose frequency of OTC medications was the single best predictor of past-week emotional distress. This finding underscores the clinical importance of knowing the frequency with which college students use these products. Interestingly, across all participants, increasing dose frequency of both pain relievers and sleep aids was significantly associated with the presence of anxiety. This finding suggests that one reason students use these products is to self-manage the experience of anxiety. Further study is needed to understand these relationships.

Last, we examined the relationship between the dose frequency of a particular drug and self-reported anxiety. Among the pain relievers, only ibuprofen was meaningfully related to self-reported anxiety. One explanation for this may be that ibuprofen, a nonsteroidal anti-inflammatory agent, better relieves somatic symptoms associated with anxiety (eg, neck and back pain). Among the drugs with psycho- tropic effects, use of both psuedoephedrine and valerian was significantly related to reports of anxiety in the past week. This is an interesting finding, particularly because pseudoephedrine is a stimulant and may mimic or increase symptoms associated with anxiety. Although the explanation for this finding is unclear, one may speculate that because anxiety and sleep disturbances often co-occur, some students self-medicate to increase daily alertness and promote sleep. Researchers should investigate whether the use of stimulants and sleep aids are etiologically related to the development of sleep disorders among college students.

Limitations and Future Directions

There were limitations to the current study. One involved the characteristics of the sample. The sample size here was diminutive compared with studies of the US population. Nevertheless, our sample size was relatively comparable to those in previous investigations of college student samples. Another general limitation is that unknowns exist with respect to how and why participants chose these products. For instance, some participants may have chosen a store- brand sleep medication on the basis of price but without knowledge of the active ingredients. In addition, participants may have experienced anxiety secondary to physical pain and discomfort and thus used analgesics appropriately for such physical symptoms. Researchers should address these issues in future work in this area.

Another drawback involves the unknown clinical specificity of the presence of physical or personal distress. We asked participants to indicate (yes or no) whether they had experienced various types of problems in the past week. Although this method is acceptable given the scope of our study, researchers in further investigations of causal links between OTC medication use and emotional distress must use reliable and valid measures of constructs, such as anxiety and depression.

The format of the questionnaire shows promise, particularly as a measure of dose frequency for OTC medications and herbal or dietary supplements. However, investigators must conduct reliability and validity studies to evaluate how useful a tool this measure would be to college health professionals. Researchers in any thorough reliability study should examine the effect of administering the survey using a traditional self-monitoring procedure (eg, participants would take the measure home and enter doses for each day of the following week, instead of the backward estimation procedure we used). Last, because we found links between the use of OTC stimulants and self-reported anxiety and sleep problems, it is reasonable to include the use of stimulant and performance drinks in future investigations.

Conclusion

A greater percentage of students in this study used OTC medications and herbal or dietary supplements than has been reported for previous samples drawn from the United States. We assert that these findings reflect an increasing trend toward self-medication among college students, but the findings also could represent idiosyncratic features of this particular sample. We also demonstrated that knowing the dose frequency of OTC medications is the single best predictor of self-reported distress among college students. One potentially relevant clinical finding is that higher doses of products containing either pseudoephedrine or valerian were associated with self-reported anxiety. The survey we used shows promise as a measurement tool, but more studies are needed to establish its utility to college health professionals.

Acknowledgment

The authors thank Dr Melenda Smith and Sasha Ward for their early contributions to this project.

References

1. Kennedy J. Herb and supplement use in the US adult population. Clin Ther. 2005;27:1847-1858.

2. Yussman SM, Wilson KM, Klein, JD. Herbal products and their association with substance use in adolescents. J Adolesc Health. 2006;38:395-400.

3. Stein RA, Strickland TL. A review of neuropsychological effects of commonly used prescription medications. Arch Clin Neuropsychol. 1998;13:259-284.

4. Mochizuki H, Tashiro M, Tagawa M, et al. The effects of a sedative anithistamine, d-chlorheniramine, on visual spatial discrimination and regional brain activity as measured by positron emission tomography (PET). Hum Psychopharmacol. 2002;17:413-418.

5. Newberry H, Beerman K, Duncan S, McGuire M, Hillers V. Use of nonvitamin, nonmineral dietary supplements among college students. J Am Coll Health. 2001;50:121-129.

6. American College Health Association. Healthy Campus 2010. http://www.acha.org/info_resources/hc2010.cfm. Accessed August 6, 2006.

7. American College Health Association. American College Health Association National College Health Assessment (ACHA- NCHA) spring 2005 reference group data report (abridged). J Am Coll Health. 2005;55:5-16.

8. Grant BF, Stinson FS, Dawson DA, et al. Prevalence and co-occurrence of substance use disorders and independent mood and anxiety disorders. Arch Gen Psychiatry. 2004;61:807-816.

9. Mischoulon D. The herbal anxiolytics kava and valerian for anxiety and insomnia. Psychiatric Ann. 2002;32:55-74.

10. Singh YN, Singh NN. Therapeutic potential of kava in the treatment of anxiety disorders. CNS Drugs. 2002;16:731-743.

11. US Food and Drug Administration Center for Drug Evaluation and Research. Office of Nonprescription Products Web site. http://www.fda.gov/cder/Offices/OTC/default.htm. Accessed August 6, 2006.

12. Rizzo JA. Prescription to over-the-counter switching of drugs. Dis Manag Health Outcomes. 2005;13:83-92.

13. Shader RI, Greenblatt DJ. The safety of over-the-counter drugs: some reflections and unanswered questions. J Clin Psychopharmacol. 2003;23:111-112.

14. Lo A. Patient characteristics associated with non-pre- scription drug use in intentional overdose. Can J Psychiatry. 2005;48:232-236.

15. Burak LJ, Damico A. College students' use of widely advertised medications. J Am Coll Health. 2000;49:118-120.

16. Steinman KJ. High school students' misuse of over-the- counter drugs: a population-based study in an urban county. J Adolesc Health. 2006;38:445-447.

17. Wazaify M, Shields E, Hughes CM, et al. Societal perspectives on over-the-counter (OTC) medicines. Family Practice. 2005;22:170-176.

18. Howland J, Weinberg J, Smith E, et al. Prevalence of allergy symptoms and associated medication use in a sample of college seniors. J Am Coll Health. 2002;51:67-70.

19. Simons L, Klichine S, Lantz V, et al. The relationship between social-contextual factors and alcohol and polydrug use among college freshmen. J Psychoactive Drugs. 2005;37:415-424.

20. Reid GJ. Pain medication in junior high. Arch Ped Adolesc Med. 1997;151:449-455.

21. Pilitteri JL, Kozlowski LT, Person DC, et al. Over-the- counter sleep aids: widely used by rarely studied. J Subst Abuse 1994;6:315-323.

22. Charlton BG. Self-management and pregnancy-safe interventions for panic, phobia and other anxiety disorders might include over-the-counter (OTC) "SSRI" antihistamines such as diphenhydramine and chlorpheniramine. Acta Psychiatrica Scandinavia. 2005;112:323.

23. Wilson KM, Klein JD, Sesselberg TS, et al. Use of complimentary medicine and dietary supple-

ments among US adolescents. J Adolesc Health.. 2006;38:385-394.

24. Fennell D. Determinants of supplement usage. Prev Med. 2004;39:932-939.

25. Haller CA, Benowitz NL, Jacob P, et al. Hemodynamic effects of ephedra-free weight-loss supplements in humans. Am J Med. 2005;118:998-1003

26. Bents RT, Tokish JM, Goldberg L. Ephedrine, pseudoephed- rine, and amphetamine prevalence in college hockey players. Phys Sportsmed. 2004;32:30-34.

27. Beaubrun G, Gray GE. A review of herbal medicines for psychiatric disorders. Psychiatr Serv. 2000;51:1130-1134.

28. Unutzer J. Over-the-counter psychotropics. Gen Hosp Psychiatry. 2000;22:221-223.

29. Van Rijswijk E, van de Lisdonk E, Zitman FG. Who uses over-the-counter psychotropics? Characteristics, functioning, and health profile. Gen Hosp Psychiatry. 2000;22:236-241.

30. Hart KE, Hill AL. Generalized use of over-the-counter analgesics: relationship to premenstrual symptoms. J Clin Psychol. 1997;53:197-200.

31. Gravetter FJ, Wallnau LB. Statistics for the Behavioral Sciences. 7th ed. Belmont, CA: Thomson Wadsworth; 2007.

32. Keith TZ. Multiple Regression and Beyond. Boston, MA: Allyn & Bacon; 2005.

33. Dusselier L, Dunn B, Wang Y, et al. Personal, health, academic, and environmental predictors of stress for residence hall students. J Am Coll Health. 2005;54:15-24.

34. American Psychiatric Association. Diagnostic and Statistical Manual of Mental Disorders. 4th ed. Washington, DC: APA; 1994.

Drug Use of the Incarcerated

By Cyndee Howell, R.N.

If "necessity is the mother of invention" then incarceration could be considered the father. Despite the best efforts of custody officials and medical staff, intoxicating agents are frequently acquired by imprisoned individuals. Drugs and alcohol can be smuggled into jails and prisons by friends and family, staff, or the inmates themselves.

Packages of drugs can be hidden in body cavities or ingested in balloons or condoms to be excreted and unwrapped for use later. Should the balloons disintegrate while still in the smuggler's digestive track, death from accidental overdose can be imminent. Drugs have been found concealed in food items or engineered into the adhesives of stamps and paper goods. In 2011, corrections officers in New Jersey discovered a children's coloring book sent to an offender had a controlled substance mixed in the crayon scribbling. Regardless of the method, each instance of passing such items is considered trafficking contraband and is an offense punishable by law.

Contraband does not necessarily need to be imported behind the prison walls. Thousands of pills are dispensed to offenders each day by medical staff to treat a wide variety of health issues. A significant percentage of incarcerated offenders suffer from chronic mental health conditions and receive psychotropic medications under the guidance of qualified medical personnel. Additionally, the prison population mirrors other national aging trends with a larger percentage being over the age 65 than ever before. Therefore, the need to dispense medicine to treat chronic health conditions such as hypertension, cardiovascular disease and diabetes is growing.

Prescription medications are frequently trafficked by inmates. Offenders will "palm" or "cheek" their medication; a tactic where the offender only pretends to ingest a tablet or capsule but in actuality hides it somewhere on their person or in their cheek. The pills can then be sold to other inmates, hoarded to be taken in larger doses than prescribed, or crushed or combined to obtain a psychoactive effect. Inmates will go to great lengths to facilitate cheeking including working in groups to create a diversion or placing a dollop of petroleum jelly or hemorrhoid ointment in their mouth so the pill will stick to the roof of their mouth without being detected. Others swallow their pills, but use self-induced vomiting or laxatives to recover the pills whole leaving them available for sale or trade. To most people, taking a pill that has been stored in the rectum or vomited up by another person seems an unsavory idea to say the least. But offenders are willing to overlook these details of how the contraband arrived as they feed an addiction or simply look for a way to break up the monotony of incarceration.

When taken other than directed, a wide variety of common drugs have the potential for abuse including those that treat high blood pressure, pain, asthma, even allergies and or diarrhea. Some anti-depressants have a euphoric effect when modified, while others sedate. Respiratory inhalers can be altered and some cough syrups contain a significant percentage of alcohol. Even innocuous items such as fruit, table sugar, or bread can be fermented, turning simple carbohydrates into jailhouse moonshine.

Diverting medication for use other than its prescribed use however, is a dangerous game. The inmate-patient misses a dose of what they need to treat their medical or mental health condition putting them at higher risk for complications. The person taking contraband medication is almost always unaware of the risks, side-effects and interactions the medication may have. When taken incorrectly, drugs used to treat high blood pressure can induce hypovolemic shock or coma. Antidepressants and pain medications misused for their sedative effects can halt breathing entirely. Others drugs can cause tachycardia, palpations and paranoia. Further complications arise when the inmates suffers a severe reaction from ingesting contraband. They often cannot—or will not—identify the substance ingested which hampers treatment options.

To Legalize or Not To Legalize?
Economic Approaches to the
Decriminalization of Drugs

By Anne Line Bretteville-Jensen, SIRUS, Oslo, Norway

Drug legalization is gaining ever-widening support in most Western societies. A liberalization of current drug laws will most probably lead to a fall in drug prices. The present article focuses on recent economic studies examining the effects of a fall in prices on quantities consumed and recruitment. Estimates of price elasticities indicate that a substantial increase in consumption by current drug users should be expected if prices decrease, whereas estimates of participation, elasticities suggest an increase in the number of users. Tests of the so-called gateway theory (i.e., whether the use of a less harmful drug increases the risk of future use of more harmful drugs) offers less unambiguous results.

Keywords: *consumption; decriminalization; gateway theory; harm reduction, legalization; participation elasticity, price elasticity*

Introduction

After decades of the "war on drugs" and optimism regarding the effect of enforcement and strict drug policy regimes, liberalistic attitudes to drugs and drug-related concerns along with increased support for harm reduction strategies are gaining in popularity across much of Europe and the North American continent. Canada, for instance, announced in July 2003 an interim law allowing cannabis for medical purposes. A survey revealed that 47% of Canadians are in favor of legalizing cannabis (Bibby, 2001). Despite a higher prevalence of cannabis users, the United States has fewer advocates of legalization. Nevertheless, a survey published in USA Today revealed that 34% were in favor, which is an all time high. From 2003, it is no longer illegal in Belgium to possess amounts up to 5 grams of cannabis, though sale and consumption in public are still prohibited. Similar changes are on the way in Switzerland. In 2004 England reclassified

Anne Line Bretteville-Jensen, "To Legalize or Not To Legalize? Economic Approaches to the Decriminalization of Drugs," *Substance Use & Misuse*, vol. 41, no. 4, pp. 555-565. Copyright © 2006 by Informa Healthcare. Reprinted with permission.

cannabis from a category B to a category C drug, which in practice means decriminalization. The Netherlands has had its coffee shops for some time where cannabis in amounts of up to 5 grams could be sold to people no younger than 18 and consumed in public. They have argued for a strict separation of, on the one hand, "soft" drugs like cannabis and, on the other, "hard" drugs like cocaine and heroin (Korf, 1995). We shall return to one of the Dutch arguments for their policy choices when discussing the "stepping-stone hypothesis" later on. Some countries in southern Europe have, in practice, decriminalized cannabis, though only Portugal has removed penal sanctions for possession of small amounts of any kind of drugs, which it did in July 2001. The Scandinavian countries have so far not liberalized their drug laws and impose stricter penalties for drug offenses than most other Western countries. Still, more Norwegians are in favor of legalizing cannabis buying and selling now than a decade ago (Bye, 2003).

The effect of liberalizing current drug policies may be extensive both for individuals and society. This article aims at examining some of the more significant consequences and to demonstrate that an economic approach to liberalization could represent an important contribution to the ongoing discussion. We argue that although an economic tool like cost- benefit analysis, designed to take all consequences into account, may not be very useful in guiding political decisions in this particular case, recent economic studies examining drug users' price responses and the validity of the "gateway theory" may be highly pertinent. We focus on two possible consequences of a price fall, namely whether it could lead to increased consumption by current users and whether the number of users could rise. Recent economic research is presented and discussed. To prepare the ground, we start by discussing from an economic perspective the

arguments put forward for criminalizing narcotic drugs in the first place.

The term "legalization" is commonly used in a heterogeneous manner. For some it means, for instance, the decriminalization of consumption and possession of drugs like cannabis while leaving the penalties for selling and distributing unchanged. Others have a full decriminalization of a range of drugs in mind and want to treat drugs much as we do alcohol, by means of a detailed regulatory regime for consumption and sale. The most extreme use of the term is when legalization implies letting the market forces alone decide price setting and quantities to be traded. In the following we use the terms legalization and decriminalization synonymously and have in mind a system much like the current one for alcohol.

Why Were Drugs Criminalized in the First Place?

There are many types of activities that impose negative externalities on others (passive smoking, pollution, etc.). Drug use can impose negative externalities on the users' family, friends, and society. When such side effects are not accounted for in individual decision making, the consumers and sellers, left to themselves, will not generate the optimal level of the activity involved. Such "market failures" are usually solved by taxing the harmful activities and compensating those who are negatively affected. When drug use emerged as a social problem in the 1960s, however, most Western societies decided to prohibit the use, possession, and sale of narcotic substances, treating it differently from the legal intoxicant, alcohol. Anthony Culyer (1973) set up a list of frequently used arguments for prohibiting drug use:

1. Drug users may physically harm others. Drug use may induce addicts to be violent and commit crimes—mostly acquisitive crimes for

income-generating purposes. One can argue that the illegality of drug use itself is what causes outlays on drugs to exceed normal salaries, forcing addicts into criminality as their only option to feed the habit. Interview data indicate, however, that many addicts were petty criminals before they started on drugs, and many seem in addition to perpetuate their criminal career after quitting "the habit." That apart, drug use does impact on individuals' crime involvement and is one of the corollaries of drug use that harms nonusers. Economic theory argues, though, that the mere existence of negative externalities by itself is not enough to prohibit an activity. A parallel can be drawn to industrial pollution: Zero tolerance would not be optimal. Instead, one aims to find a level of pollution that is "acceptable." Economic textbooks tell us that an acceptable level of pollution is where the marginal cost of further reduction equals the marginal willingness to pay for reduced pollution. Is there an optimal level of illicit drug use that is acceptable for society?

2. Drug use causes increased public spending on health. Drug users consume more of public health services than nonusers, and drug treatment is expensive. But there are many other activities that increase the risk for illness and bad health. Smoking, driving, and mountaineering are three examples, and one could ask why drug use should be treated differently. Again, from the economic viewpoint, the solution is not prohibition of all risky activities but rather prevention and harm reduction strategies.

3. Drug use upsets even people not personally in contact with drug users. The question of whether or not this so-called informational externality should be taken into account has been discussed among economists, but even if one decides to include this type of externality, prohibition would probably not be the welfare maximizing solution.

4. Drug use is contagious, and potential users should be protected from exposure. Drug use can probably not be said to be contagious in a medical or literal sense, but because users commonly start at a young age and young people may not foresee all possible consequences of their actions, there may be reason to enforce special protective measures for these high-risk groups. The same applies to future generations whose utilities are not usually currently accounted for in political decision making. Protection of individuals not able to fulfill the requirements of rational agents may be seen, also in terms of economic theory, to be acceptable reasons for prohibiting sale and consumption of certain goods.

5. Drug users are less productive and have a higher risk of premature death. This argument only holds as an argument for intervention when there is a persistent scarcity of labor in an economy.

6. Drug users must be protected against themselves as they obviously act in a self-destructive manner. This argument cannot be evaluated in relation to economic theory as microeconomics assumes that every individual is rational and able to consider what is best for him or herself. If addicts' preferences for consuming drugs are not taken as representing their "real" preferences, other mechanisms are needed to evaluate social welfare.

Drugs like cocaine and heroin are special commodities and differ from other goods in that they are potentially addictive. Prohibition is, however, an unusual means of handling externalities, and, as is well known, one unintended effect of this policy has been the development of enormous illegal drug markets. To reduce the problems caused by the drug industry, governments have targeted both the supply and the demand side of the illegal market with an array of interventions. The question being asked by more and more people is whether the costs to society and the individual users are not starting to outweigh the benefits of a prohibitive drug policy. The amount of resources spent by society on drug control (police and customs) and on the legal system (prison administration and administration of justice) and the cost paid by the individual drug user in terms of harassments, stigmatizing, imprisonments, increased health risks, and so on are substantial. To what extent the prohibitive policy achieves the aims of reduced drug use and recruitment of drug users is being discussed.

In principle, a cost-benefit analysis (CBA), which sums up the costs and benefits of a given project/policy and examines whether or not the net benefit is positive, could provide an answer. Also, when it comes to comparing the current drug policy regime with an alternative, a CBA could systematically evaluate both the negative and the positive effects of both regimes and tell which drug policy option would generate the best results for the society. The problem, of course, is actually to quantify the relevant variables for the analysis. Although economists have suggested various methods for quantifying factors, like the value of a life saved or lost, these methods are not as straightforward as they sometimes are presented. Quantification problems cause the method of CBA to be of little help when discussing drug legalization, and, consequently, the objective of this article is not to give a clear "yes" or "no" to the question. Here we focus on recent economic studies of the possible effects of a price decrease on consumption and the number of users and on articles examining the gateway theory.

To What Extent Will Addicts Respond to Price Changes?

Legalization will most probably lead to a substantial fall in drug prices. The relatively high current price levels reflect dealers' compensation for risk taking. The basis for this compensation will fall if the penal sanctions directed against dealers are removed. The lower price level may, however, to some extent be offset by taxation of the goods, but the black market would reemerge if taxation was considered too high. Therefore, a fall in drug prices should be expected. How would current drug users respond to decreasing prices?

Data derived from interviews with Norwegian drug injectors over a 10-year period may illustrate the diverging trends in average prices and consumption of heroin (Figure 1). The reported price level of heroin has fallen dramatically over the years, whereas the average monthly consumption has more than tripled.

One way of measuring the relationship between drug consumption and price is by estimating price elasticities for drugs. An elasticity estimate shows the percentage change in quantity consumed resulting from a 1% change in price. When rising prices reduce consumption, the estimate has a negative sign, and thus an elasticity of — 1 means that a 1% increase in price results in a 1 % reduction in quantity demanded. Conventional wisdom has it that the "demand" for addictive goods will not be responsive to price as the addiction itself would force addicts to regularly consume a certain amount of the drug in question regardless of price (Koch and Grupp, 1971, 1973; Rottenberg, 1968). This argument suggests that the elasticity of demand for an addictive good should be close to zero. Economists first rejected this claim for cigarettes and alcohol (Chaloupka and Warner, 2000; Cook and More, 2000). Studies have confirmed that "heavy" drinkers/smokers were price responsive, often more so than less heavy users.

Even though scarcity of data has resulted in fewer empirical studies for illegal substances than there are on legal addictive substances like alcohol and tobacco, a number of works have been published over the last decade. One of the first elasticity studies for drugs dates back to

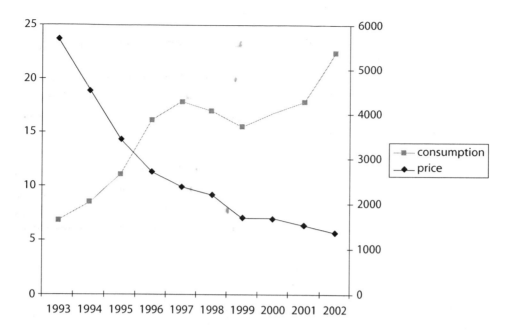

FIGURE 1. Average monthly consumption in grams and gram prices of heroin among drug injectors in Oslo from 1993 to 2002.

1972 when Nisbet and Vakil (1972) estimated the price response for marijuana among UCLA students and reported elasticities in the range of —0.4 to —0.5. Grossman and Chaloupka (1998), using a large panel data set (also initially based on students), estimated price elasticity for cocaine of —0.3, whereas Silverman and Spruill (1977) obtained, in an indirect manner, an elasticity estimate for heroin of —0.27. In Bretteville-Jensen and Bi0rn (2004), interviews with people attending a needle-exchange service in Oslo offered elasticity estimates of —1.20 for heroin. Based on aggregated time series data for the Dutch East Indies (now Indonesia) and Taiwan, van Ours (1995) and Liu et al. (1999), respectively, reported opium price elasticity estimates in the ranges —0.7 to —1.0 and —0.27 to —1.17.

In these studies other factors in addition to price are assumed to influence drug consumption, such as age, sex, education, income, and use of other intoxicants, and these were taken into account when available. The estimates cover a wide range of values. Price elasticities cannot be assumed to be constant parameters because they vary according to type of substance, type of data, time period, country, user subgroup, econometric model applied, and so on. They may also vary depending on rising or decreasing prices in the marketplace. For cigarettes, Pekurinen (1989) revealed asymmetry in price responses indicating that consumption changed twice as much when the prices fell as when they rose. There is no study of asymmetry in response to changes in drug prices.

Bretteville-Jensen and Bi0rn (2004) also looked for "kinks" along the demand curve for heroin (i.e., segments with elasticities of different sizes). According to theories of drug "demand" listed in Wagstaff and Maynard (1988), they tested whether there were vertical segments, reflecting elasticities equal to zero, in the demand curve. No vertical segments were located, however. As for ordinary goods, their findings show that the price elasticity of demand for heroin rises with rising prices, suggesting that people respond relatively more to price changes from initially high levels compared with price changes from initially low levels. Further, they found that an increased price of amphetamine would reduce the consumption also of heroin. Estimates of cross-elasticities (i.e., the percentage change in quantity consumed of drug A resulting from a 1% change in the price of drug B) may prove important if the legalisation of all drugs leads to changes in relative drug prices.

In contrast to most consumption goods, drugs may cause addiction that, ideally, should be factored in when estimating the price effect. This requires panel data (i.e., information regarding the same individuals recorded at different points in time). Grossman and Chaloupka (1998) and Bretteville-Jensen and Bi0rn (2003) are two studies that aimed at taking account of potential addictiveness by using panel data and included previous consumption of the drug as a separate variable.

Although the price elasticity estimates for drugs vary in size, they seem to point in the same direction: Heavy drug users curtail consumption when prices increase and increase consumption in response to falling prices. The claim that addicts would be nonresponsive to changes in prices has therefore been rejected also in the case of narcotic drugs. However, the wide rage of elasticities is mirrored in less precise predictions of possible consequences of legalization. Further, when assessing the various consequences of legalisation, the negative side effects of increased consumption would have to be balanced against the increased utility a drop in prices would mean for the drug consumers.

Increased Number of Drug Users?

Legalizing drugs could affect the number of users through several channels. First, we have the price effect. Cheaper drugs may induce some nonusers to take up "the habit" if high expenditures previously prevented them from doing so. Also, if drugs become relatively cheaper than alcohol, heavy drinkers may replace alcohol with drugs. Second, legalization could affect the availability of drugs, both physically and culturally. The "contagion model" claims that more drug use in public and more people using drugs would "contaminate" more nonusers to start consuming drugs. Third, restricting legalization to "soft drugs" like cannabis could still affect the number of "hard drug" users if the stepping stone hypothesis or the gateway theory is right. In what follows we review some studies from economists that explore these potential effects.

As said, falling drug prices would probably affect the number of users as drugs would become more "accessible" economically. Estimations of the so-called participation elasticity indicates whether changes in drug prices also influence the initiation of drug use and is defined as the response in reported drug use prevalence to a 1% increase in prices. If increased prices reduce prevalence, elasticity has a negative sign, van Ours (1995) estimated participation elasticity for opium from —0.3 to —0.4, whereas Liu et al.'s (1999) opium estimate was slightly lower (—0.2). Grossman and Chaloupka (1998) reported the corresponding elasticity for cocaine of —1.0. Pacula et al. (2000), using the same data set as Grossman and Chaloupka (1998) (Monitoring the Future), obtained an estimate of —0.3 for marijuana. Saffer and Chaloupka (1999) found that a fall in cocaine or heroin prices had a positive effect on the likelihood of starting to consume these drugs; they estimated the participation elasticities as —0.28 for cocaine and —0.94 for heroin. Hence, there seems to be empirical support for the claim that prices affect drug use initiation. As in the case of the consumption elasticities, the range of estimates is pretty broad.

As mentioned, protecting people from becoming addicted was cited as one important reason for prohibiting narcotic substances in the first place. Indeed, a past director of Norway's criminal investigation unit stated the following in the late 1960s: "Every new abuser lures or persuades about 3-4 of his acquaintances to try the drug. Each of these makes 3-4 others to join and so on, thus creating geometrical increment: 3-9-27-81." If he is right, we will all become drug addicts in time. That aside, his opinion illustrates the general concern about the assumed ease with which drug use could spread at a time when the spread of infectious diseases was a leading proliferation model. Of course, the infectious disease model no longer attracts much of a following, not least because the mechanisms behind proliferation are so much more complicated and social rather than physical. Although microeconomic theory embraces the atomistic individual or household, some theoretical contributions have taken cognisance of the effect people have on each other. Schelling (1998) and Manski (2000), for instance, emphasize the importance of social interaction in economics, and Moene (1999) applies social interaction theories to drug use and addiction. The empirical studies of Jones (1989, 1994) support the significance of social interaction in the consumption of cigarettes, and good data in relation to other addictive goods would be of great value.

The so-called stepping-stone hypothesis or gateway theory represents yet another attempt at explaining how people start using illegal drugs, and perhaps hard drugs in particular.

The idea is that the use of a less harmful substance increases the risk of using other more harmful substances at some later point in time. Is, for instance, cannabis a gateway to harder drugs like cocaine and heroin? The answer to this question is important for whether the law should distinguish sharply between soft drugs and hard drugs. Recent articles from economists discuss this matter.

Empirically, there seems to be sound support for the stepping-stone hypothesis because most heroin users report to have started using heroin after first having consumed cannabis, pills, and amphetamine. Pudney (2003) lists three possible effects that could induce cannabis users to try harder drugs: (1) consumption of cannabis opens up contacts with the criminal world and hence with users of hard drugs, (2) cannabis use may create an urge for stronger experiences of the same type, and (3) experience with cannabis may weaken the fear of possible adverse effects of hard drugs.

If there is such a slippery slope from soft to hard drugs, it would make legalization of soft drugs more "expensive" and would undermine Dutch policy's strict separation of drug types, as it would, indeed, the recent British reclassification of cannabis. The prevalence of hard drug use in the Netherlands is, however, not higher than in other countries in central Europe (EMCDDA, 2003), and the stepping-stone hypothesis is disputed. For instance, one of the questions raised concerns what the first step on the staircase to hard drug use actually is: Is it cannabis use or rather starting to drink or smoke that is the real problem? Another concerns whether the theory itself holds true. The empirical association between the initiation of cannabis and later heroin use could be spurious because they both may be influenced by a third unobserved variable. It may be that unobserved individual heterogeneity, let's call it antisocial behavior, affects both cannabis and heroin use and that the reason most heroin users come from a cannabis-using background is simply because cannabis is more available than heroin, physically, economically, and culturally to very young people. Pacula (1998a,b), Fergusson and Horwood (2000), and Beenstoch and Rahav (2002) find empirical support for gateway effects, whereas these effects, appear small in both Pudney (2003) and van Ours (2003). Only some of the gateway studies have aimed to control for the possible effects of unobserved factors.

Another recent empirical finding is that the "staircase" is actually not much of staircase anymore. Young people today may start their illegal drug careers with substances other than cannabis. In the wake of the house and rave party phenomenon, many young people were introduced to ecstasy, a pill that often contains amphetamines and sometimes also small quantities of hallucinogenic drugs like LSD. Many ecstasy users say they had never tried other illegal drugs before ecstasy. If this pattern is widespread among current users of hard drugs, it undermines the stepping-stone hypothesis further.

Discussion

Some Western societies have already liberalized their drug policy, and in many others legalization is attracting widening support. Of course, more people favor decriminalizing use and possession only and do not go in for a totally liberalized regime. Similarly, more people support legalizing a soft drug like cannabis than cocaine or heroin. At times, the legalisation debate has been heated, with strong feelings in evidence among both proponents and opponents. The present article attempts to show that economics can make a contribution to the legalization debate through empirical studies on the consequences of a fall in drug prices and through testing the gateway theory. Subsequent to a discussion of the reasons for initially criminalizing drugs and a brief description of the principles of CBA, we focused on two possible effects of a price decrease that are probably more vital than others: the effect on drug consumption and the effect on the number of users.

Drug-related harm is closely related to the amounts consumed. Therefore, consumption responses to changes in drug prices are important inputs when assessing the possible consequences of legalization. Economic studies seem to indicate that falling prices would cause a substantial increase in consumption by current users. Extrapolation of current findings, however, must be done with caution because legalization could affect many variables simultaneously. Further, the elasticity estimates for heroin confirm that the size of the elasticity is smaller for lower price levels. If legalization leads to large price cuts, the response of drug users may be less significant than suggested by the estimates referred to above because they are based on high price levels. On the other hand, a large price fall may in part be counteracted by taxation. Also, a high consumption level does not necessarily mean increased health risks. Lower prices of heroin could, for instance, make people switch from injecting to smoking heroin, a route of administrating the drug that would lower the risk of overdoses and blood-borne diseases.

Drug consumption is affected by availability in several senses of the term. Legalization would probably make drugs more available economically, physically, and culturally. Empirical findings suggest that lower prices would boost the number of users. A priori, the cultural and the physical effects are more difficult to estimate. Easy access, removal of penal sanctions, reduced stigma associated with use, and so on may encourage nonusers to try the drug. According to the contagion model, increasing number of users should lead to further increases over time. On the other hand, if the attraction of illegal drugs lies in the "forbidden fruit" character, then legalization may reduce the user population. The stepping-stone hypothesis underpins policies that distinguish between soft and hard drugs. Pudney (2003) and van Ours (2003) report little support for the hypothesis and point to the possibility that a strict drug policy may in fact cause an increase in heavy drug use if the policy encourages contact between users of different substances.

The empirical studies cited above seem to indicate a rise in consumption by regular users and in the number of users all told in the wake of a liberalized drug policy. The full effect of the increase is difficult to assess, however. For the users, the health effects will, for instance, depend on the initial level of use, methods of administrating the drug (e.g., whether heroin is injected or smoked), the consumption of additional intoxicants, initial health status, and so on. For friends and families, increased consumption could mean additional problems in their relations with the addict. Society may experience fewer drug-related crimes if drugs become cheaper, though that effect may be offset by a rise in the number of users. Health expenditures will probably increase. Given the quantification problems related to CBA, a more pragmatic but less formal approach for assessing drug legalization would be a social experiment. As the number of countries implementing some form of decriminalization or legalization seems to be increasing, the opportunity to conduct proper evaluations of the effects of policy changes is improving too. Analyses of cross-national data must be conducted with care, however, as the scope for problems with endogeneity and unobserved heterogeneity are pronounced. Dissimilar developments of, for example, prevalence rates of drug use between country A (with legalized drug use) and country B (without legalized drug use) after a drug policy change may be affected by many factors other than just the change in drug laws, and it will be a challenge to adequately control for the relevant variables when a legalization is to be assessed. Still, such social experiments are of special interest for a discipline like economics where the scope and relevance of laboratory experiments are limited.

One could also study markets for other intoxicants to gain a better understanding of the prospective effects of legislative amendments. Many Western countries prohibited the sale of wine and spirits in the first part of the previous century. America, in particular, went through a difficult time with the growth of professional criminal organizations, the American mafia, as depicted in films like The Untouchables. There is probably general agreement that the revocation of the Prohibition Act was a wise move. Whether the consequences of the legalization of alcohol would be replicated for cannabis, for instance, is another matter, however. Although cannabis might be a less harmful intoxicant than alcohol, there are important differences between them, historically and culturally, that would affect the legitimacy of any policy revision. It remains to be seen whether legalisation will make the use of cannabis more common, for instance, among people in older age groups, or whether it will remain a subgroup activity as it is today. Decriminalization or legalization will probably not change adults' choice of intoxicants overnight, but who's to say how drug-using habits will be in 50 years time?

Anne Line Bretteville-Jensen has a Ph.D., in Economics from the University ofBergen (2003). She is currently are- searcher at the Norwegian Institute for Alcohol and Drug Research (SIRUS), Oslo, and at Programme for Health Economics in Bergen (HEB), University of Bergen. Her areas of interest are the economics of addiction and health economics in general. She has published in journals like Addiction, Journal of Health Economics, Health Economics, European Addiction Research, Scandinavian Journal of Economics, and Empirical Economics. She has received the IVO-award 2000. The prize is provided every 2 years by the Addiction Research Institute Rotterdam to a researcher under the age of 35 who is conducting research into the use of substances such as alcohol, tobacco, and illegal drugs as well as research into problems associated with substance use. The prize has had candidates from all over the world.

Glossary

Cost-benefit analysis (CBA): Sums up the costs and benefits of a given project/policy and examines whether or not the net benefit is positive.

Cross-price elasticity: The percentage change in quantity consumed of good A resulting from a 1% change in the price of good B.

Drug decriminalization: Removal of penal sanctions directed against sellers and consumers of currently illegal drugs. However, often used only for the removal of sanctions directed against the demand side of the drug marked.

Drug legalization: Includes decriminalization as well as regulations concerning legal availability of drugs.

Externality: When the actions of one person directly affect the utility of another person.

Elasticity estimate: Indicates the percentage change in consumption resulting from a 1% increase in price of the good.

Gateway theory: Simply states that the use of one drug increases the risk of starting to consume another and possibly more harmful drug later on and that the risk increases with frequency of use (dose-response).

Harm reduction strategies: A set of practical strategies that reduce negative consequences of drug use, incorporating a spectrum of strategies from safer use, to managed use to abstinence. Harm reduction strategies is said to meet drug users "where they're at," addressing conditions of use along with the use itself.

Informational externality: The effect on other people's utility created by the pure knowledge of a certain incident or condition.

Participation elasticity: The percentage change in prevalence rate resulting from a 1% increase in the price of the good.

Social interaction theories: Theories of how economic agents/decision makers (persons, firms, or nonprofit organizations) interact. Agents' chosen actions may affect other agents through the pref-erences, expectations, or constraints faced by the others.

Stepping-stone hypothesis: Used more or less synonymously with gateway theory defined above.

Unobserved heterogeneity: Unobserved differences between observations.

References

Beenstock, M., Rahav, G. (2002). Testing gateway theory; do cigarette prices affect illicit drug use? Journal of Health Economics 21:679-698.

Bibby, R. W. (2001). Canada's Teens: Today, Yesterday, Tomorrow. Canada: Stoddart.

Bretteville-Jensen, A. L., Bi0rn, E. (2003). Heroin consumption, prices and addiction: evidence from self-reported panel data. Scandinavian Journal of Economics 105:661-679.

Bretteville-Jensen, A. L., Bi0rn, E. (2004). Do prices count? A micro-econometric study of illicit drug consumption based on self-reported data. Empirical Economics 29:673-695.

Bye, E., ed. (2003). Alcohol and Drugs in Norway. Annual report. Oslo: Norwegian Institute of Alcohol and Drug Research.

Chaloupka, F. J., Warner, K. (2000). The economics of smoking. In: Culyer, A. J., Newhouse, J. P. eds. Handbook of Health Economics. Amsterdam, The Netherlands: Elsevier, pp. 1539-1627.

Cook, P., Moore, M. (2000). Alcohol. In: Culyer, A. J., Newhouse, J. P. eds. Handbook of Health Economics. Amsterdam, The Netherlands: Elsevier, pp. 1629-1673.

Culyer, A. J. (1973). Should social policy concern itself with drug "abuse"? Public Finance Quarterly 1:449-456.

EMCDDA (2003). The State of the Drugs Problem in the European Union and Norway. Annual report. Lisbon, Portugal: European Monitoring Centre for Drugs and Drug Addiction.

Fergusson, D. M., Horwood, L. J. (2000). Does cannabis use encourage other forms of illicit drug use? Addiction 95:505-520.

Grossman, M., Chaloupka, F. J. (1998). The demand for cocaine by young adults: a rational addiction approach. Journal of Health Economics 17:427-474.

Jones, A. M. (1989). A double-hurdle model of cigarette consumption. Journal of Applied Econometrics 4:23-39.

Jones, A. M. (1994). Health, addiction, social interaction and the decision to quit smoking. Journal of Health Economics 13:93-110.

Koch, J. V., Grupp, S. E. (1971). The economics of drug control policies. The International Journal of the Addictions 6:571-584.

Koch, J. V., Grupp, S. E. (1973). Police and illicit drug markets: some economic considerations. British Journal of Addiction 68:351-362.

Korf, D. J. (1995). Dutch Treat. Formal Control and Illicit Drug Use in the Netherlands. Thesis Publishers, Amsterdam.

Liu, J.-L., Liu, J.-T., Hammitt, J. K., Chou, S.-Y. (1999). The price elasticity of opium in Taiwan. 1914-1942. Journal of Health Economics 18:795-810.

Manski, C. F. (2000). Economic analysis of social interaction. Journal of Economic Perspectives 14:115-136.

Moene, K. O. (1999). Addiction and social interaction. In: Elster, J., Skog, O.-J., eds. Getting Hooked. Rationality and Addiction. Cambridge, United Kingdom: Cambridge University Press, pp. 30- 46.

Nisbet, C. T., Vakil, F. (1972). Some estimates of price and expenditure elasticities of demand for marijuana among U.C.L.A. students. The Review of Economics and Statistics 54:473-475.

Pacula, R. L. (1998a). Does increasing beer tax reduce marijuana consumption? Journal of Health Economics 17:557-585. National Bureau of Economics Research, Cambridge, USA.

Pacula, R. L. (1998b). Adolecent Alcohol and Marijuana Consumption: Is There Really a Gateway Effect? NBER Working Paper No. 6348. National Bureau of Economic Research, Cambridge, USA.

Pacula, R. L., Grossman, M., Chaloupka, F. J., O'Malley, P. M., Johnston, L., Farrelly, M. C. (2000). Marijuana and Youth. NBER Working Paper No. 7703. National Bureau of Economic Research, Cambridge, USA.

Pekurinen, M. (1989). The demand for tobacco products in Finland. British Journal of Addiction 84:1183-1192.

Pudney, S. (2003). The road to ruin? Sequences of initiation to drug use and crime in Britain. Economic Journal 113:182-198.

Rottenberg, S. (1968). The clandestine distribution of heroin, its discovery and suppression. Journal of Political Economy 76:78-90. Saffer, H., Chaloupka, F. J. (1999). The demand for illicit drugs. Economic Inquiry 37:401-411.

Schelling, T. C. (1998). Social mechanisms and social dynamics. In: Hedstrom, P., Swedberg, R. eds.

Social Mechanisms. Cambridge University Press. Silverman, L. P., Spruill, N. L. (1977). Urban crime and the price of heroin. Journal of Urban Economics 4:80-103.

van Ours, J. (1995). The price elasticity of hard drugs: the case of opium in the Dutch East Indies. Journal of Political Economy 103:261-279.

van Ours, J. (2003). Is cannabis a stepping-stone for cocaine? Journal of Health Economics 22:539- 554.

Wagstaff, A., Maynard, A. (1988). Economic Aspects of the Illicit Drug Market and Drug Enforcement Policies in the United Kingdom, Home Office Research Study 95, London.

Treatment and Prevention

By Howard Abadinsky

New York, June 17, 1988. The four junior high school girls came down West End Avenue grinning, their book bags on their backs. At the corner of West 94th Street, they stopped in front of a boy not much older than they were. Without a word, he pulled up his red T-shirt and took a large clear-plastic bag out of the front of his pants. He extracted four smaller packets from it, handing them to the girls for four $5 bills, which he added to a big wad of money in his right hand.

—Fox Butterfield (1988, p. 10)

"Just Say No!"
—Anti-drug campaign spearheaded by
First Lady Nancy Reagan

There are probably as many approaches to treating and preventing drug abuse as there are theories to explain the phenomenon. But unlike diseases whose etiology and, thus, treatment and prevention, appear to be clearly physiological, drug abuse has no such clarity. As with other chronic diseases, however, the National Institute on Drug Abuse (NIDA) recommends speaking in terms of "remission" and "improvement" rather than "cure" when discussing the treatment of substance abuse ("Drug Abuse," 1987), since the problem has proved quite intractable. Then there are the incongruities described in chapter 1: the moderate use of psychoactive substances—from nicotine to cocaine—may be the focus of a treatment response. These "treatments" are not based on the properties inherent in the chemicals themselves but are dependent upon the societal definition of "abuse." Thus, in the United States the moderate use of alcohol, tobacco, or coffee is seen as acceptable behavior, while even the occasional use of heroin or cocaine is seen as requiring "treatment." The difficulty is apparent: people who do not feel ill and who do not want treatment are coerced into a "treatment" situation by their families, their employers, or the criminal justice system.

In this chapter we will examine the variety of treatment and prevention strategies used to

Howard Abadinsky, "Treatment and Prevention," *Drug Abuse: An Introduction*, pp. 137-178. Copyright © 1989 by Rowman & Littlefield Publishers, Inc. Reprinted with permission.

respond to the problem of substance abuse. Often several treatment approaches are used simultaneously or sequentially because drug abusers usually suffer from a complex of medical and social problems. First, we will look at approaches to treatment based on some of the theories discussed in chapter 4; then we will examine specific treatment programs that, although they appear under separate topical headings for pedagogical purposes, may in practice use a mix of treatment modalities based on psychological and sociological theory.

The Cure Industry

Like the quest for an explanation of drug abuse, the search for a cure, particularly a magic bullet in the form of a chemical cure, has a history that cautions us to be skeptical. At one time morphine was offered as a cure for opiate addiction; cocaine was offered as a cure for morphine addiction (patients become habituated to cocaine while remaining addicted to morphine); heroin was proposed for the cure of morphine addiction; and methadone was presented as a cure for heroin addiction. In fact, the "cure industry" has a long and often less than honorable history.

The medical profession, notes H. Wayne Morgan (1981), "often shared the distaste for drug users that permeated the society" (p. 65). The problem of addiction was only peripheral to the practice of most doctors, who usually tried to avoid association with the failure so common to treating the problem of drug abuse. This left a fertile field for the charlatan, and toward the turn of the century the quest for a cure led to the development of an industry similar to that of patent medicines. Unregulated nostrums were widely advertised as "cures[95] for drug abuse, and they frequently contained alcohol, cocaine, and opiates. In 1906, these compounds came under

regulation, followed by a significant decline in sales. In response, drug sellers portrayed themselves as outsiders who were feared by a medical establishment centered In the eastern part of the United States. This approach had strong appeal, particularly in the South and Midwest, where anti-Eastern Establishment feelings ran deep.

A number of (self-proclaimed) doctors operated clinics for addicts and grew quite wealthy from their "cures." The most famous was Charles B. Towns, a Georgia farmer, insurance salesman, and stockbroker. David Musto (1973) refers to Towns as the "king of the cure proclaimers." Arriving in New York City in 1901, Towns spent several years as a partner- in a stock brokerage firm that failed in 1904. Shortly thereafter, he began advertising a cure for drug addiction, gaining patients who used his "secret formula," The medical profession was skeptical, but Towns and his cure were widely accepted and promoted even by federal agencies; a 1909 article in the Journal of the American Medical Association was also favorable. The Charles B. Towns Hospital proclaimed a cure rate of between 75 and 90 percent. Determining "success" was rather simple— if the patient never returned, he or she was "cured". Eventually it was revealed that Towns's secret formula contained three ingredients: prickly ash bark, extract of Hyoscyamus (a poisonous plant), and belladonna (deadly nightshade—a poisonous plant).

At the same time, however, sanitariums existed where the approach to drug addiction was similar, if not identical, to many contemporary inpatient programs. The addict was withdrawn from narcotics, sometimes with the aid of nonaddicting drugs that kept the patient more comfortable. Prior to 1914, treating addiction was especially difficult because morphine was available in a pure form so the withdrawal process was more severe (Morgan, 1981). The patient was given frequent soothing baths, and as soon as the person's body began to function more normally, a regimen of nourishing food and exercise was followed. The patient, now withdrawn from drugs, was engaged in such tasks as reading and gardening and was given a great deal of supportive reassurance.

The extent of the treatment often depended on a person's ability to pay for services (Morgan, 1981). In more recent times, the profit that can accrue from treating certain types of substance abusers—such as those with appropriate health insurance—has led to the expansion of a private cure industry often based in health/hospital settings (Freudenheim, 1987); they will be discussed later in this chapter.

Heroin Antagonists

As part of the search for a "magic bullet" to cure addiction, scientists developed a number of heroin antagonists, substances that block or counteract the effects of opiates. Some, such as cyclazocine and naloxone, have significant side-effects. While cyclazocine taken orally effectively blocks the effects of heroin for twelve to twenty-four hours, It also produces nausea, sweating, a feeling of intoxication, anxiety, and hallucinations. Users suffer withdrawal symptoms when the substance Is discontinued, although they do not develop a craving for it. A dose as small as ,25 mg of naloxone will block the effects of heroin for ten hours, but it is effective only when administered intravenously. Neither of these substances reduces the "drug hunger" of heroin addicts (DeLong, 1972).

Naloxone is recommended for testing of opiate dependence prior to admission to a methadone program (Judson and Goldstein, 1986). The substance is administered to persons seeking methadone because these people may not be opioid dependent or may have only minimal dependence. "Treatment of these addicts with methadone raises important ethical and legal questions in view of the likelihood of producing physical dependence in previously nondependent persons" (Peachey and Lei, 1988, p. 200). The antagonist nalorphine (Nalline) counters the depression of the central nervous system caused by opiates and is administered as an antidote for heroin overdoses.

The National Institute of Drug Abuse (NIDA) was instrumental in the development of naltrexone, a long-acting, orally adminstered narcotic antagonist first synthesized in 1965 and marketed as Trexan by DuPont. This nonaddicting drug defeats the effects of opiates by occupying their receptor sites in the brain. The substance will displace any agonists (substances capable of combining with a receptor) that are present, causing severe withdrawal in those persons who are opioid dependent. Given to patients after detoxification two or three times a week, naltrexone will block any euphoric response from the use of opiates, and it is relatively long-lasting with few side-effects.

Naltrexone is effective only with persons who are motivated to give up the feeling of euphoria that opiates can provide. The manufacturer clearly states its recommended use as an adjunct in the treatment of opioid abusers (Ginzburg, 1986): "Treatment failure cannot be blamed on the failure of naltrexone to block opioids nor is treatment success likely to be the consequence of a use of naltrexone alone" (p. 5).[1]

Detoxification

As in the past, contemporary treatment programs typically begin with detoxification, "a term left over from an obsolete theory that addicts suffer from an accumulation of toxins" (Dole, 1980, p. 138). Antagonists are sometimes used as an aid in heroin detoxification. Withdrawal from maintenance doses of methadone, because of its potency, is generally accomplished by decreasing dosages. The antihypertension drug clonidine has been used to relieve many of the symptoms of opioid withdrawal, particularly those involving autonomic nervous system hyperactivity; the substance is nonaddicting ("Drug Abuse," 1987). Clonidine has been recommended by some physicians for the detoxification of methadone patients being maintained on relatively low dosages. Whereas methadone can be found in the patient more than a week after the last dose, clonidine has a shorter life. Thus, a clonidine patient can be placed on naltrexone immediately upon detoxification, whereas a methadone patient would experience unpleasant withdrawal symptoms under similar treatment (Ginzburg, 1986).

Cocaine detoxification presents a serious problem because of a craving for the drug; this may be associated with the depletion of dopamine, which, as noted in chapter 4, is essential to life. While withdrawal from opiates and cocaine can be accomplished without using other chemicals—although the patient may feel quite uncomfortable—detoxification from sedatives can lead to seizures and cardiac arrest and, therefore, must be accomplished by prescribing decreasing amounts of the substance.

The use of chemicals to facilitate a comfortable withdrawal can serve to attract drug abusers into treatment and increases the probability that they will complete detoxification. However, at least with respect to heroin users, there are troubling aspects. Addicts typically enter treatment when their habit is too expensive to support and they have to work hard simply to prevent the onset of withdrawal symptoms because their high tolerance level denies the achievement of the "high." Under such conditions, notes David Bellis (1981), addiction is no longer fun. "Then [the addict] enters a detoxification ward and is comfortably withdrawn from heroin. Detoxification is made so easy compared to 'cold turkey': that addicts are not confronted with negatively enforcing pharmacological and physiological aspects of

addiction" (p. 139). Detoxification reduces the addicts level of tolerance so that the high can be enjoyed once again at an affordable price. Bellis (1981) cautions drug program staffs that they should not be surprised or miffed when addicts leave the detoxification ward and inject heroin withm a few minutes or hours" (p. 140).

Opioid Agonists

There are synthetic substances that have a chemical makeup similar to opioids, such as levo-alpha-acetylmethadol, better known as LAMM (or LAM: Long-Acting Methadone). LAMM acts more slowly than heroin or methadone (it does not yield a quick high) and has been used experimentally for detoxification and maintenance (Schecter, 1980). But the most widely used agonist is methadone, a wholly synthetic narcotic that was developed as a substitute for morphine by German scientists during the Second World War. Somewhat less powerful than heroin, methadone produces virtually the same-analgesic and sedative effects as heroin and is no less addictive. After World War II, methadone was used in hospital settings to systematically detoxify persons addicted to opiates. Methadone has distinct advantages over opiates: It can be administered orally, and it is delivered to the bloodstream over a period of two hours or more with effects lasting up to twenty-four hours (Dole, 1980).

The first clinical use of methadone to treat narcotic addiction occurred at the United States Public Health Hospital at Lexington, Kentucky, where It was substituted for morphine and heroin to help detoxify addicted patients. Withdrawal from heroin was made relatively painless by first administering doses equivalent to the patient's use of heroin on the streets; the doses of methadone were then lowered until the patient was no longer addicted, a process that took seven to ten days (Blackmore, 1979). During the early 1960s, when narcotic addiction once again emerged as a major national concern. Dr. Vincent Dole and Dr. Marie Nyswander of Rockefeller University reported on their successful use of methadone to treat heroin addicts in a dramatically new way—maintenance. In 1964, Dole and Nyswander provided twenty-two hospitalized heroin addicts with increasing doses of methadone until they reached a "stabilized state," meaning the patients had neither withdrawal symptoms nor a craving for further increases in the dosage. "With repeated administration of a fixed dose, methadone loses its sedative and analgesic powers. The subject becomes tolerant" (Dole. 1980, p. 146). The patients were then released, and they returned each day for an oral dose of methadone. The following year a research report by Dole and Nyswander (1965) revealed extraordinary results from this approach, which they ascribed to methadone's ability to provide a "pharmacological block" against heroin.

It was theorized that heroin abuse in certain addicts results in a metabolic disorder that requires the continued ingestion of narcotics if the person is to remain homeostatic. With such disorders, methadone acts to normalize the patients functioning. Continuing research with additional patients provided further support for methadone maintenance: addict patients refrained from heroin use, secured employment, and avoided criminal activity. In 1966, Dole and Nyswander established a large outpatient methadone program at Beth Israel Hospital in New York City. Other programs followed. Dole and Nyswander (1966) intimated that they had discovered the "magic bullet": methadone blocked the effects of heroin.

The typical methadone program begins with a period of inpatient care and substitution of low doses of methadone for heroin (the patient is not Informed of the dosage he or she receives). The methadone is usually mixed with orange juice (which helps to reduce its bitter taste) and consumed in front of a nurse. Slow increases in dosage reduce the "high," which disappears once tolerance develops. Addicts subsequently report daily on an outpatient basis and are permitted take-home doses for weekends. As they progress, less-than-daily pickups are permitted. Patients usually provide a urine specimen before they are given methadone. James DeLong (1972) outlines the dosage levels:

> The general rule of thumb is that a daily dose of 100 mg will block any effect of heroin for almost all addicts. Most programs administer a minimum of 80 mg, although a few may go as high as 300 mg in selected cases. A program that administers 80 mg or more is probably aiming at a blockage dose. A lower dose will not block the effect of heroin—an addict can achieve euphoria if he tries. However, the lower dose will block the narcotic hunger and thus remove some of the pressure for heroin use. For most addicts, a dosage of 40 or 50 mg is enough to eliminate this craving, but an even lower dose may be enough if the addict has a light habit. (p. 215)

"The actions of chronic methadone treatment are to prevent withdrawal symptoms, prevent so-called 'drug hunger,' whatever the basis of that is; chronic methadone treatment also 'blocks' by cross-tolerance, the euphoric effects of other short-acting narcotics" (Kreek, 1987, p. 53).

By the late 1960s a few thousand addicts were being maintained on methadone; by early 1973 there were approximately 73,000 (Danaceau, 1974). This change was brought about by the Nixon administration, which was convinced that methadone could help reduce the crime rate—a cornerstone of the "law and order" presidency of Richard Nixon. Experts who knew better, argues Edward Jay Epstein (1974), "chose not to deflate the unrealistic claim that methadone would substantially reduce crime" (p. 22). They hoped that such programs would lure otherwise recalcitrant hard-core heroin addicts into treatment.

Eventually, the bad news came out. Methadone was not the "magic bullet." Indeed, there was no blockade, but simply cross-tolerance—the patient maintained at significantly high doses of methadone would not experience the "high" from heroin. Moreover, methadone did not affect the euphoric experience of the "rush" In fact, it was discovered that methadone patients, even those taking high daily doses, were often abusing heroin as well as other drags. And, while methadone maintenance was designed for heroin addicts, the problem was often one of polydrug use.

It was further revealed that the figures given out by Dole and Nyswander were deceptive: the rate of "cure" attributed to methadone was better explained by the screening mechanism used—older and more motivated addicts were preferred—and the fact that unsuccessful cases were simply dropped from the program and the final tabulations. Methadone clinics came under severe attack by those associated with the drug- free therapeutic communities, and-by 1979 methadone clinics were operating at about 90 percent of their capacity (Blackmore, 1979). Robert Newman (1977) states that "proponents of specific treatment approaches rarely missed an opportunity to make exaggerated claims for their own modality and to vilify publicly other therapeutic efforts" (p. xx). There was also very strong resident opposition to methadone treatment centers in most communities.

This is not to say that methadone maintenance is without a role in the treatment of heroin addiction. For certain persons in the heroin- abusing population, methadone maintenance appears to be quite beneficial. It can act as a cratch for persons motivated to give up heroin. The programs also attract addicts seeking a chemical cure, although

the provision of counseling and job assistance may be the actual "cure." But even without such services, notes James DeLong (1972), methadone may have a placebo effect—the addict who believes that methadone is beneficial will find it so.

To the extent that heroin addiction is explained by physiology for example, persons with abnormal endorphin levels compensate for this distressed state by ingesting heroin—methadone maintenance is the equivalent of providing insulin to diabetics. If psychoanalytic theory is accurate, methadone may serve as an anti-aggression chemical for those heroin addicts whose drug abuse is based on a need to control the rage and aggressive tendencies, originating in a problematic anal stage of development (Khantzian, 1980).

In a review of evaluations of methadone maintenance programs, M. Douglas Anglin and William McGlothlin (1985) conclude that "methadone maintenance has been shown to effectively reduce drug use, dealing, and income-generating crime, and to a lesser extent to increase employment and family reponsibility." Furthermore, methadone maintenance "appeals to a portion of the addict population that has not been amenable to other social intervention strategies" (p. 274).

There is some concern that older addicts on methadone maintenance, who might have gone into remission without any intervention, become addicted to methadone. On the other hand, "patients who terminate before they have achieved stable social functioning are very unlikely to remain abstinent." And, "even patients who terminate under the best of circumstances still may have less than a 50 percent chance of remaining abstinent as long as "three years" (Hargreaves, 1986, p. 70). Mary Kreek (1987) reports that only 20 to 30 percent of former "hard-core" heroin addicts are found to remain heroin-free for three years or more following discharge from a methadone maintenance program, which is about the same success rate reported for other treatment modalities, Including residential drag-free or short-term methadone detoxification programs. Anglin and McGlothlin (1985) state that while it has not produced the wonderful results anticipated by early researchers, methadone maintenance makes a "real and beneficial contribution to reducing the social and individual costs associated with addiction" (pp. 274-75).

The methadone maintenance program at Beth Israel Medical Center in New York has continued to operate since its establishment by Dole and Nyswander. Beth Israel treats more than eight thousand patients who make more than 1 million visits annually to the center's twenty- three outpatient clinics. Approximately 70 percent of the patients have been in continuous treatment for more than two years and 48 percent for more than five years. Treatment is voluntary—the program will not take coerced patients—and patients can remain on methadone for as long as they wish or can opt for detoxification. For the past ten years, the program has operated above capacity. At any point In time more than a thousand eligible applicants cannot be admitted.

Chemical Responses to Cocaine Abuse

Medication may be used as an adjunct to treating cocaine abusers, either as a method for dealing with the deleterious effects of cocaine use itself or in response to the underlying motivations for using cocaine. Medication may be needed to deal with patients who are suicide risks during the post-cocaine "crash" period or who exhibit transient psychotic states. Delusional states and paranoid reactions from excessive cocaine, if they are severe enough, require medication. As noted in chapters 3 and 4, it has been hypothesized that cocaine use may be a form of self- medication for those suffering from certain chemical deficiencies, particularly neurotransmitters that effect mood and activity levels. In fact, note Henry Spitz

and Jeffrey Rosecan (1987), some cocaine abusers have been successfully treated with prescribed antidepressants. Rosecan and Nunes (1987) have outlined the drugs used to treat cocaine abusers, and they emphasize that medication should be used only as an adjunct to a comprehensive cocaine abuse treatment program:

1. **Tricyclic antidepressants (TCAs).** Used for the treatment of cocaine depression, particularly in patients whose use of cocaine appears to be a form of self-medicating efforts to ward off depression, "they [TCAs] appear to reverse some of the neurochemical effects of chronic cocaine administration" (p. 260). It is believed that TCAs act as cocaine antagonists by displacing or blocking cocaine receptors In the CNS and help to reduce the craving for cocaine.

2. **Lithium.** Lithium, a standard drug for psychotic disorders, particularly depressive states, is used for patients whose cyclothymia (mild mood swings) or manic-depression or bipolar (extreme) mood swings preceded cocaine use.

3. **Stimulants.** In patients with a history of child or adolescent attention-deficient disorder (ADD)—Inattention, impulsivity, hyperactivity—cocaine may be a self-medicating effort to deal with this disorder if it continues into adulthood. Such patients respond well to methylphenidate (Ritalin), a stimulant that in ADD patients has a sedating effect. It does not appear to have any positive results in non-ADD cocaine abusers.

4. **Bromocriptine.** Marketed as Parodel, bromocriptine is a dopamine agonist used in the treatment of Parkinson's disease. As noted in chapters 3 and 4, chronic cocaine use may deplete the

neurotransmitter dopamine, causing a craving by dopamine receptors that is satisfied by further Ingestion of cocaine. Bromocriptine appears to bind to the receptors, thus reducing the cocaine craving. It does have serious side-effects, including nausea, headaches, dizziness, abnormal Involuntary movements, and psychosis. Its use, according to Rosencan and Nunes (1987), is justified only in treatment-resistant cases where recovery is hampered by severe craving.

While many of these substances have been used for decades in medical treatment, Rosecan and Nunes (1987) caution that their use for treatment of cocaine abuse remains experimental.

Treatment Using a Psychoanalytic Approach

To the psychoanalyst, symptoms of neurotic behavior such as drug abuse are tied to repressed material of early life—the developmental stages examined in chapter 4.[2] The symptoms will disappear when the repressed material is exposed under psychoanalytic treatment. Psychoanalysis and the therapies based on it aim at "inducing the patient to give up the repressions belonging to his early life and to replace them by reactions of a sort that could correspond better to a psychically mature condition." To do this a psychoanalyst attempts to get the patient "to recollect certain experiences and emotions called up by them which he has at the moment forgotten—repressed (Reiff, 1963, p. 274). This is accomplished through dream interpretation and free association. In a relaxed state, the patient is asked to say what comes to mind about any given element in a dream, or the therapist may ask the patient to let a proper name or even a number occur to him or her. The train of associations stirred up by the dream, the

name, or the number becomes an entry point for the release of repressed material. In order to recreate the emotional state originally attached to these associations, the therapist takes advantage of transference: the development of an emotional attitude, positive or negative, by the patient toward the therapist. Thus, the psychoanalyst may be emotionally (and unconsciously) experienced by the patient as a paternal or maternal figure in a re-creation of the emotions tied to very early psychic development.

Psychoanalysis requires highly skilled therapists and articulate patients, since psychoanalysis and the therapies based on it are "talking therapies." They Involve a long period of costly treatment; psychoanalysis typically involves four or five fifty-minute sessions a week for as long as seven years. There are few published reports of the successful treatment of serious drug abusers using psychoanalytic approaches. As Clifford Yorke (1970) notes with respect to heroin addicts, "the number of confirmed addicts seeking psychoanalytic treatment is almost certainly very small, the number of analysts prepared to accept them even smaller, and the number of addicts who pursue their treatment to conclusion smaller still" (p. 156).

Psychology, notes Jame DeLong (1972), has not found a consistent pathology among drug addicts: "No psychiatric diagnosis can be shown to apply to all heroin addicts or even to a majority of them" (p. 224). George E. Woody and his colleagues (1983) argue, however, "Recent studies indicate that the types of psychiatric problems observed in addicts are similar to illnesses that are often treated with psychotherapy when they occur in nonaddicted populations" (p. 639).

In practice, therapists treating drug abusers, while they may be steeped in psychoanalytic theory, generally avoid the psychoanalytical goal of effecting personality changes. Instead, they focus on improving the ego level of functioning.

Therapists attempt to help patients maintain constructive reality-based relationships, solve problems, and achieve adequate and satisfying social functioning within the client's existing personality structure. The stress of treatment is on the functions of the ego and its ability to adapt to changes in the environment, despite inadequacies experienced during early stages of development. (For a comparison of the effectiveness of different forms of psychotherapy with opiate addicts, see Woody et al, 1983.) This is accomplished through encouragement and moral support, persuasion and suggestion, training and advice, re-education and counseling—not psychoanalysis. The drug therapist typically focuses on identifying specific needs rather than intrapsychic processes.

Anne Jamieson, Alan Glanz, and Susanne MacGregor (1984) describe the approach used at City Roads, a short-term drug treatment program in London:

> The aims of counseling are to clarify needs and to build up the residents' motivation to do something about their needs. The first phase involves getting to know the resident, building up confidence and trust in City Roads. The very fact of sitting down and talking to a staff member who takes an interest in the resident is in itself fruitful. The resident starts to feel that someone cares. This [is] a very positive experience, which many drug abusers are not used to. The next step is "getting to the root of the problem," exploring the personal strengths and weaknesses and their origin. ... The needs or problems under investigation are seen as psychological ones. People are seen as being unable to take responsibility, unable to form relationships, depressed, bitter, angry, frustrated,- and lacking in trust. The

causes of these problems are thought to lie in past experiences, most commonly in an emotionally unstable childhood characterized by lack of parental care, alcoholism in the home, and institutional upbringing, which are thought to lead to deprivation of warmth, care, and stability. (pp. 116-117)

Treatment Using Behavior Modification

The strength of psychoactive substances as positive reinforcers and the negative reinforcement associated with abstinence provide conditioned responses in a drug addict. The major difficulty in treating drug abusers is finding reinforcers that can successfully compete with these substances. For behavior modification to be effective, negative or positive reinforcement, according to classical operant conditioning, must follow immediately after the behavior is exhibited. This is what makes drug use so reinforcing—instant gratification—and why it is so difficult to use behavior modification techniques with chronic drug abusers.

Behavior modification can also include the use of punishment or aversive stimulation to shape behavior. (The latter was popularized in the Stanley Kubrick motion picture A Clockwork Orange.) In drug treatment, Anectine (succinylcholine), a muscle relaxant that causes brief paralysis but leaves the patient conscious, is injected into the subject immediately following the heroin cook-up ritual. The addict remains conscious but is unable to move or to breathe voluntarily, a sensation that simulates the onset of death. The dangers of heroin use are cited while the patient remains paralyzed. Drug antagonists can serve a similar function by rendering the use of opiates or other substances Ineffective (lacking positive reinforcement) or extremely unpleasant (negative reinforcement or punishment). Another technique Is electric shocks self- administered by the addict whenever a craving for the chemical arises. Anna Childress, Thomas McLennan, and Charles O'Brien (1985) found that with drug abusers, imagined aversive stimuli were superior to real aversive stimuli (although this appears to run contrary to a great deal of research in operant conditioning). They report that the use of chemical or electrical stimuli has not proven effective in producing a conditioned aversion in drug abusers, while success has been reported with verbal aversion techniques in which "a patient is asked to imagine strongly aversive stimuli (usually vomiting) in association with imaginal drug-related cues, scenes, and/or behavior" (p. 951).

Other behavioral therapies use biofeedback and relaxation training, and sometimes assertiveness training, to prepare drug abusers to better cope with stress and anxiety believed to be linked to drug use. Researchers have found that certain environmental cues can serve as triggers to activate drug cravings (Dole, 1980). And desensitization has been used: "Patients are usually first relaxed, then given repeated exposure to a graded hierarchy of anxiety-producing stimuli (real or imaginal)" In order to provide a form of immunity (Childress, McLennan, and O'Brien, 1985, p. 957).

In a variant of classical behaviorism, social learning theory places the stress on cognitive mediational processes. According to this view, human beings are active participants in their operant conditioning processes—the individual determines what is and what is not reinforcing. As noted in chapter 4, the actor must learn that ingesting certain chemicals is desirable. Human behavior is complex and reinforcement often abstract. Thus, notes Albert Bandura (1974), "human beings can cognitively bridge delays between behavior and subsequent reinforcement without impairing the efficacy of incentive operations" (p. 862). Humans have a unique capacity to use abstractions—symbols—that can serve as important reinforcers. In using operant conditioning with drug abusers, the social learning theorist stresses the need to analyze the patient in order to discover the variables that are reinforcing.

Much of the success of behavior modification has occurred in the controlled setting of a total institution (Goffman, 1961) such as a prison or hospital. In such environments, important reinforcers can be manipulated by the therapists, often in the form of contingency contracting.

Contingency management and contracting. Sometimes referred to as the token economy, contingency contracting rewards residents for behavior classified as "therapeutic" by providing them with points or tokens that can be redeemed for items valued by the patient, anything from snacks to television time to weekend passes. Roy Pickens and Travis Thompson (1984) describe the program utilized in a drug treatment ward at the University of Minnesota Hospital, where point transactions—added or subtracted—are recorded by staff members in a small booklet that each patient is issued daily. Points can be earned for personal care activities such as cleaning the room or washing clothes, for work chores such as preparing meals, for participation in ward activities, for attending classes that are designed to help residents think rationally about themselves, and for assertiveness and problem-solving that improve Interpersonal skills. Extra points can be earned for the quality of participation and are provided to the resident at the end of each activity: 'At this time a staff person marks the points earned in the patients point booklet and briefly describes how the quality of their participation earned them extra points, or how they might Improve their participation in the class to earn extra points" (p. 55). Points earned are exchangable for various goods or services, for example, snacks, soft drinks, cigarettes, or personal care items. It is obvious that contingency management is not designed to directly affect drug-using behavior but is a means of getting patients to participate in the therapeutic activities that have abstinence as a goal.

The Minnesota program also utilizes contingency contracting a formalized agreement between a staff person and the patient that specifies the manner In which learning principles are applied to the modification of the patient's behavior." The contingency contract is drafted and signed by the parties and "details the specific behaviors to be changed, how such behaviors are to be monitored, and the contingencies [rewards or punishments] to be placed on the behaviors" (Pickens and Thompson, 1984, p. 57). Contingency contracts are also used with patients during the first several weeks after discharge, when they return to their home environment following their hospital stay. The contracts are designed to allow for the implementation of behavioral contingencies in the patient's own home environment to reduce the likelihood of a return to drug use.

Contingency management has been used by methadone clinics to deal with patients who use opiates and other drugs while on methadone maintenance or methadone withdrawal programs. Rewards for drug-free urine include a cash payment and methadone take-home privileges. Negative contingencies include the loss of cash payments or take-home privileges, daily urinalysis, and counseling (Stitzer, Bigelow, Liebson, and McCaul, 1984; see also Magura, Casriel, Goldsmith, Strug, and Lipton, 1987). Stephen Magura and his colleagues (1988, p. 117) report that contingency management utilizing take-home privileges did not have a significant effect on most methadone patients whose polydrug use included cocaine. Cocaine "seems especially attractive to patients and thus was resistant to behavioral modification" (p. 117). Contingency contracting with negative reinforcement has been used to ensure abstinence in cocaine treatment programs: "For example, a patient participating in such a contract will agree that, in the event of relapse, a previously drafted letter will be sent to his employer informing the latter of the patient's cocaine problem" (Kertzner, 1987, p. 145). Robert Kertzner states that negative contingency contracting has been found very effective with patients who agreed to participate. Limitations of this strategy, he adds, are the large number of patients who decline to participate. "Others have modified this technique to Include positive sanctions for continued abstinence, such as returning patients' money held In escrow" (1987, p. 146).

Opposition to behavior modification. There has been considerable opposition to behaviorism in theory and practice (that is, using behavior modification on humans). Opponents argue that it conceives of human beings as equivalent to animals—classical behaviorists refer to all species as organisms—and the techniques used are reminiscent of animal training. It is sometimes described by opponents as "brainwashing." Behavior modification proceeds on the premise that whatever has been learned can be unlearned and replaced by a more suitable behavior. Drug use is seen as the result of inappropriate reinforcement that supports its continuance—drugs are obviously powerful reinforcers to those who enjoy their use. The behavior modifier looks for the reinforcers that maintain the maladaptive behavior and designs strategies to change environmental conditions so that contingencies are placed on behavior patterns that are accepted by society. As opposed to other forms of therapy that require the cooperation of their subjects, behavior modification can be accomplished without the knowledge of the patient. In programs that use contingency management, failure to participate or conform results in punishment. Opponents have argued that the real purpose of such programs is to guarantee docile residents eager to earn what is important in a total institution—which has no important reinforcing value in the freedom of the outside world.

Behaviorists respond that they recognize differences between animals and humans—the term organism is simply a semantic convenience. And while brainwashing does rely on many operant procedures, it involves more than changing behavior. Brainwashing seeks to change attitudes, opinions, and beliefs. And the failure to inform patients that they are being treated by operant techniques would not only be unethical but contrary to sound treatment practice: change occurs more rapidly, behaviorists argue,' when the patient knows the rules and what behavior is being targeted for modification.

Group Treatment

Treatment using psychotherapeutic techniques or behavior modification may utilize casework (one-to-one counseling) or group approaches. According to Helen Northern (1969), one of the advantages of the uses of the group approach is that "stimulation toward Improvement arises from a network of interpersonal influences in which all members participate" (p. 52). The basic theory underlying this approach is that the impact provided by peer interaction is more powerful than therapist–patient interactions within the one-to-one situation. In casework, the relationship between therapist and patient may remain distant because the therapist typically lacks the all-important personal experience with drug abuse. In the group approach, it is the group, not the group leader- therapist, that is the helping Instrument, and this obviates the lack of a personal drug experience by the therapist.

Treatment groups may be formed around one basic trait that all members share and from which the group derives its descriptive label, or they may be formed around a single trait, such as cocaine abuse, with a subtrait being age or gender, for example, adolescents, young adults, female, male, and so on. In general, notes Henry Spitz (1987), the more heterogeneous the group elements, the more intragroup tension is generated that prompts Interaction; the more homogeneous the group elements, the greater the bases for intermember trust and group cohesion. Groups may also be organized at different points in the treatment process, for example, intake, detoxification, inpatient, and outpatient. There also may be groups for important family members such as parents, siblings, and spouses. No matter how the group is organized, commonalities not only form the basis for group cohesiveness and support, but also facilitate the emergence of shared themes which serve as a focal point for group interaction" (Spitz. 1987. p. 168). While group approaches have many advantages over casework, there are considerably fewer therapists trained to work with groups.

Drug Treatment Programs

Treatment can be accomplished in a variety of settings, voluntary and involuntary inpatient and outpatient. We will review some drug programs, the settings, and the treatment that they offer.

Civil and Criminal Commitment

Civil commitment, or the nonpunitive incarceration of addicts for purposes of treatment, began in 1935 when a federal narcotic "farm" was opened in Lexington, Kentucky; a second farm opened in Fort Worth, Texas, in 1938. Addict-patients who requested commitment and Involuntary patients who had been prosecuted for criminal offenses spent six months at these facilities. The facilities followed a standard course of withdrawal, physical restoration, psychological therapy in the form of individual and group counseling, and vocational counseling, after which patients were returned to their communities. The physical structure of these facilities, however, resembled that of a modified prison with walls and bars, and security was strict (Morgan, 1981). Reviews of the program were either mixed or inconclusive, and the federal government chose not to expand civil commitment. In 1961, however, California enacted a program built on the Lexington model.

California Civil Addict Program. In 1961, the state legislature established the California Rehabilitation Center within the Department of Corrections for the compulsory care of persons addicted to narcotics. In 1962, the United States Supreme Court ruled (in Robinson v. California 370 U.S. 660) that drug addiction was an Illness, and therefore a state could not make this status a crime. In that decision the Court also suggested that the Constitution would not be offended by involuntary civil commitment procedures for the purpose of treating the illness of addiction.

A later decision gave further support to the commitment for treatment approach, and in 1963, the legislature amended certain sections of the California Rehabilitation Act to emphasize treatment.

The California statutes provide three methods of commitment (Ryan et al., 1966):

1. After conviction for a misdemeanor or felony but prior to sentencing, a separate superior court proceeding determines if the person is addicted or is in imminent danger of becoming addicted. A positive finding can result in placement with the California Rehabilitation Center for an indeterminate period not to exceed seven years. After treatment, the individual is returned, to the committing court, and criminal proceedings are again activated.

The statutes permit the court to dismiss the criminal charges if the civil addict has responded satisfactorily to the program.

2. Any interested party may report to the district attorney under oath the belief that another person is addicted to narcotics or is in imminent danger of becoming addicted. If sufficient evidence (probable cause) is present, the district attorney may petition the superior court for commitment to a term not to exceed seven years. After discharge this individual is shown in official documents as having no criminal conviction.

3. Any person who believes himself or herself to be addicted or about to become addicted may report such belief to the district attorney, who can then petition the superior court for commitment not to exceed two-and-a-half years. However, most patients are involuntary commitments who have been convicted of crimes (DeLong, 1972).

After commitment, residents must remain in treatment for at least six months. Then they can be released to-after-care/parole supervision. Release to after-care means supervision in the community by a parole agent who has the authority to order a return to the Institution for reversion to the use of drugs or other misbehavior such as associating with addicts, falling to seek employment, or absconding (not reporting). Research into the performance of released patients indicates that they did no better than addicts who received drag therapy in California prisons (DeLong, 1972).

The addict must spend three consecutive years in outpatient status before he or she can be certified by the Narcotic Addiction Evaluation Authority as having successfully completed the program. At any time during the three years of after-care, if his or her behavior requires it, the patient may be returned to the institution for further treatment. In 1970, the required period was reduced to two years, except for methadone maintenance patients. By the end of 1972, nearly eighteen thousand persons had been admitted to the program (McGlothlin, Anglin, and Wilson 1976-77). At the end of 1985 there were 1,362 residents in the California program and 905 on outpatient status (Good et al.. 1986).

Although the stated intent of the enabling legislation was nonpunitive, the program was placed under the Department of Corrections and not a more appropriate treatment agency (such as the Department of Mental Hygiene). As William McGlothlin, Douglas Anglin, and Bruce Wilson (1977a) note, there is little doubt that the political climate in 1961 favored strong measures to suppress narcotic addiction and that the intent of the civil commitment legislation was at least equally as much for control as for treatment (p. 5). Nevertheless, they report that the program clearly reduced daily narcotic use and related behavior among outpatient clients, and. to a lesser extent, the program also appeared to have had lasting benefits subsequent to discharge (1977b, p. 198).

The main center at Corona, about fifty miles from Los Angeles, houses up to two thousand four hundred residents who stay a minimum of six months (the average patient residency is about fourteen months), after which they are released to an after-care program (parole supervision). Release to after-care depends on performance in therapy groups and other parts of the institutional program: one-hour group meetings of each sixty-bed unit five days a week, plus groups of fifteen meeting for one to two hours, two or three times per week.

> The large group generally deals with problems in the day-to-day living in the institution, and the small groups focus more on individual problems. The

overall process is viewed as a modified therapeutic community, and a primary goal is to cause the individual to assume greater responsibility for his/her behavior. From time to time other specialized therapy programs have been initiated. In particular, two dorms have employed more intensive group therapy for four or more hours per day. About 20 to 25 percent are engaged in formal academic training at any given time and around 20 percent are in vocational training. (McGlothlin et al., 1977, p. 7)

New York State Narcotic Addiction Control Commission. In 1966, New York adopted a program similar to that in California. While it incorporated most of the elements of the California program, instead of assigning it to the department of corrections, an independent agency called the Narcotic Addiction Control Commission (NACC) was established on a mental health model. Addicts could be committed through the civil process, voluntarily or as a result of petitions initiated by family members, or as a result of the criminal process (in lieu of receiving a prison term). Civil commitments and those based on misdemeanors were for a maximum of three years, and a five-year commitment was imposed for felonies. Addicts were required to reside in closed institutions (some were former prisons), where they received treatment for their addiction as well as educational opportunities and vocational training. They were subsequently paroled to after-care and came under the supervision of a narcotic parole officer (as distinguished from parole officers working for the Department of Corrections). A reversion to the use of drugs could result in being returned for further institutional care, and urine testing was frequent. Unfortunately, so was absconding, as many addicts simply "jumped parole." A major factor in the demise of NACC was the cost of continuing a program when its expenses were constantly increasing, the supply of addicts seemingly unending (although politics could not be discounted).

The program was established by Governor Nelson Rockefeller, who, at the time, was making a second bid for the Republican presidential nomination—he had been rejected in 1964 for being "too liberal" (the Republicans nominated Barry Goldwater). The drug problem, argues Edward Jay Epstein (1977), provided Rockefeller with an issue that could attract conservative support without alienating liberal Republicans. In 1974, Rockefeller became vice-president under Gerald Ford, and the program was dismantled. By 1979, all NACC commitment centers were closed, a number of them being converted into correctional institutions.

Federal Narcotic Rehabilitation Program.   In 1966, Congress enacted the Narcotic Rehabilitation Act (NARA) which provides for the commitment of three groups of addicts:

1. those choosing treatment as an alternative to criminal prosecution;
2. those assigned after a criminal conviction; and
3. those choosing treatment, or commitment is requested by a relative, without having a criminal charge.

The act empowers a sentencing judge to commit drug-abusing defendants for a period of evaluation not to exceed ninety days. During that time, the offender is evaluated by NARA staff from the Bureau of Prisons at the commitment institution to ascertain his or her stability for treatment. A report is then submitted to the judge, who can commit the defendant to the custody of the surgeon general for treatment which may last up to thirty-six months. Convicted offenders may be committed to the Bureau of Prisons for drug treatment for up to ten years (but not to exceed the maximum sentence for which they were convicted), or placed on probation.

Individuals who have not been charged with a federal crime can be committed via a petition submitted by the U.S. attorney on their behalf or on behalf of a relative. Involuntary patients have a right to a hearing with counsel to determine if they are to be civilly committed. Treatment may last up to forty-two months, although the institutional phase may last only six months (Kay, 1973). Upon release from institutional treatment, patients can be required to participate in an aftercare program under the Probation Division of the United States courts, and a relapse can result in being reinstitutionalized (Eaglin, 1986).

Coercive supervision, civil or criminal, appears to have a positive outcome. George Vaillant (1970) found that while the most effective motivation for abstinence is the fact that narcotics are illegal, "the most potent treatment [is] compulsory supervision. Thus, if the addict is followed over time, external coercion of some kind appears a critical variable in facilitating abstinence" (p. 494). This was my experience when, as a parole officer (Abadmsky. 1987). 1 supervised heroin addicts in New York City—close personal contact, unannounced home visits and searches, arm-checks for needle marks, and random urinalysis provided the ego and superego strengths for addicts to remain heroin free. "Besides offering addicts compulsory support and an external superego, parole itself was probably a substitute for addiction in that it required ex-addicts to remain regularly employed" (Vaillant, 1970. p. 495). The parole officer could redirect the considerable skills and energy of the successful heroin addict into seeking and maintaining legitimate employment (see also Eaglin, 1986). From the behaviorist view, the probation or parole officer provides the basis for applying operant conditioning—rewards tor abstinence, punishment for relapse.

The Therapeutic Community

The therapeutic community (TC) Is a generic term that describes residential, self-help, drug-free treatment programs with some common characteristics, Including concepts adopted from Alcoholics Anonymous (DeLong, 1972): "the notion that there is no such thing as an ex- addict, only an addict who is not using at the moment; the emphasis on mutual support and aid; the distrust of mental-health professionals; and the concept of continual confession and catharsis. However, the TC has extended these notions to Include the concept of a live-in community with a rigid structure of day-to-day behavior and a complex system of punishment and rewards" (pp. 190-191).

According to George De Leon (1986), the primary aims of therapeutic communities are:

> a global change in lifestyle reflecting abstinence from illicit substances, elimination of antisocial activity, increased employability, and prosocial attitudes and values. A critical assumption in TCs is that stable recovery depends upon a successful integration of these social and psychological goals. The rehabilitative approach, therefore, requires multidimensional influences and training that, for most clients, can occur only after an extended period of living in a twenty-four-hour residential setting. (p. 69)

The therapeutic community becomes a surrogate family and a communal support group for dealing with alienation and the abuse of drugs that derives from it. Its purpose, notes Mitchell Rosenthal (1973). is the strengthening of ego functioning, and therapy except for time spent at sleep, is total, James DeLong (1972) notes that there is a quasi- evangelistic quality to the "TC movement," and the residences often resemble a commune, a popular aspect of the late 1950s and 1960s counterculture movement, except that there is generally a strict hierarchy and rigid adherence to norms. The model for therapeutic communities, note Jerome Piatt and Christina Labate (1976), is Synanon. founded in 1958 by Charles E. Dedench, a former alcoholic who was a participant and advocate of the Alcoholics Anonymous approach to substance abuse. The Synanon Foundation expanded rapidly into several states, with facilities run almost entirely by ex-addicts.

Other therapeutic communities, such as Odyssey House, however, have been more receptive to the use of professionals in their programs, and Phoenix House in New York was established by a psychiatrist, Mitchell Rosenthal. David Bellis (1981) is critical of therapeutic communities that resist professional involvement, using instead untrained staff and residents, "many hardly off heroin themselves" (p. 155). While Synanon requires a lifetime commitment, most TCs have abandoned or modified this aspect of the Synanon model. They frequently include vocational training and education to prepare residents to live in the community without continuous help from the TC.

A prominent feature of a TC is the stiff entry requirement: a tough initial interview that tests an applicant's motivation by focusing on his or her inadequacies and lack of success. Successful applicants must indicate a complete investment in the program, which is designed to encourage the resident to identify with the former addicts running the program and become resocialized into a drug-free existence. The new resident is isolated from all outside contacts, including family and friends, and the withdrawal process is accomplished without drugs but with support from other residents. Once the withdrawal process is over, a program of positive and negative reinforcement is implemented. The resident is assigned menial work projects, such as cleaning toilets, but there is an opportunity for more prestigious assignments and greater freedom with program conformity. Transgressions are punished with public humiliation—reprimands, shaved heads, wearing a sign indicating the nature of the violation. Shame and guilt are constantly exploited to force conformity and to change the addict's view of drugs (Piatt and Labate, 1976). Drug use, physical violence, and sexual activity between residents are strictly forbidden and result in expulsion.

Residents are kept busy in a highly structured environment with little time for idleness or boredom—they are expected to be active in all aspects of the TC program. Their failure to do so becomes the subject of individual criticism and the encounter session, a central feature of the therapeutic process. The encounter is a relatively unstructured, leaderless group session in which members focus on a particular resident (who occupies the "hot seat") and confront him or her with criticisms about attitudes and behavior. The target is encouraged to fight back—verbally—although the goal is to break the rationalizations and defenses that help to perpetuate irresponsible thought patterns and behavior (a resocialization process). "The style of the encounter, with its abrasive attacks and its permitted verbal violence ... is designed to encourage the spewing out of pent-up hostility and anger, to force the patient to confront his maladaptive emotional response and behavior patterns" (Rosenthal, 1973, p. 91). Dan Waldorf (1973) points out that the TC is an exciting, friendly, and highly moral—almost Utopian—environment. But, notes Michael Rosenthal (1984), it is not for all abusers:

Severe disturbances may be exacerbated by the TC regimen and may have an adverse effect not only on the disturbed client but also on the treatment environment and the progress of others in the treatment population. Also unsuitable for treatment are candidates whose drug involvement is of so limited a nature as to require a less rigorous intervention or who—despite the deleterious effects of drug abuse—are able to function with the help of a positive support network (e.g., family of significant others). (p. 55)

In addition to the community-based therapeutic communities, several TCs have been established in prisons in New York: the "Stay'n Out Therapeutic Community." Inmates selected for the program are recruited at state correctional facilities and are housed in units segregated from the general population, although they eat and attend morning activities with other prisoners. The program, which lasts from six to nine months, is staffed by graduates of community TCs and ex-offenders with prison experience who act as role models demonstrating successful rehabilitation. Harry Wexler and Ronald Williams (1986) describe the program:

During the early phase of treatment, the major clinical thrust involves observation and assessment of client needs and problem areas. Orientation to the prison TC procedures occurs through individual counseling, encounter sessions, and seminars. Clients are given low-level jobs and granted little status. During the later phase of treatment, residents are provided opportunities to earn higher-level positions and increased status through sincere

Daytop Village

Located on New York's Staten Island, Daytop Village (DV) is a large mansion built around the turn of the century, Both outside and inside, it conveys the atmosphere of a college fraternity house, Persons entering or leaving the facility check in with a person seated at a desk near the entrance, Depending on the time of day, people may be cleanings walking to and fro, or lounging, playing cards, checkers, or chess and listening to music. Friends and relatives of the residents are not welcome [66]as they are likely to undermine the progress that residents are making,. Relatives are likely to upset a resident's progress more from misguided good Mentions, but nonetheless, they are not free to visit except by special permission" (Sugannan, 1974, p. 2). "Open house" is held on Saturday evenings, which outsiders are encouraged to attend for a formal program. It is explained to visitors that DV should be considered not a "program" but "a family of people helping each other to overcome their problems; that drugs themselves were not their real problem but only the symptom of underlying problems of personality, and especially the problem of not feeling good about oneself" (Sugannan, 1974, p. 2).

A tour of the facility reveals that it is spotlessly clean—residents clean up after themselves immediately when smoking, drinking, or eating. Overall maintenance is a task assigned to new residents, who are responsible for the least desirable housekeeping tasks.

> One impression that may be formed in only half an hour is a well-ordered community where rules are generally respected and enforced when necessary, where people jump to carry out orders and do so quite cheerfully, and where people work hard. Considering the kind of people who live here and what they were like before, things seem to run with amazing smoothness. As one sees more, one discovers that this orderliness is only achieved at the price of constant pressure and surveillance, tough sanctions for deviance, and a high dropout rate. (Sugarman, 1974, p. 4)

While I was a parole officer, I heard heroin addicts describe DV (and similar TCs) as worse than the prison environment; some refused to stay even when faced with the alternative of farther incarceration.

The approach at DV is almost an exact replication of that at Synanon, put in place by David Oeitch, who became director in 1964. Beitch had been director of the Synanon house in Westport, Connecticut residents and staff reject the notion of a program and, instead, refer to the approach as "The Concept." In the first years of operation, the concept began when an abuser attempted to gain admittance and was told to call back at specified intervals for a number of days before being invited for an interview. Prior to the interview, the prospect was left seated for several hours In the living room and had to ask permission to go to the washroom or for anything else he or she wanted. The individual was not permitted to talk to anyone except the specially assigned resident. This experience was so nerve wracking for some addicts that they left before the interview.

The interview itself was demanding and traumatic: the addict was ridiculed and required to accept his or her situation for what It was—"Don't try to con us, we're dope fiends also"—and to admit that drug-using behavior Is a symptom of either a stupid person or a "baby." The prospective resident often was required to scream at the top of his or her lungs, "Help me" or, "I need help." Robert Brook and Paul Whitehead (1980) report that now, in contrast to the earlier intake/entry procedures, the atmosphere at DV is less threatening, and admissions are handled during a two-day period through the Screening, Induction, and Referral Unite "At this time, medical examinations are given and psychological, demographic, and drug history data are collected" (p. 33).

After the interview the prospect is welcomed into the community, given a tour, and introduced to the other residents. He or she is required to give up all personal possessions; telephone and letter-writing privileges must be earned. New residents undergoing withdrawal do so without medication and in the living room where they can interact with others, play cards, or listen to music. Exaggerations of suffering are ridiculed, while a "grin and bear it" attitude is supported by the other residents, "This sharing of experience lessens its wretchedness. We see here an interesting example of the way in which physical symptoms can be radically affected by the social context in which the person finds himself" (Sugarman, 1974, p. 15), Novices are discouraged from talking to other new residents in order to avoid reinforcing negative behavior, and they soon begin to integrate into the continuing rounds of lectures and encounter sessions. Residents are to relate to each other as family—brothers and sisters. Thus, honesty, even if confrontational, is required, while, in addition to drugs and violence, sexual activity is strictly forbidden.

involvement in the program and hard work. Encounter groups and counseling sessions are more in-depth and focus on the areas of self-discipline. sell-worth, self-awareness, respect for authority, and acceptance of guidance for problem areas. Seminars take on a more intellectual nature. Debate is encouraged to enhance self-expression and to increase self-confidence. (p. 224)

Released prison TC graduates are encouraged to become part of the extensive TC network available in the community. In an examination of the effect of the prison TC on parole success, Wexler, Lipton, and Foster (1985) found that "Stay'n Out" was effective in reducing recidivism rates.

A great deal of controversy has developed over the rate of success experienced by therapeutic communities, and most research has been inadequate or inconclusive (Brook and Whitehead. 1980). Many TCs release statistics that cannot withstand scrutiny by disinterested researchers. The imposing screening process keeps out many drug abusers who would probably fail in the program, and graduation from a TC does not provide a basis for diagnosing success. A realistic portrayal would conclude that the TC provides some ex-drug abusers with a support system insofar as they gain employment with a TC or similar program. Outside of the TC,

> drug addicts, regardless of age, sex, or race, tend to occupy low status positions, rarely have legitimate sources of income, and are vulnerable to unemployment and general economic fluctuations. Impoverished educational backgrounds further limit their chances to better their positions. Within Synanon, addicts have positions that afford them a measure of self-respect and the opportunity to earn the respect of others. These factors help to account for the many who choose to remain in Synanon and make it a way of life. (Brook and Whitehead, 1980, p. 29)

Those who need to manage in the community without the continuing support of a TC are at risk, since they will return to the same environment that led to drug abuse in the first place, and they often bring with them all of the educational and vocational deficiencies they had upon entering. Those entering the TC with a greater degree of mental health, only limited or no attachment to a criminal subculture, and employment skills are obviously better equipped to deal with the post-TC existence.

Other Treatment Programs

In the last few years there has been an enormous expansion of programs to treat substance abusers. Some are profit-making and others are nonprofit; many call themselves therapeutic communities, although they differ dramatically from the TCs discussed above. These programs typically share a number of variables. They do a great deal of outreach—most employ a marketing person—often advertising for clients likely to have health insurance, such as employed alcoholics and cocaine users, as opposed to heroin addicts, since the cost can range between $250 and $500 a day for inpatient care. Many are located in a healthcare facility, and this typically increases the cost of treatment. Adding a chemical abuse program to a health-care facility can help reduce the number of otherwise vacant beds. The treatment approach usually includes individual and group counseling, and the model tends to be eclectic rather than doctrinal. Virtually all of the many programs that I have examined throughout the country utilize an Alcoholics Anonymous (AA) or Narcotics Anonymous (NA) approach, despite the paucity of research on the efficacy of the AA approach.[3]

Alcoholics Anonymous and Narcotics Anonymous. Alcoholics Anonymous (AA) is a fellowship founded by William ("Bill W") Wilson (1895-1971), a financial investigator and alcoholic, and Robert ("Dr. Bob") Holbrook Smith (1879-1950), a physician and alcoholic. Bill W. earlier had joined the Oxford Group (renamed Moral Re-Armament in 1939), an international religious movement, because of the influence of another alcoholic whose religious experience appeared to act as a "cure," Bill W. was influenced by the work of William James (1842-1910), a psychiatrist and philosopher, particularly his Varieties of Religious Experience (1902). As part of the Oxford Group, he began dedicating his activities to curing alcoholics, an effort that was quite unsuccessful until he met another member of the Oxford Group, Dr. Bob, in 1935 while on a business trip. He helped Dr. Bob become abstinent, and the two recognized that success in helping alcoholics was not to be found in preaching abstinence but in a fellowship where each alcoholic simply relates his or her story of drunkenness and conversion to a nonalcoholic lifestyle. The "listening" is as Important as the "telling." "There could not have been just one founder of AA," notes Robertson (1988b) "because the essence of the process is one person telling his story to another as honestly as he knows how" (p. 34). The group became known as Alcoholics Anonymous after the title of Wilson's 1939 book of the same name, often referred to by AA members as "The Big Book" (it was quite bulky when originally published). Wilson was supported by the substantial royalties the book eventually generated.

The AA program requires an act of surrender—an acknowledgment of being an alcoholic and the destructiveness that results—a bearing of witness, and an acknowledgement of a higher power. While AA is non- denominational, there Is a strong repent-your-sins revivalism spirit, and some groups begin their meetings with the Lord's Prayer (Robertson, 1988b). (In 1987, a Maryland resident, convicted for drunken driving, was placed on probation and ordered to attend AA. In 1988, the American Civil Liberties Union brought suit on his behalf arguing that requiring AA attendance violated their clients right to freedom of religion [Ayres, 1988b].) AA recognizes the potency of shared honesty and mutual vulnerability openly acknowledged. The AA group serves to support each member in his or her effort to remain alcohol free. "Maintenance of sobriety depends on our sharing of our experiences, strength and hope with each other, thus helping to identify and understand the nature of our disease" (AA literature).

The AA conceptual model is that alcoholism is a disease that cannot be cured—thus, there are no ex-alcoholics, merely recovering alcoholics. AA members are encouraged to accept the belief that they are powerless over alcohol, that they cannot control their intake, that total abstinence is required. New members are advised to obtain a sponsor who has remained abstinent and who will help them work through the "Twelve Steps," which are the essence of the AA program. Those who are successful twelfth steppers" carry the AA message and program to other alcoholics—they become "missionaries" for AA.

AA and groups based on the AA-approach, notes Henry Spitz (1987), "attempt to instill the substitution of more adaptive attitudes to replace habitual dysfunctional ones. The extreme use of denial and projection of responsibility for chemical dependency onto other people, circumstances, or conditions outside oneself is an example of a target behavior strongly challenged in the substance abuse self help groups The familiar opening statement of "I'm an alcoholic and/or drug addict" epitomizes the concrete representation that defense mechanisms of projection and denial run counter to the group culture and norms" (p. 160).

"There is a minimum of formal organization, no power of punishment or exclusion in AA, and the only authority is shared experience" (Norris, 1976, p. 737). The basic AA unit is the local group, which is autonomous except in matters affecting other AA groups or the fellowship as a whole. "No group has powers over its members and instead of officers with authority, groups rotate leadership" (AA literature). A secretary chosen by the members plans the meetings and sets the agenda. In most local groups the position is rotated every six months. Delegates to the General Service Conference serve two years. There are twenty-one trustees, of whom seven are nonalcoholics who are often helping professionals in social work or medicine and who may serve for up to nine years—alcoholic trustees may serve only four years. There are no entry requirements or dues: "the hat is passed" at most meetings to defray costs. Some of this money goes to support a local service committee and the General Service Office in New York. While AA does not engage in fund-raising, and no one person is permitted to contribute more than $1.U0Q. considerable income is generated from the sale of publications.

The Twelve Steps of Narcotics Anonymous

1. We admitted that we were powerless over our addiction, that our lives had become unmanageable.
2. We came to believe that a Power greater than ourselves could restore us to sanity.
3. We made a decision to turn our will and our lives over to the care of God as we understood Him.
4. We made a searching and fearless moral inventory of ourselves.
5. We admitted to God, to ourselves, and to another human being the exact nature of our wrongs.
6. We were entirely ready to have God remove all these defects of character.
7. We humbly asked Him to remove our shortcomings.
8. We made a list of all persons we had harmed, and became willing to make amends to them all.
9. We made direct amends to such people whenever possible, except when to do so would injure them or others.
10. We continued to take personal inventory and when we were wrong promptly admitted it.
11. We sought through prayer and meditation to improve our conscious contact with God as we understood Him, praying only for knowledge of His will for us and the power to carry that out.
12. Having had a spiritual awakening as a result of these steps, we tried to carry this message to addicts and practice these principles in all our affairs.

SOURCE; *Narcotics Anonymous World Service Office, PO Box 9999, Van Nuys, CA 91409; telephone (818) 780=3951.*

The financial affairs of the General Service Office are handled by nonalcoholics: "The reason is that Bill Wilson and the early AAs were afraid that if anybody running AA fell off the wagon, that would be bad enough, but if he were handling finances as well, the results could be disastrous' (Robertson. 1988a. p. 57).

Because of their fear of losing employment, recovering alcoholics are often unwilling to admit their problem in front of others—hence strict anonymity became part of the AA approach. AA never uses surnames at meetings or in its publications. According to an AA publication: "Individual anonymity is paramount. No AA member has the right to divulge the identity or membership of any other member. We must always maintain personal anonymity at the level of press, radio, TV and film" (hence the use of "Bill W. and "Dr. Bob"). AA members typically attend tour meetings a week for about five years, after which they attend less frequently or they may drop out completely when capable of functioning comfortably without alcohol. "The movement works in quiet and simple ways. Members usually give of themselves without reservation: exchange telephone numbers with newcomers: come to help at any hour when a fellow member is in crisis: are free with tips on how to avoid that first drink" (Robertson, 1988a. p. 47).

Robertson (1988b) notes that some AA groups are less than accepting of persons addicted to substances other than alcohol. However, now there are groups for drug abusers based on the AA approach, for example, Cocaine Anonymous (CA). These are generally referred to as Twelve-Step Groups; one is Narcotics Anonymous (NA).

In the last ten years, reports Nan Robertson (1988a), young people, "most of them addicted to other drugs as well as alcohol," have streamed Into AA. "It is common now at AA meetings." she points out, "to hear a young speaker say. My name is Joe, and I'm a drug addict and an alcoholic." A number of AA groups resent and resist the entry of drug abusers into AA, which helps explain the existence of CA and NA.

The two programs that follow are typical of those utilizing an AA/NA approach. The first is an outpatient program for young persons; the second, an inpatient one for adults.

Straight, Inc.[4] Straight, Inc., is a nonprofit organization for the treatment of young drug abusers, founded in 1976 by a group of business leaders and concerned parents in the St. Petersburg, Florida, area. The program now operates in eight cities. Straight receives no government funding; operating expenses are covered by client fees (70 percent) and private donations (30 percent). The average length of treatment is one year, and the treatment staff consists of professionals and paraprofessionals (persons without a bachelor's degree). Clients range in age from twelve to early twenties; the average age is seventeen. Sixty percent are male. The program currently treats about eight hundred people nationwide, and more than five thousand five hundred persons have been treated since the program began. Straight accepts only voluntary clients, and each must be accompanied by a parent. Most clients have abused a variety of substances, but rarely heroin.

The therapeutic approach utilized at Straight Is a combination of the "Twelve Steps" and cognitive therapy. The program is drug-free and operates on an out-patient basis, although each client at admission is required to spend at least two weeks with a "host" family that has a child in an advanced stage of the program. After these first two weeks, the client returns home to begin a twelve-hour daily participation in the program, Monday through Saturday, and seven hours on Sunday. Satisfactory performance reduces the number of hours and days until the program is completed. In the final stage, the client helps the staff with group sessions, and some clients receive training to become part of the program staff.

The program uses peer pressure in an effort to instill a more positive attitude toward behavior. The peer group is activated as a helping tool through "rap sessions"; some are confrontational (such as those used in the therapeutic community) while others are instructional or idea- developing: "Different types of raps are scheduled throughout the day, although all focus on drug use and recovery through self-change using the program tools. Led by two rap leaders (staff members), raps have topics that involve the group in working together on a single rap theme and also working individually on different therapeutic tasks within the treatment process. There are also groups in which parents and siblings participate. After completing the Straight program, the young person is urged to participate in an Alcoholics Anonymous or Narcotics Anonymous group in the community.

Powell III Inpatient Treatment Programs[5] The Powell III Inpatient Treatment Program was established in 1973 and is based at the Iowa Methodist Medical Center in Des Moines. Treatment is "oriented to Alcoholics Anonymous and Narcotics Anonymous." On admission the patient is given a preliminary examination, temperature and blood pressure are taken by a nurse, and he or she "may begin standard detoxification procedure." A physician takes a complete medical history and orders blood and urine tests and x-rays. A counselor/case manager is assigned to meet with the patient periodically to discuss his or her progress. During the second week of residence, patient and counselor develop an individual treatment plan, set a discharge date, and coordinate any post-release referrals that are necessary. A social worker is assigned to the patient and the patient's family to make an assessment of the family unit to help guide the staff team during the treatment process. A psychologist administers the Minnesota Multiphasic Personality Inventory (MMPI) and may initiate additional tests if there is a question of brain dysfunction, learning disabilities, or stress disorders. A significant part of the program involves a healthy, balanced diet and recreation—"to learn how to have fun and to use leisure time in healthy ways."

During the first week, the patient has written assignments involving essay-type questions about certain behaviors, for example, "What happened during the last few days before entering the program that led you to seek treatment? Provide an inventory of negative behavior resulting from your use of psychoactive chemicals." The patient must also memorize the first three steps of the twelve-step AA program and is introduced to AA meetings, which become an important part of the program for the remainder of inpatient treatment (generally thirty days). There are also lectures and films on the medical, psychological, and social aspects of drug abuse.

Throughout the inpatient stage there is a daily mix of individual and group counseling, lectures, films, meals, and recreation. There are special group meetings that are attended by family members and other sessions that are attended by both patients and family members. Out-patient care consists of referral to AA or NA, and there are services provided by Powell III in the event of relapse.

Success Rate of Drug Treatment Programs

Patrick Biernacki (1986) notes that there are serious problems with respect to gauging the success of drug treatment programs. He asks, for example. What does a 50 percent rate of success mean? Would some, most, or all of the persons who were "successful have abandoned drug addiction without treatment? He points out that drug treatment programs may be successful only with those addicts who have already resolved to stop using

drugs: "Once addicts voluntarily have resolved to stop using drugs, treatment programs may then be able to help them realize their resolutions to change" (p. 191).

Prevention of Drug Abuse

Efforts at prevention attempt to reduce the supply of or the demand for illegal drugs. The former is the goal of drug law enforcement (which will be examined in chapter 7); the latter has been the goal of coercive legislation and education. "Considering the difficulty and cost of treating individuals with substance abuse problems, the prospect of developing effective substance abuse prevention programs has long held a great deal of appeal" ("Drug Abuse," 1987, p. 35). But effective prevention has proven to be as elusive as effective treatment (and effective law enforcement).

Educating persons, particularly elementary, high school, and college students who are seen as the primary population at risk, about the dangers of drug use would seem to be an idea devoid of controversy and a sound response to the problem of drug abuse. After all, Richard Brotman and Frederic Suffet (1975) point out, this appears to be quite rational: Provide valid information about the harmful consequences of drug abuse, and most persons will elect to avoid them. However, Patricia Wald and Peter Hutt (1972) note, "there Is substantial uncertainty and confusion in the area of drug education and prevention" because "there is no real evidence that such educational efforts are successful" (p. 18). Research by Isidor Chein and his colleagues (1964) among adolescents revealed that those youngsters with greatest knowledge of drags are also those most susceptible to abusing drugs. Informational programs typically suffer from major weaknesses that may actually encourage drag use: "The unfortunate result is that young people may become more rather than less likely to experiment with drags" (Goodstadt, n.d., p. 2).

Providing greater knowledge of drugs may serve the unintended (or latent) function of piquing interest in or arousing greater curiosity about drugs, and it may possibly encourage the more daring among adolescents to seek out drug experiences. In New York, heroin is seemingly everywhere in black and Puerto Rican ghettos, where young people are exposed to it at an early age: they know about heroin and drug addicts through close first-hand exposure; they witness the purchase of drugs, the addicts nodding on the streets, clustering in doorways, communal washrooms, and rooftops to "get off." They experience the addicts' theft of family belongings in an effort to secure funds for drugs. The real question, Dan Waldorf (1973) states, is not why so many ghetto residents become drug abusers, but why a majority avoid becoming addicted to such a powerful substance that provides relief from an oppressive environment. However, even though there is evidence that drug users possess much greater knowledge of drugs than nonusers, "there is no evidence that increases in such knowledge stimulate use" (Hanson, 1980, p. 273).

The standard educational approach has involved a presentation of factual information concerning the dangers of substance abuse, because it was assumed that increased knowledge served as an effective deterrent to use—that students would make rational decisions not to use drugs. "Such information has frequently been laden with ethical and moral judgments so that the 'proper' decision for the individual has been preordained" (Zinberg, 1984, p. 204). An integral part of this approach has often been scare-type lectures, presented by physical education teachers or nonschool personnel such as police officers, that are supposed to frighten students into avoiding dangerous substances. Often filled with misinformation or exaggeration, these lectures raise the skepticism of students and place all educational efforts in jeopardy. In more recent years the antidrug public-service message has often been delivered by well-known entertainers or athletes —a questionable approach, given the level of substance abuse reported in these groups. A 1987 "Stop Substance Abuse" film featured athletes, including basketball star Orlando Woolridge of the New Jersey Nets, urging youngsters to avoid drugs; in 1988 the Nets announced that Woolridge was entering a drug rehabilitation program.

The American Social Health Association (1972) states that drug education "must avoid overconcentration on the drug problem.' Many youngsters, knowing more about drugs than their parents and teachers, will not accept moralization but will respect realistic, valid information derived from a credible source" (p. 5). The dangers of exaggeration or misinformation in an antidrug effort are emphasized by Brotman and Suffet (1975), who state that "if a program's audience disbelieves information on drugs which in their experience are not terribly dangerous, they may also discredit information on drugs whose dangers are more certain, and thus be induced to try them (p. 60). A better approach to educating young persons about certain dangerous chemicals avoids exaggeration and scare-tactics and, instead, relics on a factual presentation about dangerous substances and the body's reaction to them—euphoric qualities as well as dangers. The goal is to provide information so that students can make informed decisions, and not the prevention of drug use, which is seen as too much to expect from any educational program.

There are some problems with this approach:

1. It may encounter opposition from public officials and/or parents who believe in the need for schools to teach proper behavior, that is, to preach the evils of drug use.

Project DARE

Project DARE (Drug Abuse Resistance Education) is a joint project of the Los Angeles Police Department (LAPD) and the Los Angeles Unified School District It is designed to help fifth-, sixth-, and seventh-grade children resist peer pressure to use drugs, alcohol, and tobacco. Uniformed police officers serve as instructors. All are veteran officers and serve full time on the project as volunteers. They are carefully selected by DARE supervisory staff and receive training from school district specialists.

> A DARE police officer is assigned to teach in every elementary school under the LAPD's jurisdiction, offering the seventeen-session core curriculum to either fifth- or sixth-grade students. A junior-high program for seventh- graders, which includes early intervention with students deemed at risk, is also at full implementation in fifty-eight junior high schools.
> In bringing the core curriculum to the elementary schools, DARE officers are assigned to five schools per semester, and they visit each classroom once a week. Beyond this, the officers conduct one-day visits at other schools for an assembly program and follow-up visits in individual classrooms; hold formal training sessions on drug abuse for teachers; and conduct evening parent meetings. (Belong, 1987, p. 4)

The use of uniformed police officers as instructors, notes William Dejong (1987), is seen as a key element in the program's success: "Police have a knowledge of the drug scene and its impact on both individuals and society as a whole that regular classroom teachers cannot match. Indeed, many classroom teachers frankly admit their discomfiture in teaching lessons on drug abuse. For children this age, police hold a mystique. Kids respond to them" (p. 7). And since the program "involves police officers in positive, non-punitive roles, students are more likely to develop positive attitudes toward police officers and greater respect for the law" (p. 17).

Curriculum. The DARE curriculum consists of seventeen lessons:

1. **Personal safety.** This lesson acquaints students with the role of the police officer in the classroom and reviews various safety practices to protect students from harm. There are discussions about the rights of students that are printed in their DARE notebooks—for example, the right to be protected from harm, the right to say no to another person when asked to do something they know is wrong, the right to say no to being touched in unacceptable ways. Students discuss the 911 emergency number and, through role-play, leant how to summon help.

2. **Drug use and misuse.** The harmful effects of drugs when misused are highlighted, and a film, "Drugs and Your Amazing Mind," explains the positive and negative effects of a number of drags on the body, why people use drugs, and how to say no.

3. **Consequences.** The officer assigns a work sheet that requires students to list positive and negative consequences of both using and choosing not to use alcohol and marijuana. The students report their answers, which the officer places on the blackboard under "positive" and "negative." The officer points out that most of the negative consequences are listed under use of alcohol and marijuana, while most of the positive consequences refer to choosing not to use these substances.

4. **Resisting pressure to use drugs.** This key lesson introduces four major influences on people's behavior: personal preferences, family expectations, peer expectations, and the mass media. After defining peer pressure, the officer explains the different types of pressure that friends will exert to get others to use alcohol or drugs, ranging from friendly persuasion and teasing to threats—"If you won't, I won't be your friend." Students then complete two exercises, "Saying No to Friendly Pressure" and "Saying No to Teasing Pressure" The first requires students to respond to a cartoon showing two children pressuring a third to drink some beer in a friendly way, while the second does the same with a cartoon with' the caption, "Don't be chicken. It's only a joint!" Students are to write down a way to say no.

5. **Resistance techniques: Ways to say no.** In order to reinforce lesson 4, students practice effective ways of responding to peer pressure. In groups, students come before the class and rehearse one of these resistance techniques, and the officer explains how certain techniques work better in certain situations.

6. **Building self-esteem.** After reviewing completed homework assignments on the topic, "Why Some Kids Use Drugs," the officer establishes that poor self-esteem is one of the most important factors associated with drug use. The importance of giving and getting compliments is stressed; students put their names at the top of a work sheet entitled, "Giving a Compliment," which they exchange with classmates. Students write compliments about each student as the sheet is passed, and they are eventually returned to their owners. Each student then writes a self-compliment.

7. **Assertiveness: A response style.** Through role play, an assertive response is contrasted with both passive and aggressive styles. Students then list situations that call for an assertive response; then they work with a partner to develop a skit on being assertive using one of the situations listed by the class—or they invent one. These skits are evaluated by the students. The officer emphasizes that assertiveness is appropriate when turning down offers to use drugs.

8. **Managing without taking drugs.** The officer discusses stress and constructive ways of dealing with it. Students generate a list of stressful situations and note how much stress they live with on a work sheet titled "My Stress Level" Working in groups, students choose two stressors and devise strategies for preventing these stressors from

operating or for relieving stress when they do. The strategies are shared with the class. The officer presents numerous ways to manage stress that include learning how to relax, exercise, talking to a friend.

9. **Media influences on drug use.** This lesson examines the strategies employed by mass media to promote certain products. Based on these strategies, students work in groups to develop an anti-alcohol or anti-drug commercial, which is performed before the class.

10. **Decision making and risk taking.** Students list typical risk-taking behaviors, and the officer identifies steps to follow when faced with a choice involving risk. Students practice decision making through role play and several written exercises, some involving hypothetical offers of alcohol or drugs from friends.

11. **Alternatives to drug use.** Referring back to earlier lessons on why some young people use drugs, the officer asserts that these are reasons that are experienced by all young persons and that there are healthier ways of responding. Students fill out a work sheet on activities they enjoy and are asked to explain why these activities are more fun than taking drugs.

12. **Role modeling.** Older students who are school leaders and have resisted peer pressure to use drugs discuss their experiences with the class.

13. **Forming a support system.** The officer Introduces the concept of a support system by asking, "Why do people need other people?" and, "What do other people do for us?" The officer points out that everyone has needs that can be met only through positive relationships with other people. Students complete a work sheet on "Choosing Friends," which requires that they list the qualities they look for in choosing friends. Students share their responses and discuss barriers to friendship and how to overcome them. The officer notes that all students already belong to two support systems—the class and the family—and the officer draws a diagram of his/her support systems. Students do the same as part of a homework assignment.

14. **Ways of dealing width pressure from gangs.** Students name the social activities they enjoy and the people with whom they share them. The officer notes their relationships with people and how these people enable them to satisfy their need for recognition, acceptance, and affection. Some people join gangs, the officer notes, to meet these same needs, and the negative consequences of gang membership are discussed. The officer discusses ways to avoid gang approaches; this is followed by reading vignettes involving bullying behavior by gang members. Students discuss the choices they have and their consequences.

15. **Project DARE summary.** Students summarize and assess what they have learned from participating in the program.

16. **Taking a stand.** Students complete a homework assignment work sheet, "Taking a Stand," which articulates how they will keep their body healthy, control their feelings when they are angry or under stress, decide whether to take a risk, respond when

a friend pressures them to use alcohol or drugs, and respond when they see people on television using alcohol or drugs. This assignment becomes the student's "DAME Pledge," which they read to the class. The student whose pledge is voted the best by the class reads it at a school assembly.

17. **DARE culmination.** A school-wide assembly includes the reading of the winning "DARE Pledges," and each student who completed the program receives a certificate of achievement signed by the chief of police and superintendent of schools.

2. A great deal is still unknown about drugs of abuse.

3. Depending on their age. students may not be able to understand the information being provided.

Furthermore, "some experts believe that giving specific factual knowledge reinforces the antidrug propensities of persons not likely to abuse drugs anyway but actually contributes to the 'seduction' of vulnerable high-risk groups by romanticizing the negativism that motivates their conduct" (Wald and Abrams, 1972, p. 133). Research by Richard Stuart (1974) indicates that a fact-oriented drug curriculum may actually increase the danger of involvement with drugs.

Research indicates that drug addicts are quite familiar with the effects and dangers of the substances they abuse, but they either discount the risks or view them as minor and part of the "game" (see, for example, Hendler and Stephens, 1977). Troy Duster (1970) reports that the prospective addict sees himself as an exception to the pattern of addiction around him: "It is typical of the early experience of the addict-to-be that he knows of people who use narcotics and who get away with it ... [in that] they are neither addicted nor are they known to the police. This double victory is witnessed by probably every individual who knowingly used heroin illegally for the first time" (p. 192). Good- stadt (n.d.) suggests

acknowledging the positive reinforcements of drug use: "Drug use consequences are not all negative; if they were, nobody would continue to use drugs. Moderate use of some drugs offers physical, psychological, and social benefits for some people. Drug education programs that do not take into account this important aspect of the decision to start or continue using drugs diminish their credibility and effectiveness" (p. 3).

Norman Zinberg (1984), a psychiatrist and well-known researcher on drug use, recommends educational programs that parallel the approach so often used with respect to adolescent sexual behavior: "Although our society does not condone teenage sexual activity, it has decided that those who are unwilling to follow its precepts should be given the basic information needed to avoid disease and unwanted pregnancy." Accordingly, drug education should provide information on how to avoid the effects of destructive drug combinations (for example, barbiturates and alcohol), the unpleasant consequences of using drugs of unknown purity, the hazards of using drugs with a high dependence liability, the dangers of certain modes of administration, and the unexpected effects of various dose levels and various settings" (p. 207). Some people, however, notes Goodstadt, believe that responsible use of drugs is not an acceptable objective tor education programs, especially for the young, but this position ignores the realities of drug use:

First, use of alcohol and medications with parental supervision is usually neither harmful nor illegal. Second, it is unrealistic to talk to illegal drug users as if they do not, and would not, use drugs. Efforts to prevent drug abuse by reducing the most risky forms of drug use (for example, drinking and driving, cannabis use and gymnastics) need not condone illegal drug use. Third, it may be unrealistic to counsel immediate abstinence for chronic drug users; more responsible use of an illegal drug may be an appropriate intermediate objective for such a population. (p. 3)

And an eight-year study of adolescent drug use revealed that the vast majority of teen-agers who occasionally use drugs suffer no long-lasting negative effects and cannot in later years be distinguished from those who abstained from drug use (Blakeslee, 1988b).

A broad approach to prevention involves "affective" or "humanistic" education (although the use of this term is likely to trigger negative responses from persons holding certain religious and social views). These efforts are designed to enhance self-esteem, to encourage responsible decision making and to enrich the personal and social development of students. The bases of this approach are the following assumptions ("Drug Abuse," 1987, p. 35):

1. Substance abuse programs should aim to develop prevention- oriented decision making concerning the use of licit or illicit drugs.
2. Such decisions should result in fewer negative consequences for the individuals.
3. The most effective way of achieving these goals is by increasing self-esteem,

interpersonal skills, and participation in alternatives to substance use.

These assumptions are generally implemented through communication training, peer counseling, role playing, and assertiveness training.

In the Los Angeles school system, this approach has been implemented through Project DARE.

Similar programs have focused on various areas of social functioning:

1. **Social Influence Approach.** "Inoculating students" against using dangerous substances by making them aware of the social pressures they are- likely to encounter and teaching skills that promote refusal.
2. **Social Learning Approach.** Chemical abuse is seen from the perspective of learning theory, that is, like other behavior, it is learned through modeling and reinforcement. Through instruction, demonstration, feedback, reinforcement, behavioral rehearsal (classroom practice), and extended practice through homework assignments, the youngster is taught life-coping skills that have a broad range of applications beyond the specific goal of preventing drug abuse. There is considerable variation in age groups and program length, and some use adults, while others use peer leaders.

In an extensive review of research into drug education, David Hanson (1980) concludes:

Research has demonstrated that while it is relatively easy to increase drag knowledge, it is more difficult to modify attitudes. A number of students have reported greater changes in knowledge and attitude, or have reported changes in knowledge unaccompanied by changes in attitude. Clearly the most rigorous test of educational effectiveness involves subsequent drag usage. By far the largest number of studies have found no *effects* of education upon use. A few have found drug usage to be reduced while others have found it to be increased following drug education. (p. 273, emphasis added)

Harith Swadi and Harry Zeitlin (1987) state: "It must be our conclusion that the available methods of drug education that aim at preventing drug abuse are at best ineffective, if not counterproductive" (p. 745). The National Institute on Drug Abuse (1987) says that "substance abuse prevention research remains in its infancy" and that "we are still far from having a range of prevention strategies whose long-term efficacy is in little doubt" (p. 50). Although the General Accounting Office (1987) reported to Congress that drug prevention efforts have been unevaluated or have shown little or no impact, in 1987 Congress allocated almost $250 million to continue such efforts.

The difficulty experienced in producing and implementing effective drug abuse prevention programs may be related to some of the technical aspects of such programming. It may be—and there is evidence to support such a hypothesis— that drug abuse prevention programs are too often "put together" and implemented by well-meaning but limited persons—a "happy hands at home" approach to a complex problem. For example, Patricia Bush and Ronald Iannotti (1987) note that efforts designed to educate elementary-school-age children about drug abuse often fail to consider Cognitive Development Theory (originally developed by Jean Piaget), and lessons may be inappropriate to the child's developmental stage: "Health education programs which are produced by adults who are unaware of children's developmental stages may be, while not necessarily counterproductive, a waste of resources" (p. 70). "Strategies which are adequate for preventing experimentation among those at low risk of engaging in serious antisocial behaviors may be wholly inadequate for preventing initiation and use by those who exhibit a deviance syndrome. On the other hand, well-founded strategies for preventing drug abuse among those at highest risk tor abuse may be inappropriate for those at risk of only becoming experimental users (Hawkins, Lishner, and Catalano, 1987, p. 78).

Thus, a rational prevention program needs to establish and explain its goals:

> If the goal … is to prevent serious maladaptive behavior associated with drug abuse in adolescence, then it may be desirable from an etiological perspective to focus prevention efforts on those youth who manifest behavior problems, including aggressive and other antisocial behaviors during the elementary grades. On the other hand, if the goal is to prevent experimentation with drugs, or to delay the age of experimentation in the general population, such highly focused efforts may be inappropriate. (Hawkins et al., 1987, p. 80)

Diana Baumrind (1987) offers a caution: "When socially deviant youths are required to participate in the school setting in peer-led denunciation of activities they value, they are more likely to become alienated than converted" (p. 32). And, an eight-year study reveals that once an adolescent decides to use drugs in response to internal problems, peer- based prevention programs will not work (Blakeslee, 1988b).

Despite the lack of evidence supporting current drug prevention efforts, Michael Goodstadt (n.d.) believes that when judging the impact of educational programs, there is some promising evidence based on smoking-prevention studies "which offer approaches that can be applied to education about other drugs" (pp. 1-2). In fact, "Americans are smoking and drinking less ... not because the army imprisoned North Carolina tobacco farmers or bombed stills in Scotland, but because attitudes have been changing with the help of education and treatment programs" (May, 1988 p. 12).

Notes

1. For a thorough discussion of agonist and antagonist analgesics, see the -December 1987 issue of Drug and Alcohol Dependence 20: 289-409.

2. "Psychoanalyst" is not a restricted title such as that enjoyed by psychiatrists, who must be physicians, or clinical psychologists, who must hold a doctorate in psychology. While there are certifying bodies for psychoanalysts, they do not have a government-supported monopoly on the use of the title. There is a great deal of acrimony between psychologists and psychiatrists over who is qualified to practice psychoanalysis (Goleman, 1988).

3. William R. Miller and Reid K. Hester (1980), in a review of AA evaluation literature, state: Attempts to evaluate the effectiveness of AA have met with considerable, if not insurmountable methodological problems, among them the very anonymity of members which precludes systematic follow-up evaluation. Most studies have failed to include control groups (a near impossibility because of the availability of AA to all who are interested), have relied almost entirely upon self-report (often via mailed questionnaires) and upon abstinence as the sole criteria for success, have been plagued by sizable attrition rates and large selection confounds, and have failed to use single-blind designs, thus remaining open to criticisms of interviewer bias (particularly when the investigators have been "insiders'— members of AA themselves). (p. 47) Nan Robertson (1988a), a Pulitzer Prize-winning reporter for the New York Times and a longtime member of Alcoholics Anonymous, writes: "About 60 percent of those coming to AA for the first time remain in AA after going to meetings and assiduously 'working the program' for months or even years. Usually, they stay sober for good. But about 40 percent drop out." On February 22, 1988, 1 wrote to Nan Robertson asking her to provide the basis for her statistics on the success of AA, but she has not yet responded. In his careful research, Geary Alford (1980) found that a residential treatment program for alcoholics that used the AA approach was highly effective: Approximately 50 percent of the patients completing inpatient treatment were essentially abstinent, employed or productively functioning, and exhibited stable, adaptive social relationships at two years post-discharge. This figure increases to 56 percent if very light-moderate drinking is allowed." As with the research reviewed by Miller and Hester (1980), Alford's study did not utilize a control group.

4. Information based on Straight, Inc., publications. Straight, Inc., is being used here for illustrative purposes. Arnold Trebach (1987) presents a portrait of the program that is far from flattering: untrained workers utilizing "brain washing," physical and psychological intimidation, and unlawful restraint.

5. Information based on Powell III publications.

Treatment Implications of Chemical Dependency Models

An Integrative Approach

By Kirk J. Brower, MD, Frederic C. Blow, PhD, and Thomas P. Beresford, MD

Abstract: *Five basic models of chemical dependency and their treatment implications are described. The moral model, although disdained by most treatment professionals, actually finds expression in over half the steps of Alcoholics Anonymous. The learning model, albeit the center of the controlled drinking controversy, is also utilized by most abstinence-oriented programs. The disease model, which enjoys current popularity, sometimes ignores the presence of coexisting disorders. The self-medication model, which tends to regard chemical dependency as a symptom, can draw needed attention to coexisting disorders. The social model emphasizes the importance of environmental and interpersonal influences in treatment, although the substance abuser may endorse it as a justification to adopt a victim's role. A sixth model, the dual diagnosis model, is presented as an example of how two of the basic models can be integrated both to expand the treatment focus and to increase treatment leverage. Whereas the five basic models are characterized by a singular, organizing treatment focus, the dual diagnosis model is viewed as an example of a multifocused, integrative model. It is concluded that effective therapy requires (a) flexibility in combining elements of different models in order to individualize treatment plans for substance abusers, and (b) careful assessment of both the therapist's and the substance abuser's beliefs about treatment models in order to insure a treatment match based on a healthy alliance.*

Keywords: *Substance abuse, alcoholism, treatment models, treatment matching, dual diagnosis.*

Kirk J. Brower, Frederic C. Blow, & Thomas P. Beresford, "Treatment Implications of Chemical Dependency Models: An Integrative Approach," *Journal of Substance Abuse Treatment*, vol. 6, issue 3, pp. 147-157. Copyright © 1989 by Elsevier B.V. Reprinted with permission.

INTRODUCTION

The purpose of this paper is to describe and examine various models of chemical dependency and their implications for treatment. A model provides a means to conceptualize chemical dependency for the purposes of enhancing our understanding of the problem and of suggesting solutions to the problem. A model is a representation of reality. The validity of a treatment model, the extent to which it accurately represents reality, can best be judged in terms of its usefulness in clinical work.

Models of chemical dependency can be divided, for the purpose of classification, into basic and integrative models (Table 1). The five basic models are the moral model, the learning model, the disease model, the self-medication model, and the social model. Each of these basic models will be described in terms of the assumptions they make about the etiology of chemical dependency and the goals and strategies they suggest for treatment. The advantages and disadvantages of each model for treatment are also examined (Table 2).

Integrative models combine or integrate elements from the basic models. Alcoholics Anonymous, the dual diagnosis model, and the biopsychosocial model are all examples of integrative models. In contrast to the basic models, which concentrate primarily on a single treatment focus, integrative models are multifocused. For example, whereas the disease model focuses primarily on substance abuse and the self-medication model focuses primarily on underlying psychopathol- ogy, the dual diagnosis model focuses on both substance abuse and coexisting psychopathology.

Other classifications of chemical dependency models have been described (Brickman, Rabinowitz, Ka- ruza, Coates, Cohn, & Kidder, 1982; Kissin, 1977; Ludwig, 1988; Marlatt, 1985a). In this paper, however, the purpose is not to advocate for one particular model (Brickman et al., 1982; Marlatt, 1985a), nor to describe only models of alcoholism (Donovan, 1986; Kissin, 1977; Ludwig, 1988, chap. 1). Rather, our descriptions are designed to help practitioners take advantage of the best elements of each model, while avoiding the disadvantages of each, in order to optimize treatment of substance abuse in general.

The major thesis of this paper is that clinical work is enhanced by being flexible enough to integrate or combine the most relevant elements of each model in order to individualize treatment for substance abuse. Conversely stated, clinical work may be compromised by rigid adherence to any one model at all times for all patients, because each of the models has distinct disadvantages as well as advantages when applied to treatment. Different patients may benefit by emphasizing one model over another (Kissin, 1977). Likewise, the same patient may benefit by emphasizing

TABLE 1. Classification of Chemical Dependency Treatment Models

Basic Models (Single Focus)	Integrative Models (Multifocus)
Moral	Alcoholics Anonymous
Learning	Dual diagnosis
Disease	Biopsychosocial
Self-medication	Multivariant
Social	

TABLE 2. Basic Models of Chemical Dependency

	Model				
	Moral	Learning	Disease	Self-Medication	Social
Etiology	Moral weakness; lack of willpower; bad or evil character	Learned, maladaptive habits	Idiopathic; biological factors important	Symptom of another primary mental disorder	Environmental influences
Treatment goal	Increased willpower against evil temptations	Self-control via new learning	Complete abstinence to arrest disease progression	Improved mental functioning	Improved social functioning
Treatment strategy	Religious counseling or conversion; punishment	Teaching of new coping skills and cognitive restructuring	Focus on chemical dependency as primary problem; reinforce identity as recovering alcoholic/ addict	Psychotherapy and/or pharmacotherapy of causative mental disorder	Altering of environment or coping responses to it
Advantages	Moral inventory and amends beneficial; holds users responsible for consequences; gauges countertransference	Neither blaming nor punitive; emphasizes new learning; holds users responsible for new learning	Neither blaming nor punitive; disease implies treatment-seeking as appropriate response; does not focus on hypothetical etiologies	Neither blaming nor punitive; emphasizes importance of diagnosing and treating coexisting mental disorders	Emphasizes need for social supports and skills; easily integrated into other models
Disadvantages	Blaming and punitive; willpower ineffective	Undue emphasis on control	Underestimates coexisting mental disorders; cannot explain return to asymptomatic drinking	Implies that treatment of mental disorder is sufficient	Facilitates projection of blame; implies treatment of social problems is sufficient

different models during different phases of treatment. Thus, the critical question for both treatment providers and researchers is how to match substance abusers during their treatment course to the various models in order to maximize treatment outcome (Glaser, 1980; Marlatt, 1988). The matching process will be seen to require an assessment of both the substance abuser's and the therapist's beliefs about treatment models. Moreover, proper assessment requires the clinician to view the substance abuser from the various perspectives offered by the various models (Shaffer, 1986a).

We will first discuss the five basic models. We will then present the dual diagnosis model, both as an example of an integrative model and as an example of treatment matching on the basis of beliefs. Finally, we will describe other integrative models of chemical dependency.

MORAL MODEL

We start with the moral model of chemical dependency because, historically, it is the oldest. A recent Supreme Court decision in which alcoholism was interpreted as resulting from "willful misconduct," however, demonstrates that the moral model is still current and operative (Seessel, 1988). The characteristics of the moral model are presented in Table 2. In this model, chemical dependency results from a moral weakness or lack of willpower. The substance abuser is viewed as someone with a weak, bad or evil character. Accordingly, the goal of rehabilitation is to increase one's willpower in order to resist the evil temptation of substances. The user is expected to change from evil to good and from weak to strong. The strategies for change include both a "positive" reliance on God through religious counseling or conversion and a "negative" avoidance of punishment through criminal sanctions or damnation.

The major treatment disadvantage of the moral model is that it places the helping professional in an antagonist relationship with the substance abuser by adopting a judgemental stance that is blaming and punitive. The substance abuser is at fault in this model. If he or she does not change, then punishment is deserved. These attitudes are generally countertherapeu- tic. The other major disadvantage for treatment is that willpower for many, if not most substance abusers seen in treatment settings, is ineffective against chemical dependency. Although we are all aware of histories in which alcoholic persons made a decision to quit and did so on their own, most individuals seen in treatment centers have already tried willpower with little success. A treatment strategy that depends solely on willpower, therefore, sets the stage for failure and decreases a substance abuser's sense of self-esteem.

The moral model is often embraced by patients themselves who enter treatment feeling that they are bad and weak-willed. As a result, some patients ask for our help to make them strong enough to resist substances. Once they feel strong enough, however, they can easily reason that they are strong enough to use substances again. A treatment goal of strength, therefore, can paradoxically lead to relapse. This is why Alcoholics Anonymous (A.A.) and other twelve step programs stress the concept of powerlessness. Nevertheless, it is important to determine which model the patient believes in, a point to which we will return during our discussion of treatment matching.

Despite the disadvantages of the moral model, it correctly focuses attention on the importance of moral concerns during the process of recovery for some substance abusers. A.A., for example, has long recognized that making a moral inventory of wrongdoing, coupled with making amends when possible, can be beneficial for recovery (Alcoholics Anonymous, 1976). In fact, steps 4 through 10, constituting over half of A.A.'s twelve steps, are devoted to moral concerns, even though A.A. ostensibly subscribes to the disease model of alcoholism. Three important points can be made here. First, A.A. is an example of an integrative approach, by combining elements of both the moral and disease models. Second, A.A. does not emphasize the moral elements of its program until step 4, exemplifying the principle of emphasizing different models during different phases of recovery. Third, A.A. and other twelve step programs actually refer to themselves as spiritual, rather than moral, programs.

However, the spiritual model can be considered a variant of the moral model. It attributes chemical dependency to the substance abuser's misalliance with God and the universe. The substance abuser is viewed as someone who is alienated from God, stubbornly self-willed, and who attempts to dominate and control the outside world. Accordingly, the goal of treatment is to help substance abusers develop their spirituality by discovering and following God's will and by seeking a more "complementary" relationship with the universe (Brown, 1985).

Another treatment advantage of the moral model is that it holds people responsible for the consequences of their substance use. Although blaming people for having chemical dependency is seen as a disadvantage, holding people responsible for consequences is useful in overcoming denial and increasing motivation for change. Protecting substance abusers from the consequences of their use often "enables" them to continue using.

Finally, the moral model can be used to advantage by clinicians in order to gauge the status of their treatment relationships with substance abusers and even to screen for psychopathology. We have all had the experience of finding ourselves in an antagonistic relationship with a substance abuser, feeling angry, blaming him or her for lack of motivation, and pushing for an administrative

discharge from the treatment program. This experience should serve as a signal that we are operating under the moral model, regardless of our consciously espoused treatment model. The wise clinician will then ask why he or she has shifted to the moral model. One reason may be diagnosis. Substance abusers with an antisocial personality disorder, for example, really do have "bad characters" in addition to chemical dependency. We naturally respond to our perceptions of badness with moral indignation. Thus, our countertransference to the antisocial character may manifest by unconsciously shifting to the moral model in terms of our treatment responses. By monitoring our treatment responses for their congruence with the various models of chemical dependency, we can gain important diagnostic information and be vigilant to our countertransference. Once aware of our countertransference, a psychiatric consultation for the substance abuser can be obtained and treatment more specific for the antisocial personality, if present, can be recommended (Woody, McLellan, Luborsky, & O'Brien, 1985).

LEARNING MODEL

According to the learning model, chemical dependency and other addictive behaviors result from the learning of maladaptive habits (Marlatt, 1985a). The substance abuser is viewed as someone who learned "bad" habits through no particular fault of his or her own. Accordingly, the general goal of therapy is to teach new behaviors and cognitions that allow old habits to be controlled by new learning (see Table 2). Whether the specific goal of therapy is "controlled drinking" (to use alcohol as the example) or complete abstinence, the emphasis is on self-control. In this model, a "relapse" can be thought of as a loss of self-control resulting in harmful use of substances. The user is expected to change from a miseducated creature of maladaptive habits to a reeducated individual capable of self-control. The major strategy for change is education, including the teaching of new coping skills and cognitive restructuring (Marlatt, 1985a).

The salient advantages of the learning model are that it is neither punitive nor blaming for the development of maladaptive habits and that it stresses new learning and education as a treatment strategy. We should state our belief, however, that all legitimate treatment approaches value new learning, whether in the form of lectures, skills training, conditioning techniques, or psychotherapy. Another advantage of the learning model, like the moral model, is that it holds people responsible for obtaining and implementing the new learning (Marlatt, 1985a).

Its prominent disadvantage is its emphasis on control. This disadvantage, from our point of view, is not related to the controversy surrounding controlled drinking (Miller, 1983), because the learning model allows flexibility in choosing a treatment goal of either complete abstinence or controlled substance use. However, the model's emphasis on control ignores (a) the complex and hidden meanings this word can have for the substance abuser and (b) the therapeutic value for many substance abusers in admitting their loss of control. When a substance abuser and therapist agree that the goal of treatment will be self-control, even for the purpose of abstinence, the substance abuser may harbor a hidden goal based on the fantasy that one day the use of chemicals will be possible again once self- control is established. In this way, a treatment agreement for self-control may foster collusion with the substance abuser's denial of the need for abstinence. Alternatively, some substance abusers recover very well by internalizing the beliefs that they cannot control their chemical use and, therefore, that they cannot use chemicals. (The belief in loss of control is also stated in step 1 of A.A. as "We admitted we were powerless over alcohol and that our lives had become unmanageable.") Therapists need to be aware that for some substance abusers, the concept of control is paradoxical; that is, in order to gain control, they must admit their loss of control (Brown, 1985). Therapists who can appreciate this paradox of control are in the best position to integrate, as needed, the models that emphasize loss of control with models that emphasize self-control. Indeed, the practical techniques of relapse prevention, which are based on a learning model of self-control (Marlatt, 1985a), are paradoxically utilized by many disease model programs that are based on the concepts of powerlessness and loss of control. We will now discuss the disease model in more detail.

DISEASE MODEL

The disease model of alcoholism and other chemical dependencies is probably the dominant model among specialized treatment providers at present. Alcoholism as a disease, for example, has been officially endorsed by the American Medical Association, the American Psychiatric Association, the National Association of Social Workers, the World Health Organization, the American Public Health Association, and the National Council on Alcoholism. According to this model, the etiology of chemical dependency is unknown, but genetic and other biological factors are considered important (Schuckit, 1985). The substance abuser is viewed as someone who is ill or unhealthy, not because of an underlying mental disorder, but because of the disease of chemical dependency itself. The sine qua non of the disease is considered to be an irreversible loss of control over alcohol (Alcoholics Anonymous, 1976) or other substances. Once present, the disease is regarded as always present, because there is no known cure. Accordingly, the goal of treatment is complete abstinence (see Table 2). Without complete abstinence, the disease is regarded as progressive and often fatal. The user is expected to change from using to not using, from ill to healthy, and from unrecovered to recovering. The major treatment strategy is to focus on chemical dependency as the primary problem, rather than on lack of willpower, lack of self-control, or lack of mental health. The substance abuser is guided to develop a positive identification as a recovering alcoholic or addict who is powerless over substances. In addition, most disease model programs (as with the learning model) teach new behaviors to substitute for the substance use (such as going to A.A.), while family education and therapy are directed to eliminate "enabling" by significant others.

The advantages of the disease model are that it is neither punitive nor blaming and that it implies the importance of seeking treatment and help, as one would with any other disease. Guilt is alleviated because people are not held responsible for developing chemical dependency any more than for developing high blood pressure or diabetes. Blame can be directed towards the disease rather than towards the person with the disease. On the other hand, having a disease implies a responsibility for taking care of oneself by seeking treatment. In contrast to the learning model, then, the disease model emphasizes self-care rather than self-control. Another advantage is its clear focus on the chemical dependency as a problem to be treated in its own right. This focus prevents the dangers inherent in other models that focus primarily on postulated etiologies, which we will explore further with the self-medication and social models.

One disadvantage of the disease model is that it fails to account for those alcoholics who actually return to asymptomatic drinking (Shaffer, 1986b). The proportion of alcoholics who return to asymptomatic drinking has been estimated on

the basis of a number of studies to be about 5-15% (Miller, 1583; Vaillant, 1983). These alcoholics tended to be less dependent on alcohol in terms of symptoms and duration, younger in age, and did not regard themselves as having a disease (Miller, 1983; Vaillant, 1983). Miller (1983) has even argued that these alcoholics were more likely to relapse when exposed to abstinence-oriented disease models, although only one study is cited to support that conclusion (Polich, Armor, & Braiker, 1981). Certainly, more research is needed to determine which alcoholics do best with which treatments because rigid adherence to one model for all alcoholics may be detrimental to some.

The other major disadvantage of the disease model is that some of its proponents fail to appreciate the possible independence of coexisting psychopathology. Many if not most alcoholics, for example, experience depressive symptoms during the first year of abstinence (Schuckit, 1986). Brown (1985) has concluded that "the high percentage of respondents reporting depression suggests that it may be a necessary part of recovery" (p. 51). Unfortunately, the tendency to normalize depressive symptoms during early recovery by attributing them to the disease of alcoholism may inhibit efforts to diagnose and treat a coexisting "major depression" as defined by DSM-III-R (American Psychiatric Association, 1987). From our point of view, waiting through the first year of alcoholism treatment to allow symptoms of major depression to subside may work, but is unnecessarily cruel and potentially dangerous. The reason that it may work is because untreated major depressive episodes typically last about 6 months to 1 year (Kaplan & Sadock, 1988, p. 295). The reason that it is cruel is because major depression is responsive to appropriate pharmacotherapy within 4-6 weeks (Brotman, Falk, & Gelenberg, 1987). Regarding dangerousness, major depression is an unusually painful psychic state that can cause significant psychosocial disruption, if not relapse and suicide.

In contrast to the disease model, which tends to minimize coexisting psychopathology such as depression, the self-medication model primarily focuses on the psychopathology of substance abusers, as we discuss next.

SELF-MEDICATION MODEL

According to this model, chemical dependency occurs either as a symptom of another primary mental disorder or as a coping mechanism for deficits in psychological structure or functioning (Khantzian, 1985). The substance abuser is viewed as someone who uses chemicals as a way to alleviate the painful symptoms of another mental disorder such as depression, or as a way to fill the void left by deficiencies in psychological structure or functioning. Consequently, the goal of treatment is to improve mental functioning. The user is expected to change from mentally ill to psychologically healthy. The strategies for change include psychotherapy and pharmacotherapy of the underlying mental disorder (see Table 2).

Like the learning and disease models, the self-medication model is neither punitive nor blaming. Another major advantage is that it stresses the importance of diagnosing and treating coexisting psychiatric problems when present. The importance of this is highlighted by treatment outcome studies that reveal different (usually worse) prognoses for addicts with additional psychopathology who enter traditional chemical dependency treatment programs (McLellan, Luborsky, Woody, O'Brien, & Druley, 1983; Rounsaville, Dolin- sky, Babor, & Meyer, 1987).

The major disadvantage of this model stems from its emphasis on psychopathology as etiology. Although retrospective studies provide support for the idea that psychopathology causes chemical dependency, prospective studies do not (Vaillant, 1983). In many cases, psychopathology is the result, not the cause, of chemical dependency. In other cases, it is difficult to determine what is cause and what is effect when chemical dependency coexists with other psychopathology (Schuckit, 1986). Nevertheless, psychopathology may still be the cause of chemical dependency in some individuals. However, it does not necessarily follow that treating the cause in these individuals will provide sufficient treatment for the chemical dependency. This is because perpetuating factors of chemical dependency may develop in addition to the psychopathology that initiated the dependency (Brower, 1988). Optimal treatment, therefore, requires attention to both the initiating and perpetuating factors of substance abuse.

Unfortunately, the model implies that treatment of initiating psychiatric problems will provide sufficient treatment for chemical dependency. Therapists and substance abusers alike can easily believe that once the underlying cause is discovered and treated, then the problem with chemicals will disappear. For the substance abuser, postulating a treatable etiology allows for the hope that chemical use will one day be possible once the underlying cause is treated.

For the therapist, focusing treatment on underlying psychological factors can facilitate collusion with the substance abuser's denial of chemical dependency. The problem of colluding with denial can be highlighted by examining the various configurations of denial commonly encountered in substance abusers (Table 3). The four configurations listed depend on whether the denial is directed towards the chemical dependency, towards associated problems, towards both, or neither. Substance abusers who are in complete denial recognize neither their chemical dependency nor their other problems. They often have character disorders whose symptoms are ego-syntonic and disturbing to others but not themselves. They tend not to seek treatment unless forced by external pressures. Through the use of projection, they generally see others as having the problem rather than themselves. Substance abusers without character disorders may also adopt this configuration at times, especially when feeling threatened. Clearly, this configuration is difficult to treat and has resulted in the commonly heard clinical imperative to "break through the denial."

However, the other extreme is represented by those substance abusers who present in no denial. These substance abusers are often suicidal because they are painfully aware of their chemical dependency, of the many relapses, of their depression and shame, of the many conflicts—about work or unemployment, with family, with the law —and of the medical sequelae of their chemical dependency. Despite the clinical imperative to "break through" denial, we do not recommend this configuration because substance abusers are at high risk for completed suicide, especially when feeling the full impact of their interpersonal losses and conflicts (Murphy, 1988).

It is the configuration of partial denial, type 1 that poses the greatest challenge to the self-medication model (and to the social model, discussed below). These substance abusers have denial for their chemical dependency but not for their other problems. Accordingly, they may seek treatment for their other problems such as depression, stress on the job, or interpersonal conflicts. If in the course of their evaluation or treatment, the therapist becomes aware of their harmful chemical use but adheres to the self-medication model, then collusion with the substance abuser's denial could occur. By covert agreement, the substance abuser and therapist will exclude the chemical dependency as an important focus of treatment. In effect, the substance abuser will be supported for focusing on the other problems, and the chemical use, if it is explored at all, will be interpreted as a coping mechanism. The disadvantage is that the substance abuser, significant others, and therapist will all have the illusion of treatment while the substance abuse continues.

The preferable configuration, in our opinion, at least for the initial stages of treatment, is the configuration of partial denial, type 2. In this configuration, the substance abuser is encouraged to focus on the chemical dependency while denying or minimizing the significance of other problems. Rather than breaking through or eliminating denial, the therapist acts to redirect the denial away from the chemical dependency and towards the other problems (Wallace, 1978). When appropriate, the other problems can be interpreted as consequences of the chemical dependency. In addition, the substance abuser is presented with the rationale that the other problems are more likely to improve if the chemical dependency is treated first and that a period of abstinence is required in order to assess better the other problems.

SOCIAL MODEL

In this model, chemical dependency results from environmental, cultural, social, peer, or family influences (Beigel & Ghertner, 1977). The substance abuser is viewed as a product of external forces such as poverty, drug availability, peer pressure, and family dysfunction. Accordingly, the goal of treatment is to improve the social functioning of substance abusers by altering either their social environment or their coping responses to environmental stresses (see Table 2). In other words, users are expected to change either their environments or their coping responses. The strategies for changing the environment include family or couples therapy, attendance at self-help groups where one is surrounded by nonusers, residential treatment, and avoidance of stressful environments where substances are readily available. The

TABLE 3. Configurations of Denial in Substance Abusers

Configuration	Chemical Dependency	Other Problems
Complete denial	I am not an alcoholic or addict	I have no other problems
No denial	I am an alcoholic and/or addict	I have all these other problems
Partial denial (type 1)	I am not an alcoholic or addict	It's just that I have all these other problems
Partial denial (type 2)	I am an alcoholic and/or addict	All my other problems are related to my substance use

strategies for changing substance abusers' coping responses include group therapy, interpersonal therapy (Rounsaville, Gawin, & Kleber, 1985), social skills or assertiveness training, and stress management.

The major advantages of this model are its emphases on interpersonal functioning, social supports, environmental stressors, social pressures, and cultural factors as critical elements to address in treatment. The importance of addressing interpersonal functioning is underscored by data indicating that over one-half of alcoholic relapses are attributable to interpersonal conflicts (Marlatt, 1985b). Treatment interventions for alcoholics that are directed towards increasing social skills or environmental support have been shown to produce better outcomes 6-12 months after treatment (Eriksen, Bjornstad, & Gotestam, 1986; Page & Badg- ett, 1984). In general, treatment studies have consistently revealed better outcomes for alcoholics who are more socially stable, although the effect is strongest in short-term studies (Vaillant, 1983).

Cultures that introduce children to the ritualized use of low-proof alcohol during meals with others, discourage drinking at other times, and discourage drunkenness have lower rates of alcoholism (Vaillant, 1983). In short, cultures that teach their children how to drink responsibly have lower rates of alcoholism, a conclusion which is also consistent with the learning model. While this conclusion has greater ramifications

for primary prevention than for treatment of alcoholism, other cultural factors such as ethnicity and the socialization of women may have important implications for those entering treatment. Treatment programs which are "culturally sensitive" to ethnicity and to women's social roles may produce better outcomes for specific ethnic groups and for women, although treatment outcome studies that specifically address this issue are unfortunately lacking (Amaro, Beckman, & Mays, 1987; Reed, 1987).

Another advantage of the social model is that it is readily compatible with, and easily integrated into, other models. We will give three examples. First, the learning model encourages both the enlistment of social support during treatment (Marlatt, 1985c) and the teaching of alternative coping responses to environmental stresses and interpersonal conflicts (Marlatt, 1985a). Indeed, the learning model is sometimes referred to as the social-learning model, because learning describes a process that occurs in an environmental and interpersonal context. In other words, people learn from their experiences with their environment and with other people. Second, the self-medication model conceptualizes substance abuse as a way of coping with psychological deficits resulting from frustrating and damaging relationships during early development (Khantzian, 1985). In this model, individual psycho- dynamic psychotherapy is viewed as a primary treatment (Khantzian, 1984) that focuses on relationships with other people in terms of the transference relationships that develop with the therapist (Kohut, 1971; Schiffer, 1988). Third, many proponents of the disease model view the entire family as both affected by the disease and suffering from the parallel "disease" of co- dependence (Cermak, 1986). Treatment is aimed at helping the family embark on its own recovery. Thus, most of the other models incorporate the social model to some extent in their treatment approaches, and they also regard improved social functioning as an important measure of successful treatment outcome. Conversely, we see a disadvantage in using the social model as an exclusive treatment mode because the etiology of substance abuse is multifactorial, implying a need for multiple treatment strategies (Donovan, 1986; Kissin, 1977).

The major treatment disadvantage of the social model is that it may facilitate projection of blame onto others and the environment. The substance abuser may come to feel victimized by others or by circumstances that do not seem changeable and thus renounce responsibility for solutions. Substance abusers who see themselves as victims require the therapist's empathic guidance towards taking an active role in changing their environment or their coping responses to it. The substance abuser is similarly guided by the Serenity Prayer of A.A. which encourages each person "to accept the things I cannot change," by learning to cope with them, and "to change the things I can."

A related disadvantage of the social model occurs when the therapist focuses exclusively on social problems, while minimizing the chemical dependency itself. Substance abusers, for example, may seek treatment for problems with their marriage or job. The therapist's questions about substance use during early interviews may be met with statements such as "I drink because my job is stressful" or "You would use drugs too if you were married to my spouse." Such statements represent rationalizations or projections that are expressed in the form of beliefs in the social model. The substance abuser with these complaints may tempt the inexperienced therapist, who also endorses the social model, to focus on the job or marital problems, while mutually denying the importance of the substance abuse problem. This disadvantage was described above in terms of the type 1 partial denial configuration. A clinical approach to avoiding this disadvantage is provided below in our discussion of the dual diagnosis model.

DUAL DIAGNOSIS MODEL

Substance abusers who present with depression or social problems are commonly encountered, as discussed above. Some of these individuals will insist that their depression or other problems should be the focus of treatment, rather than their substance abuse. Their belief is in either the self-medication model or the social model. In order to simplify the following discussion, we will use as an example those substance abusers who complain primarily of depression, while minimizing their substance abuse. These are substance abusers who believe in the self-medication model. Essentially, they state that they use substances because they are depressed. Their treatment will depend on the beliefs of their therapists.

If the therapist also believes in the self-medication model, then treatment will focus primarily on the depression. The potential pitfall here is a treatment match based on collusion (see Table 4), in which both the therapist and substance abuser believe in depression as a focus of treatment but mutually deny the importance of substance abuse. By contrast, if the therapist believes in the disease model, then statements such as "I use substances because I am depressed" are interpreted as rationalizations. Substance abusers may become defensive when their use of substances is explored. The therapeutic task is then formulated by the disease model therapist in terms of breaking through the defensiveness and denial. The potential pitfall here is a mismatch of beliefs resulting in an antagonistic relationship, instead of an alliance in which treatment can occur (Table 4).

The way out of this clinical dilemma is first to assess carefully everyone's beliefs in order to guard against either collusion or a mismatch, both of which are countertherapeutic. Next, the substance abuser is invited into an alliance without collusion by the following intervention: "I agree that you appear depressed and this is certainly a problem for you. We need to address that. It is also true from what you have told me that you have a diagnosis of chemical dependency. We need to address that too and let me tell you why. Any attempt I make to determine the type of depression you have will be confounded by further chemical use. Also, any treatment that I can give you for your depression will be sabotaged by further chemical use. This is because we know that regardless of which came first (the depression or the chemicals) and regardless of why you use, chemicals make depression worse over long periods of time. In short, you have two problems, they both require treatment, and the best way I can treat your depression right now is to give you treatment for chemical dependency. After that

treatment is begun, we will be better able to see if other treatments for your depression are needed."

In essence, the substance abuser is invited to believe in the dual diagnosis model (see Table 5) in which the argument about what is the primary problem requiring treatment is replaced by the idea that treatment is required for both problems. In this way, the therapist and substance abuser can build an alliance around a common goal, which is to treat depression, without denying the importance of treating chemical dependency.

Like the self-medication model, the dual diagnosis model views the coexisting mental disorder as a primary problem that may require its own psychotherapeutic or pharmacotherapeutic intervention. This helps to build an alliance with the substance abuser and prevents the minimization of coexisting mental disorders by the therapist. Like the disease model, the dual diagnosis model also views substance abuse as a primary problem requiring its own treatment. This helps to prevent collusion with the substance abuser and insures that the importance of substance abuse treatment will not be overlooked. Properly applied, the dual diagnosis model integrates elements of both the self-medication and disease models in a way that avoids the disadvantages of adhering to only one or the other.

In the dual diagnosis model, substance abuse and other mental disorders can be seen as coexisting without necessarily attributing one etiologically to the other. Both are considered

Table 4 Typology of Treatment Matches

Type of Match	Therapist and Substance Abuser	Treatment Effect
Match	Believe in same model	Variable
Collusion	Mutually deny problems that do not fit model	Countertherapeutic
Alliance	All problems addressed over time	Therapeutic
Mismatch	Do not believe in same model	Countertherapeutic unless mismatch is addressed and resolved

TABLE 5 Models of Chemical Dependency and Co-Existing Depression

Model	Primary Disorder	Secondary Disorder	Relationship Between Disorders	Treatment Strategy
Disease model	Chemical dependency	Depression	Depression = withdrawal symptom, response to losses due to chemical use, or physiological response to chemical	Treat chemical dependency, depression will remit
Self-medication model	Depression	Chemical dependency	Chemical dependency = symptom of depression, or coping response to depression and losses associated with depression	Treat depression, chemical dependency will remit
Dual diagnosis model	Both depression and chemical dependency	Neither	Each may exacerbate the other, but neither is a symptom of the other	Treat both

primary disorders that can exacerbate one another. The strategy for treatment is to focus on both disorders, although substance use must first stop in order to diagnose and treat the co-existing mental disorder. If an initial period of abstinence proves to be sufficient treatment for the coexisting mental disorder, then a shift from the dual diagnosis model toward other models can be made, as appropriate.

In this discussion, we have alluded to the value of assessing the respective beliefs of the therapist and the substance abuser regarding treatment models. When both the therapist and substance abuser believe in a common explanatory system that does not deny important problems requiring treatment, then a treatment match based on a healthy alliance has been achieved (Table 4). Obviously, this type of match is preferred, but cannot be expected to occur by accident. Only by carefully monitoring our own beliefs and those of the substance abusers we treat can we insure this type of match. Furthermore, substance abusers may require the use of integrative models in order

to establish a therapeutic alliance, as exemplified by this discussion of the dual diagnosis model. In other words, integrative models may provide the optimal clinical strategy for bridging discrepant belief systems between therapists and substance abusers.

OTHER INTEGRATIVE MODELS

Our thesis has been that clinicians need to be flexible enough to integrate the most relevant elements of each model in order both to individualize and to optimize treatment for substance abuse. Our thesis is not new: at least two other authors have detailed what we would refer to as integrative treatment models. First, Kissin (1977) suggested that a "multivariant" treatment model for alcoholism, which incorporated elements from other major models, would optimize treatment for individual alcoholics. Our approach, while similar, expands upon his by (a) generalizing beyond alcoholism to substance abuse as a whole,

(b) drawing attention to the advantages and treatment utility of the moral model, (c) including the relatively new dual diagnosis model and describing its integrative nature, and (d) emphasizing the potential value of matching substance abusers and therapists in terms of their beliefs about chemical dependency. Second, Donovan (1988) suggested a biopsychosocial model as an integrative model to be used with all addictive behaviors. The biopsychosocial model encourages therapists to consider biological, psychological, and social factors both in assessment and treatment. In this model, treatment of different substance abusers may require varying attention to each of these three domains, depending on the substance abuser's individual characteristics and circumstances. An advantage of the biopsychosocial model is that it facilitates the integration of three very important domains involved in the etiology, maintenance, assessment, and treatment of addictive behaviors. However, while it allows an integration of these three domains, it does not address the integration of the chemical dependency models per se that are widely used in clinical practice and that we have described.

Our conceptualization of integrative models has noted three essential characteristics. First, integrative models combine elements of the basic models. Second, integrative models are multifocused, which is to say that the multiple problems of the substance abuser are addressed rather than subjugated to the single focus of each basic model. In actual practice, we believe that the most effective therapists are multifocused regardless of the model they specifically endorse. For example, most disease model therapists incorporate the social model by addressing the family problems in terms of codependence. By thinking in terms of integrative models, however, therapists can both increase their awareness of what they do already and integrate other basic models into their work as appropriate. Third, integrative models not only allow seemingly discrepant models to be combined, but they also allow therapists and substance abusers with seemingly discrepant beliefs to be matched.

Finally, we note that integration, as we have been using the term, can occur on two complementary levels: the theoretical and the technical. When a disease model therapist, for example, finds it useful to incorporate relapse prevention techniques while disavowing the learning theory from which they came, then the integration is only at the level of combining techniques. This has been called technical eclecticism (Beitman, Goldfried, & Norcross, 1989). By contrast, when a new theoretical model is developed, as with the dual diagnosis model, that synthesizes two previously competing models, then true integration or theoretical eclecticism has occurred. The interested reader is referred to an excellent review by Beitman et al. (1989) for a detailed discussion of these concepts.

CONCLUSION

Five basic models (moral, learning, social, self-medication, and disease) of chemical dependency are all in use presently. Each of the basic models has distinct advantages and disadvantages when applied in treatment. It is important for clinicians to be aware of each of the models and to be flexible enough to exploit the advantages of each while avoiding their respective disadvantages. Integrative models, such as A.A. (moral and disease models) and the dual diagnosis approach (self-medication and disease models), can maximize treatment for some patients. Treatment can also be optimized by taking into account both the clinician's and substance abuser's beliefs about chemical dependency, because mismatched beliefs or colluding beliefs can be countertherapeutic. In summary, future research on treatment matching should focus on the use of integrative models to optimize treatment outcome.

REFERENCES

Alcoholics Anonymous (1976). Alcoholics Anonymous: The big book. New York: A.A. World Services, Inc.

Amaro, H., Beckman, L.J., & Mays, V.M. (1987). A comparison of black and white women entering alcoholism treatment. Journal of Studies on Alcohol, 48, 220-228.

American Psychiatric Association (1987). Diagnostic and statistical manual of mental disorders (rev. 3rd ed.). Washington, DC: Author.

Beigel, A., & Ghertner, S. (1977). Toward a social model: An assessment of social factors which influence problem drinking and its treatment. In B. Kissin & H. Begleiter (Eds.), The biology of alcoholism. Treatment and rehabilitation of the chronic alcoholic (vol. 5, pp. 197-233). New York: Plenum.

Beitman, B.D., Goldfried, M.R., & Norcross, J.C. (1989). The movement toward integrating the psychotherapies: An overview. American Journal of Psychiatry, 146, 138-147.

Brickman, P., Rabinowitz, V.C., Karuza, J., Coates, D., Cohn, E., & Kidder, L. (1982). Models of helping and coping. American Psychologist, 37, 368-384.

Brotman, A.W., Falk, W.E., & Gelenberg, A.J. (1987). Pharmacologic treatment of acute depressive subtypes. In H.Y. Meltzer (Ed.), Psychopharmacology: The third generation of progress (pp. 1031-1040). New York: Raven Press.

Brower, K.J. (1988). Self-medication of migraine headaches with freebase cocaine. Journal of Substance Abuse Treatment, 5, 2326.

Brown, S. (1985). Treating the alcoholic: A developmental model of recovery. New York: Wiley.

Cermak, T.L. (1986). Diagnosing and treating co-dependence. Minneapolis: Johnson Institute.

Donovan, D.M. (1988). Assessment of addictive behaviors: Implications of an emerging biopsychosocial model. In D.M. Donovan & G.A. Marlatt (Eds.), Assessment of addictive behaviors (pp. 3-48). New York: Guilford Press.

Donovan, J.M. (1986). An etiologic model of alcoholism. American Journal of Psychiatry, 143, 1-11.

Eriksen, L., Bjornstad, S., & Gotestam, K.G. (1986). Social skills training in groups for alcoholics: One-year treatment outcome for groups and individuals. Addictive Behaviors, 11, 309-329.

Glaser, F.B. (1980). Anybody got a match? Treatment research and the matching hypothesis. In G. Edwards & M. Grant (Eds.), Alcoholism treatment in transition (pp. 178-196). London: Croom Helm.

Kaplan, H.I., & Sadock, B.J. (1988). Synopsis of psychiatry: Behavioral sciences—clinical psychiatry. Baltimore: Williams & Wilkins.

Khantzian, E.J. (1984). A contemporary psycho dynamic approach to drug abuse treatment. American Journal of Drug and Alcohol Abuse, 12, 213-222.

Khantzian, E.J. (1985). The self-medication hypothesis of addictive disorders: Focus on heroin and cocaine dependence. American Journal of Psychiatry, 142, 1259-1264.

Kohut, H. (1971). The analysis of self. New York: International Universities Press.

Kissin, B. (1977). Theory and practice in the treatment of alcoholism. In B. Kissin & H. Begleiter (Eds.), The biology of alcoholism. Treatment and rehabilitation of the chronic alcoholic (Vol. 5, pp. 1-51). New York: Plenum.

Ludwig, A.M. (1988). Understanding the alcoholic's mind. New York: Oxford University Press.

Marlatt, G.A. (1985a). Relapse prevention: Theoretical rationale and overview of the model. In G.A. Marlatt & J.R. Gordon (Eds.), Relapse prevention (pp. 3-70). New York: Guilford Press.

Marlatt, G.A. (1985b). Situational determinants of relapse and skill- training interventions. In G.A.

Marlatt & J.R. Gordon (Eds.), Relapse prevention (pp. 71-127). New York: Guilford Press.

Marlatt, G.A. (1985c). Cognitive assessment and intervention procedures for relapse prevention. In G.A. Marlatt & J.R. Gordon (Eds.), Relapse prevention (pp. 201-279). New York: Guilford Press.

Marlatt, G.A. (1988). Matching clients to treatment: Treatment models and stages of change. In D.M. Donovan & G.A. Marlatt (Eds.), Assessment of addictive behaviors (pp. 474-483). New York: Guilford Press.

McLellan, A.T., Luborsky, L., Woody, G.E., O'Brien, C.P., & Druley, K.A. (1983). Predicting response to alcohol and drug abuse treatments: Role of psychiatric severity. Archives of General Psychiatry, 40, 620-625.

Miller, W.R. (1983). Controlled drinking: A history and a critical review. Journal of Studies on Alcohol, 44, 68-83.

Murphy, G.E. (1988). Suicide and substance abuse. Archives of General Psychiatry, 45, 593-594.

Page, R.D., & Badgett, S. (1984). Alcoholism treatment with environmental support contracting. American Journal of Drug and Alcohol Abuse, 10, 589-605.

Polich, J.M., Armor, D.J., & Braiker, H.B. (1981). The course of alcoholism: Four years after treatment. New York: Wiley.

Reed, B.G. (1987). Developing women-sensitive drug dependence treatment services: Why so difficult? Journal of Psychoactive Drugs, 19, 151-164.

Rounsaville, B.J., Gawin, F., & Kleber, H. (1985). Interpersonal psychotherapy adapted for ambulatory cocaine abusers. American Journal of Drug and Alcohol Abuse, 11, 171-191.

Rounsaville, B.J., Dolinsky, Z.S., Babor, T.F., & Meyer, R.E. (1987). Psychopathology as a predictor of treatment outcome in alcoholics. Archives of General Psychiatry, 44, 505-513.

Schiffer, F. (1988). Psychotherapy of nine successfully treated cocaine users: Techniques and dynamics. Journal of Substance Abuse Treatment, 5, 131-137.

Schuckit, M.A. (1985). Genetics and the risk for alcoholism. Journal of the American Medical Association, 254, 2614-2617.

Schuckit, M.A. (1986). Genetic and clinical implications of alcoholism and affective disorder. American Journal of Psychiatry, 143, 140-147.

Seessel, T.V. (1988). Beyond the Supreme Court ruling on alcoholism as willful misconduct: It is up to Congress to act. Journal of the American Medical Association, 259, 248.

Shaffer, H.J. (1986a). Assessment of addictive disorders: The use of clinical reflection and hypotheses testing. Psychiatric Clinics of North America, 9, 385-398.

Shaffer, H.J. (1986b). Conceptual crises and the addictions: A philosophy of science perspective. Journal of Substance Abuse Treatment, 3, 285-296.

Vaillant, G.E. (1983). The natural history of alcoholism: Causes, patterns, and paths to recovery. Cambridge, MA: Harvard University Press.

Wallace, J. (1978). Working with the preferred defense structure of the recovering alcoholic. In S. Zimberg, J. Wallace, & S.B. Blume (Eds.), Practical approaches to alcoholism psychotherapy (pp. 19-29). New York: Plenum Press.

Woody, G.E., McLellan, T., Luborsky, L., & O'Brien, C.P. (1985). Sociopathy and psychotherapy outcome. Archives of General Psychiatry, 42, 1081-1086.

Drug Treatment

By Clayton J. Mosher and Scott Akins

This chapter provides an overview of the numerous approaches to drug treatment that are currently in use. We address the theoretical foundations of each of these treatment approaches and assess the available empirical evidence with respect to their effectiveness. Five broad categories of drug treatment are addressed here: (1) pharmacological drug treatment, which involves the use of drugs or medications to treat substance abuse; (2) residential drug treatment programs in which patients live in a treatment facility for periods of from one month to two years; (3) compulsory drug treatment, which is treatment that is mandated in some way by the criminal justice system; (4) Alcoholics Anonymous and related "peer support" and 12-step programs; and (5) outpatient drug treatment, which involves a diverse range of treatment options that individuals can receive while they reside in the community. It is important to recognize that these programs are not mutually exclusive; there is considerable overlap among these programs. For example, treatment mandated by the criminal justice system can involve elements of pharmacological treatment, residential drug treatment, and 12-step models.

Before discussing specific drug treatment programs and research on their effectiveness, it is important to address a number of issues. First, as noted in Chapter 5, the vast majority of substance users never become substance "abusers" and are thus never compelled to seek treatment (Weil & Rosen, 1998). Further, even among the small minority of substance users who go on to have substance abuse problems, most will eventually quit or gain control of their use on their own; that is, without the assistance of any formal drug treatment program (Faupel et al., 2004). For some individuals, it may be that drug abuse is only one, and perhaps not even the most significant, of a number of problems (e.g., mental illness, homelessness, unemployment, poverty), and in order to address their substance abuse, attention must be directed to these other problems as well (United Nations Office on Drugs and Crime [UNODC], 2003).

Another central issue in drug treatment is that the motivation of the individual to change is likely the most important factor in predicting successful treatment outcomes (Jung, 2001). This fact is important to keep in mind when assessing the effectiveness of drug treatment programs because addicts who are motivated to quit using alcohol and other drugs are also more likely than other substance abusers to enter drug treatment in the first place (McCaul & Furst, 1994). Thus., many treatment programs (with the exception of compulsory programs) involve individuals who, despite their inability to quit using drugs on their own, generally want to quit. This complicates research on the effectiveness of drug treatment because the people who enter treatment are likely the most motivated to change, thereby making it impossible to conclusively determine that the drug treatment, as opposed to the motivation of the individual, is responsible for positive treatment outcomes (Faupel et al., 2004).

Despite the fact that a large portion of people in voluntary drug treatment programs are motivated to change, all of these programs have high "failure rates"; this is particularly true for individuals entering treatment for the first time (Akers, 1992; Anglin, Longshore, & Turner, 1999; Hubbard, Marsden, Rachal, Harwood, Cavanaugh, & Ginzburg, 1989). In terms of assessing the "success" or "failure" of a drug treatment program, studies have typically examined whether treatment is effective at (1) eliminating or reducing drug use; (2) eliminating or reducing criminal offending; (3) reducing risky sexual behavior, needle sharing, and other forms of behavior that are likely to increase the risk of HIV and other infectious diseases (Hubbard, Cradock, & Anderson, 2003); and (4) increasing rates of conventional employment. As will be discussed in more detail later in this chapter, research has found the success rate for most drug treatment programs to be modest to moderately effective with respect to these measures (Akers, 1992; Anglin et al., 1999; Hubbard et al., 1989). It is important to note that if any form of relapse to drug use following treatment is considered as evidence of failure, virtually no drug treatment program could be considered successful. Assessing the effectiveness of drug treatment on the basis of relapse is inappropriate, given that recovery from addiction is typically a long and "incremental process, involving perhaps several cycles of drug use, treatment, abstinence, and relapse" (Anglin et al., 1999, p. 192). Conversely, if success is measured with respect to the ability to produce some reduction in levels of substance use, a reduction in criminal activity, and positive employment outcomes, then treatment can be regarded as effective (Hubbard et al., 2003).

One final and particularly important issue must be considered in any discussion of the effectiveness of drug treatment programs. Although measured by reductions in drug use and criminal activity treatment success rates can be relatively modest, even the modest success evidenced by treatment is far superior to the typical result when drug problems are dealt with exclusively through criminal justice system sanctions.

Research has consistently demonstrated that drug offenders who are incarcerated and denied treatment have extremely high rates of subsequent

"Although addictions are chronic disorders, there is a tendency for most physicians and for the general public to perceive them as being acute conditions such as a broken leg— when relapse occurs, as it usually does, the 'treatment' is inappropriately considered a failure. Treatments for addiction, therefore, should be regarded as being long term, and a 'cure' is unlikely from a single course of treatment."

-O'Brien and McClellan (1996, p. 237)

drug use and offending (UNDCP, 2003). In addition, most individuals incarcerated for drug use will eventually return to society, and if they are denied treatment while in prison, they are likely to return to society with the same problems that contributed to their incarceration in the first place. Thus, dealing with drug use problems exclusively through the criminal justice system can be considered to be inhumane, and more importantly in a practical sense, is exceptionally expensive. Although comparisons of the costs of treatment versus criminal justice system responses to drug problems vary considerably according to the type of drug treatment being considered, numerous studies have found treatment to be a far more cost-effective option (Finigan, 1995; Holder & Blose, 1986; McCollister & French, 2003; NIDA, 1999; Roebuck, French, & McClellan, 2003; UNDCP, 2003). As an article in the Journal of the American Medical Association noted, "mounting effective treatment programs for drug addiction may cost 10 times less than putting addicts in prison" (Marwick, 1998, p. 1149).

The large cost differential between drug treatment and criminal justice system approaches to addressing drug use problems arises primarily from the fact that building prison cells and maintaining inmates in prisons is extremely expensive. Minimum security prison cells in the United States cost approximately $35,000 to build, and housing an inmate for one year costs, on average, $27,000 (UNDCP, 2003). A recognition of the relative savings associated with drug treatment programs has recently led a number of states to alter their drug policies and devote more resources to such programs. It is to a consideration of these various programs that we now turn.

Pharmacological Treatment Approaches

Pharmacotherapy involves the use of drugs and medications in the treatment of substance abuse and dependency. Somewhat ironically, then, this form of treatment involves using one drug in order to prevent the use of another. Substances in this form of treatment are typically used in one of two ways: on a temporary basis as the individual attempts to quit the use of another drug, or on a permanent or long-term basis in the belief that taking the new drug will reduce or eliminate the use of a more problematic drug (O'Brien, 1997).

These pharmacological approaches to drug treatment are by no means a new phenomenon. For example, in the late 1800s and early 1900s, a wide variety of proprietary medicines were sold as "cures" for alcoholism. These included products such as Parker's Tonic, Schneck's Seaweed Tonic, and Boker's stomach bitters. Interestingly, several of these products contained significant proportions of alcohol: Parker's Tonic, which was advertised as "pure vegetable extract" that "gave stimulus to the body without intoxicating," was found to contain 41.6% alcohol (Trice & Staudenmeier, 1989). Similarly, prior to the passage of the 1914 Harrison Narcotics Act in the United States, physicians often treated opiate addicts with other types of opiates, including heroin. As noted in Chapter 3, when Bayer laboratories introduced heroin in 1898, it was marketed as a "non-addictive" cure for morphine addiction (Askwith, 1998). Currently, a wide variety of nonpsychoactive but also psychoactive drugs—or "medications," as they are generally referred to when used in a treatment context—are available to help individuals with substance abuse problems.

Although pharmacotherapy can be used in isolation to treat substance dependency (e.g., using a nicotine patch to quit smoking), it is often used in conjunction with other treatment approaches and techniques such as psychological counseling or behavior modification (O'Brien, 1997). There is also no "typical" length of time associated with pharmacotherapy, with periods of treatment ranging from less than a day to several years. For example, drugs may be used to facilitate the body's detoxification and withdrawal from opiate drugs and to lessen the discomfort associated with withdrawal—a process that can be completed in as little as one to three days (NIH, 1998; UNDCP, 2002). Conversely, methadone maintenance for heroin addicts often continues uninterrupted for several years (DHHS-CDC, 2002).

Regardless of the length of the treatment period, there are two basic types of medications that are used to treat substance abuse and dependency: drug agonists and drug antagonists (some medications combine the properties of both). Drug agonists are psychoactive drugs themselves (although their effects may only be noticeable for "non-users"), and while they may generate dependency and be abused, these "substitute drugs" are viewed as safer, or in some way preferable, to the drug that they are being used to treat (NIDA, 1999). Conversely, drug antagonists have no psychoactive effects and do not generate dependency. Antagonists operate in one of two ways: they either make a person who is taking them very sick if he or she ingests a particular drug, or they block or limit the psychoactive effects of a drug so that

even if a psychoactive drug is ingested it has no (or a lesser) effect.

Drug Agonists

Agonists are used on either a temporary or long-term basis in the belief that consumption of the agonist will reduce or eliminate the use of a more problematic drug (NIDA, 1999). Nicotine replacement therapy (NRT) is the most commonly used form of drug agonist, and numerous NRT prodocts are currently marketed to people who are trying to quit smoking or the use of other tobacco products. Many of these products are available over the counter, and although the patch" is the most well-known form of NRT, there are other forms: nicotine-based nasal sprays, lozenges, gum, tablets, and nicotine inhalers that can be "puffed on" like cigarettes (I. Campbell, 2003). Although research has generally found NRT to be effective at helping people to quit smoking, these effects are generally quite modest (see reviews by Fiore, Smith, Jorenby, & Baker, 1994; Hughes, Goldstein, Hurt, & Shiffman, 1999). For example, Fiore and colleagues' meta-analysis of 17 studies on the efficacy of NRT found overall abstinence rates for the patch to be 27% at the end

---

The Dovzhenko Method

Alcoholism is a very serious problem in Russia. Estimates indicate that more than 50,000 people die from alcohol poisoning each year in Russia, compared to only 400 in the United States. Over the past 20 years, one method used to treat alcoholism has been the "The Dovzhenko Method." Dating to the former Soviet Union, this method involves "coding" alcoholics so that they believe if they drink again, they will die. One of the ways that this is carried out is as follows: Physicians induce hypnosis in patients and then administer a drug that reacts to alcohol and affects the respiratory system. Patients are then encouraged to taste a small amount of alcohol, which prompts a reaction. Patients are even required to sign a release form, relieving the doctor of liability should they drink and die from it The popularity of the Dovzhenko Method has waned in recent years as information about the true nature of the treatment has spread (Finn, 2005).

of treatment, as compared to 13% for placebo and 22% after 6 months compared to 9% for placebo. Thus, even though they are more effective than a placebo, these products do not work for the vast majority of people. An additional issue with NRT is that like smoking, it involves the ingestion of.a substance known to be highly addictive. Thus, people who rely on NRT to quit smoking may simply trade one form of nicotine addiction for another, albeit one that is potentially less harmful. These issues were addressed in a recent New York Times article, which noted that over one-third of Nicorette users indicate that although they are no longer addicted to cigarettes, they are now addicted to Nicorette (Bartosiewicz, 2004, cited in Center for Cognitive Liberty and Ethics [CCLE], 2004, p. 11). One Nicorette user quoted in the article revealed that she chewed approximately 12 pieces of Nicorette a day, commenting on her addiction to the gum that "I felt almost like a drug addict" (p. 11).

The most well-known drug agonist for the treatment of illegal drug use is methadone. As noted in Chapter 3, methadone is a synthetic narcotic that is used predominantly in the treatment of heroin (and other opiate) addiction. Initially, methadone was primarily used as a pain reliever due to shortages of morphine during World War II, but in the mid-1960s, methadone maintenance for heroin addicts emerged. In the ensuing years, methadone maintenance has been used to treat hundreds of thousands of people, and currently, of the estimated 600,000 to 980,000 narcotic addicts in the United States, approximately 115,000 to 160,000 are enrolled in methadone maintenance programs (Firoz & Carlson, 2004).

Methadone maintenance involves a procedure in which opiate addicts take regular doses of methadone to treat their addiction to heroin or some other narcotic. The substance is typically taken orally in the form of a pill or a liquid often consumed with orange juice. Compared to the effects of heroin, which generally last no more than three hours, the effects of orally administered methadone last for 12-24 hours. This is one of the reasons for its utility in treating opiate addicts (Gahlinger, 2001).

It is important to recognize that by definition, methadone maintenance involves substance dependency; it is precisely because the individual has developed an adequate level of tolerance to methadone that the drug "works" in the prevention of heroin use. Methadone is effective in the treatment of heroin and other opiate addiction because, being a synthetic opiate, it is cross-tolerant with these drugs. Thus, taking one drug in the opiate category (methadone) provides tolerance to all drugs in the category (e.g., heroin) (O'Brien, 1997). Accordingly, opiate addicts engaged in methadone maintenance are less likely to experience the intense craving for heroin that is commonly associated with opiate addiction, and if they "slip up" and inject heroin, their tolerance to methadone will largely prevent the reward or euphoria associated with heroin. Although the dose of methadone an individual takes varies depending on his or her previous heroin use, and thus tolerance level, maintenance doses of methadone typically range from 30-120 mg per day, with higher doses associated with better outcomes such as continued treatment and abstinence from heroin (Leshner, 1999; Marsch, 1998; NIH, 1998; UNDCP, 2002). It is also important to note that when methadone is taken orally and at stable doses, it does not produce any euphoria or high, and cognition, alertness, and higher mental functioning are not impaired (DHHS-CDC, 2002; Nadelmann, 1996; O'Brien, 1997; Rothenberg, Schottenfeld, Meyer, Krauss, & Gross, 1977).

However, because of the physical dependency generated by methadone and the fact that the substance can have psychoactive effects if taken in large doses or by injecting maintenance doses, many are staunchly opposed to methadone

> "'Addiction' to methadone looks far more like a diabetic's 'addiction' to insulin than a heroin addict's addiction to street heroin. Many methadone patients hold good jobs and are responsible parents. They can safely drive motor vehicles and operate heavy machinery. They are, when prescribed adequate doses of methadone, practically indistinguishable from Americans who have never used heroin or methadone."
>
> -Nadelmann (1996, p. 84)

maintenance on moral grounds (Blendon & Young, 1998). In large part, this criticism is derived from the fact that those engaged in methadone maintenance are still physically dependent on a drug. Similarly, Andrew Weil (1986) is critical of methadone maintenance because rather than showing addicts how to achieve highs without drugs, it is a "method of giving them drugs without highs"—exactly the wrong direction in which to change things (p. 190). Despite such concerns, it is important to recognize that the dependence generated by methadone maintenance is vastly different than addiction to heroin with respect to life outcomes and the ability of individuals to manage their day-to-day activities (DHHS-CDC, 2002; see Box). As Brecher (1972) notes, the reasons for the relative success of methadone maintenance programs in treating opiate addiction are fairly obvious. First, because methadone is a legal substance, the addict who enters a methadone maintenance program is able to relinquish the role of "hated and hunted criminal" (p. 159). Second, methadone is cheap, which means that addicts generally do. not have to become involved in crime to financially support their drug habit. At least in part because of the relative stability of addicts participating in methadone

maintenance programs, organizations such as the National Institutes of Health, the Centers for Disease Control, and the Office of National Drug Control Policy have endorsed these programs for the treatment of addiction to heroin and other opiates (DHHS-CDC, 2002; NIH, 1998; ONDCP, 2000b).

Research on the effectiveness of methadone maintenance programs using a variety of outcome measures has generally found these programs to be effective for the treatment of addiction to heroin and other opiates (Hubbard et al. 2003; Hubbard et al., 1989; Leshner, 1999; Marsch, 1998; NIH, 1998; UNDCP, 2002). For example, Marsch (1998) conducted a meta-analysis of over 40 studies examining the efficacy of methadone maintenance for reducing illicit opiate use, HIV risk behaviors, and criminality and found methadone to be effective in reducing all of these negative behaviors. Similarly, the Swiss initiated a nationwide trial of a methadone maintenance program in 1994, and a 1997 government report indicated that among those involved in the program, there were significant reductions in criminal activity and improvements in employment outcomes (Nadelmann, 2002b). Further, the National Institutes of Health convened a

> "Society must make a commitment to order effective treatment for opiate dependency for all who need it. All persons dependent on opiates should have access to methadone hydrochloride maintenance therapy under legal supervision, and the U.S. Office of National Drug Control Policy and the U.S. Department of Justice should take the necessary steps to implement this recommendation."
>
> -NIH (1998, p. 1936)

conference to discuss the treatment of opiate addiction and to disseminate this information to doctors, patients, and the general public. The NIH conference strongly supported methadone maintenance programs, as was noted in a special issue of the Journal of the American Medical Association (see Box). Despite the recommendations of the National Institutes of Health, access to methadone maintenance is still relatively limited in the United States. Several states still do not offer such programs, opting instead to address opiate addiction through criminal justice system sanctions.

Despite the extensive research that demonstrates the effectiveness of methadone maintenance for the treatment of addiction, it is important to recognize that "methadone maintenance is not a cure-all" (Rounsaville & Kosten, 2000, p. 1338). Returning to the issue of how "success" is defined in evaluating treatment programs, we must recognize that although methadone is clearly beneficial in reducing illicit opiate use, crime, and risky behaviors, a large portion of those who undergo methadone maintenance therapy relapse and/or experience numerous other problems related to their substance use. Further, while participating in methadone maintenance programs, many individuals still engage in heroin and other drug use, continue to be involved in risky sexual behaviors, and experience employment and family problems (Rounsaville & Kosten, 2000). Nonetheless, the fact that methadone maintenance programs benefit a substantial proportion of opiate addicts who participate in them suggests that such programs should be supported and expanded (DHHS-CDC, 2002; NIH, 1998). These programs are also cost effective: A study published in the Journal of Maintenance in the Addictions noted that every dollar spent on methadone maintenance saves from $2 to $4 in corrections costs (Flynn, Porto, Rounds-Bryant, & Kristiansen, 2003).

A substance similar to methadone used for the treatment of opiate addiction is buprenorphine (trade name Subutex). Buprenorphine is a "partial" opioid agonist, meaning that although it has the effects of an opioid, these effects are significantly weaker than those of full agonists such as methadone (and heroin) (SAMHSA, 2005a). Similar to methadone, buprenorphine can be used to ease opiate withdrawal and to indefinitely maintain opiate addicts (SAMHSA, 2005a). The use of buprenorphine has been increasingly advocated in recent years because, as compared to methadone, there is arguably less potential for abuse associated with it, the withdrawal associated with it is less severe, and it is more difficult to overdose on buprenorphine than methadone (Auriacombe, Franques, & Tignol, 2001; Vastag, 2003). In part because it is argued to have a lower abuse potential, buprenorphine, unlike methadone, can be prescribed to opiate addicts in a doctor's office (Mitka, 2003) by physicians who have taken an eight-hour training course and who have registered with SAMHSA and the DEA (Vastag, 2003). However, like methadone, buprenorphine is abused by a significant percentage of patients, who have reported crushing the tablets and injecting them for a more powerful psychoactive effect.

The relatively limited regulation of buprenorphine as compared to methadone is interesting, and in part reflects the need to deliver opiate treatment "outside traditional settings such as methadone clinics" (Mitka, 2003, p. 735). Specifically, buprenorphine treatment appears to be aimed more exclusively at the increasing number of middle-class opiate addicts, while methadone maintenance is predominately accessed by poor inner city residents (Mitka, 2003). As John Schneider, former president of the Illinois State Medical Society, comments,

> While heroin has traditionally been associated with inner city drug addicts,

Attempts to counteract alcohol-related problems among the homeless include the admmis tration of alcohol to chronic alcoholics residing in homeless shelters Consistent with a harm minimization approach to drug abuse, homeless alcoholics have been administered limited doses of alcohol on a hourly basis in order to determine the effect of this treatment on alcohol-related harm and disorder. Subjects' contacts with police and emergency room visits were examined for three years prior to the beginning of treatment and two years after, and results indicated that a stabilized alcohol intake program can significantly reduce police contacts and emergency room visits (Podymow, Turnbull, Coyle, Yetisir, & Wells, 2006).

today's user is more and more likely to be an employed young professional living in the suburbs.... we need to use primary care physicians more effectively to treat these patients [who] want to be treated in private settings, (as quoted in Mitka, 2003, p. 735)

Buprenorphine was approved by the FDA for treatment of opiate addicts in 2002, but it has not yet been widely prescribed (Vastag, 2003). In part, this is because many doctors are skeptical about the ability of drugs to treat narcotics addiction (Mitka, 2003) and also because physicians are currently limited to carrying a maximum of 30 buprenorphine patients, a figure many doctors have referred to as "absurd" (Vastag, 2003, p. 731). In contrast, buprenorphine has been widely used in France since the mid-1990s, and as of 2003 France had an estimated 72,000 high-dose buprenorphine patients, far exceeding the approximately 17,000 high-dose methadone patients in the country (French Monitoring Center for Drugs and Drug Addiction, 2004). Research on the use of buprenorphine in France has found it to be a safer alternative to methadone because of its milder effects; the death rate from methadone is at least three times greater than the death rate related to buprenorphine (Auriacombe et al., 2001). Studies have also found that buprenorphine is effective for the treatment of opiate dependence (McClellan, 2002; McClellan, Lewis, O'Brien, &c Kleber, 2000), although it may be less effective

than methadone for the treatment of more heavily dependent opiate addicts (SAMHSA, 2005a).

An even more controversial pharmacological program for treating opiate addicts is heroin maintenance. Sometimes referred to as the "British model" due to its origin in Britain in the 1960s, heroin maintenance involves prescribing doses of heroin to individuals identified as "hardcore junkies" who inject the drug at special injection sites. Although, given the current attitudes toward drugs in the United States, such programs are unlikely to be adopted here, in addition to Britain, heroin maintenance programs have been established in the Netherlands, Switzerland, Denmark, Australia, and Canada. A study of heroin maintenance programs in the Netherlands involving 549 participants found that heroin maintenance was more effective than methadone in terms of improving the physical and mental condition and social functioning of heroin addicts (van den Brink, Hendricks, Blanken, Koeter, van Zwieten, & van Ree, 2003). Similarly, a study of Switzerland's heroin prescription program found that although 31% of the hardcore drug users in the program had dropped out in the first 18 months, among participants who stayed in the program, there were several positive outcomes. For example, the proportion of participants with unstable housing fell from 43% on admission to 21%; the rate of employment more than doubled, from 14% to 32%; and there was a reduction of more than 50% in criminal offenses committed by those in the treat-. ment group (Wood et al.,

2003). A study of a supervised drug injection site in Sydney, Australia found that staff in the program intervened in 329 overdoses over a one-year period and estimated that at least four lives were saved (Wright & Tompkins, 2004). Perhaps more importantly, this study found that clients of the injection center were more likely than other injecting drug users to seek treatment for their drug use. There were also community benefits associated with the supervised drug injection site: Residents and business owners reported fewer sightings of public injection and syringes being discarded in public places (Wright & Tompkins, 2004). As Wright and Tompkins conclude, "[the] argument that medically supervised injecting centers promote drug use and related harm is not supported by the evidence" (p. 102).

Drug Antagonists

As noted earlier, in addition to drug agonists the other type of medications commonly used in the treatment of substance dependency are drug antagonists. These substances prevent substance abuse in one of two ways: they either make people who take them extremely ill when they ingest a particular psychoactive drug (e.g., alcohol), or they block the effects of a particular psychoactive drug (CCLE, 2004). With respect to the former, one of the most commonly used drugs in this category is disulfiram (or sulfiram), which is also known by its trade name, Antabuse. Disulfiram is used in the treatment of alcoholism, and although the substance is not toxic itself, it inhibits the body's ability to metabolize alcohol (O'Brien, 1997). Interestingly, the treatment effects of disulfiram were discovered serendipitously in the 1930s when workers at rubber manufacturing plants who were regularly exposed to the chemical became violently ill whenever they consumed alcohol (CCLE, 2004). Similarly, individuals who take disulfiram become violently sick when they drink alcohol, with symptoms including nausea, vomiting, headache, facial flushing, and high blood pressure ("Drug Treatments," 2002). These symptoms, which have been said to be analogous to those experienced in a "bad hangover," typically last between 30 and 180 minutes.

With respect to the effectiveness of Antabuse in treating alcoholism, research findings are mixed. Garbutt, West, Carey, Lohr, and Crews (1999) summarized the available research on this issue and concluded that there is modest evidence indicating that disulfiram helped to reduce the frequency of drinking, but that it did not increase rates of abstinence from alcohol among individuals using it. Such findings are not surprising, given that the drug does nothing to reduce the initial craving for alcohol, and the effects of disulfiram typically wear off within 24-48 hours (Doweiko, 1999). Thus, people who have been prescribed disulfiram can plan their drinking episodes and simply quit taking the medication a day or two in advance. Additionally, because the negative effects that result from combining disulfiram and alcohol are usually of short duration, it is possible to "drink through" disulfiram (Doweiko, 1999).

Additional substances currently being used, or proposed for use, in treating alcoholism include Acamprosate, which has been used for several years in Europe; Ondanestron, a drug whose primary use is to prevent nausea in cancer patients (Tanner, 2000); and Topirimate, a drug that is used to control seizures in epilepsy patients. Although Topirimate has not yet been approved by the FDA for alcohol abuse treatment/initial clinical trials suggest that this drug affects the brain's ability to experience the pleasure of drinking and can reduce the craving for alcohol (Vedantam, 2003).

An additional problem with disulfiram is that the drug cannot identify the source of the alcohol that is ingested. Thus, if an individual taking disulfiram inadvertently consumes or absorbs alcohol—which is present in commonly used products such as cough syrup, mouthwash, aftershave, and perfume—he or she can become very sick (CCLE, 2004). Thus, due to its relatively modest effectiveness, and because serious reactions to disulfiram and alcohol can include liver inflammation, heart-related problems, and potentially death, disulfiram is not widely prescribed for alcoholism treatment (O'Brien, 1997).

More commonly used in the treatment of substance abuse, particularly in recent years, are the types of drug antagonists that act to block or reduce the psychoactive effects associated with particular drugs. Antagonists prevent the psychoactive effects of drugs in one of two ways: (1) they bind to a drug molecule, making it too large to pass through the blood-brain barrier (thereby preventing any effect on the brain); or (2) they occupy receptor sites on brain cells or neurons, preventing the drug molecules from "docking" to these receptor sites and thus having an effect on the brain (CCLE, 2004; O'Brien, 1997).

Although there are several medications used to treat substance abuse in this fashion, among the most interesting is naltrexone, an opioid antagonist that was released in 1985 as a prescription drug for the treatment of narcotics addiction. Naltrexone was later found to be useful in the treatment of alcoholism as well (being approved by the FDA for this purpose in 1995). This substance is effective in the treatment of opiate addiction because it prevents addicts from experiencing any psychoactive effects if they "slip up" and consume heroin (or another opiate). Thus, as noted by McClellan et al. (2000), naltrexone can be seen as a type of "'insurance policy' in situations where the patient is likely to be confronted with relapse risks" (p. 1693).

Studies have found that orally administered naltrexone can effectively block both the physiological and subjective psychoactive effects of heroin and morphine for up to three days (Tai & Blaine, 1997), and research on the efficacy of administering naltrexone by injection has found that it can block the euphoric effects of heroin for up to six weeks (Comer, Collins, Kleber, Nuwayser, Kerrigan, & Fischman, 2002). Because of its ability to completely block the psychoactive effects of opiates, it was initially believed that naltrexone would be ideal for the treatment of heroin addiction (McClellan et ah, 2000). However, with the exception of "white-collar" opiate addicts such as doctors and nurses, the vast majority of addicts prefer treatment with methadone, so naltrexone is not commonly used to treat opiate addiction (O'Brien, 1997).

As noted above, naltrexone has also been used in the treatment of alcoholics. Although there is some debate regarding the efficacy of naltrexone in this capacity (Krystal, Cramer, Krol, Kirk, 8c Rosenheck, 2001), it appears that, similar to disulfiram, naltrexone is effective at reducing drinking frequency and "heavy drinking." However, naltrexone does not increase total abstinence rates among those to whom it is prescribed (Garbutt et al., 1999; Mann, 2004).

Substances have also been developed that are designed to prevent individuals from becoming addicted to tobacco products. For example, a drug made by the British company Xenova works by stimulating the immune system to make antibodies against nicotine. Once the antibody binds to nicotine, the resulting complex is too large to penetrate molecules in the brain, thus preventing the brain from activating the pleasure receptors that are involved in generating the pleasurable effects associated with tobacco use (Coghlan, 2002). A recent National Institute on Drug Abuse newsletter noted that this "nicotine vaccine ... may even prove useful as an inoculation against nicotine addiction, much like those that protect children from tetanus, measles, and polio" (Shrine, 2000).

Until recently, antagonist substances were only available for the treatment of abuse of substances that generated physiological dependence—notably alcohol, nicotine, and the opiates. For other drugs, most notably the stimulants, hallucinogens, and marijuana, the only available treatments were behavioral in nature (O'Brien, 1997). However, as research in this area continues to advance, products are being developed that may be useful in the treatment of drug abuse involving substances whose addictive potential is purely psychological. One such drug is TA-CD (also developed by the British pharmaceutical company Xenova); the substance is being promoted as a "therapeutic vaccine" designed to treat cocaine addiction (Xenova, 2004). The company's Web site claims that two separate clinical trials of TA-CD have found the drug to be effective at reducing the euphoric effects of cocaine.

The range of substances that can be "treated" with antagonists continues to expand and now even includes marijuana. The marijuana antagonist SR141716 has been found to reduce both the subjective psychoactive and physiological effects of marijuana by occupying particular receptors in the brain (Huestis et al., 2001; LeFoll & Goldberg, 2005). But the expansion of pharmacotherapy to include marijuana could be construed as troubling, especially given that, as discussed in Chapter 4, marijuana is a relatively innocuous substance that does not cause dependence, and very little is known about the long-or short-term effects of SR141716. As a publication of the Center for Cognitive Liberty and Ethics noted, "marijuana has been safely used for centuries, while the anti-marijuana drug SR141716 has no history of human use. One cannot help but question whether 'the cure' might be worse than 'the illness'" (CCLE, 2004, p. 14).

What is clear is that the United States government remains committed to reducing, and ultimately eliminating, particular forms of drug use and continues to look for methods by which to achieve this goal. Accordingly, given the general failure of interdiction and criminal justice system policies in reducing drug use, it may be that the increasing emphasis on pharmacotherapy reflects another "front" in the War on Drugs or the "American government's hope ... that the demand for drugs can be reduced, in part, by chemically eliminating the very desire to use an illegal drug" (CCLE, 2004, p. 6).

Residential Drug Treatment Programs

Residential treatment programs were among the first forms of organized drug treatment available in the United States. Dating back to the 19th century, residential treatment was provided in the homes, hospitals, and sanitariums that were primarily designed to treat alcoholism and opiate addiction (Faupel et al., 2004). However, over time, two distinct models of residential drug treatment have emerged. The first model is the more "medicalized" approach and typically involves doctor-monitored and often medication-assisted drug treatment (as discussed above) that usually takes place in a hospital or similar medical facility (Ray & Ksir, 2004). The other model, which is behavioral in nature, attempts to treat substance abuse by changing the patterns of behavior and/or characteristics of the individual that lead him or her to abuse drugs. This "resocialization" process involves long-term, round-the-clock, inpatient care lasting from as little as one month to two years or more (DeLeon, 1995).

Although there are many distinct residential treatment programs, the most notable are relatively short-term ("28-day") in-patient programs that are based on the Minnesota Model (e.g.,

Hazelden, the Betty Ford Center) and the longer-term residential programs known as "Therapeutic Communities." Most of these short-term residential programs are based on the 12-Step program of Alcoholics Anonymous (A.A.); we therefore discuss the rationale behind them in the section on A.A. below. One notable difference between exclusive A.A programs and residential programs, however, is that residential programs provide patients with a month or so "in residence" while they dry out in a drug-free environment (Faupel et al., 2004). Conversely, therapeutic communities (TCs) typically involve recommended residential stays of between one and two years. Although TCs are by no means the only form of long-term residential treatment, they have served as the model upon which most residential treatment approaches have been based, and they have also been implemented in a number of jail and prison settings.

Therapeutic Communities

The roots of the TC can be traced to "Synanon," a drug treatment program that advocated the complete separation of the addict from the broader society for a long period of time. Synanon was founded in 1958 by Charles Dederich, a former alcoholic and member of Alcoholics Anonymous who, in promoting Synanon, coined the phrase "Today is the first day of the rest of your life" (M. Clark, 1999). In the late 1950s, A.A. had not yet begun to provide significant treatment resources for those addicted to substances other than alcohol, prompting Dederich to create Synanon. Although it was developed to treat addiction to drugs other than alcohol, Dederich drew on some of the principles of A.A. in creating Synanon, including the view that an addict was never truly cured of his addiction (Ray & Ksir, 2004). Accordingly, Dederich initially envisaged "recovery" from addiction as requiring two years residence in the

Synanon program before an individual was able to "graduate" back into the larger society.

Similar to modern TC approaches, a key part of treatment in Synanon involved encouraging patients to work, pursue their academic education (within the program), and generally "better" themselves. However, perhaps the most distinctive feature of Synanon was "The Game," a form of group therapy in which aggressive verbal confrontation between members was encouraged and even required to "break down" the person's built-up defenses, excuses, and rationalizations regarding drug use (Akers, 1992). Part of this included what has been referred to as the "Synanon encounter," a process in which the whole group would turn on a particular member and make that person the focus of the verbal attack in order to facilitate his or her "growth" (Rowan, 2001). As will be discussed in more detail below, this confrontational style of group therapy and the rationale underlying it is a key feature of most TCs in existence today.

As noted above, Synanon began as a treatment program that aimed to graduate drug users back into the larger society in roughly two years. However, Dederich later came to conclude that Synanon members could never graduate, claiming that because addiction was incurable, people with this "fatal disease" would be forced to remain in the program for the rest of their lives (Ofshe, 1980). Although Synanon was initially praised by the national media as a "success story," not long after its inception Synanon began to move away from its initial focus on drug treatment and toward an overall "approach to life" (M. Clark, 1999). An increasing number of Synanon members were non-drug users who joined the organization because of the rigidly structured way of living it offered. The story of Synanon grew increasingly bizarre in the late 1960s and 1970s as it began to progressively morph into more of a "cult-like" organization in which Dederich exercised tremendous control over the members (M. Clark, 1999; Dougherty, 1996). Although the earlier version of Synanon actually "graduated" only 26 members in its first five years of existence (Lemanski, 1999), in Synanon II, as it was called, Dederich began to increasingly resist the practice of sending "patients" back into the larger society. These members became the workforce for what eventually became a multi-million-dollar corporation (M. Clark, 1999; Dougherty, 1996).

As part of his attempt to further increase his control over Synanon, and ostensibly due to the importance of the "community family," Dederich ordered married couples in the group to split up and instructed each person to take on a new partner (M. Clark, 1999). He also separated parents from their children, with the children being cared for in dorms by Synanon teachers. In 1977, shortly before the collapse of the group, all male Synanon members who had been in the group for at least five years were ordered to have vasectomies (excepting Dederich), and in 1975, Synanon declared itself a religion (Lemanski, 1999). The disintegration of the group was hastened when Dederich and other Synanon members were involved in the attempted murder of several people, including a situation in which Synanon members beat a former member (a "splittee") so severely that he went into a coma. In another incident, Dederich himself pleaded no contest to a conspiracy to commit murder charge, and although he was able to avoid prison as a result of his plea, he was forced to relinquish control of Synanon. Ironically, in his 1982 plea Dederich admitted, "I don't know how to cure a dope fiend. I never did" (as quoted in Dougherty, 1996).

Despite the problems with Synanon, several components of its basic model have been adopted by residential treatment programs and remain widely used today. Consistent with the Synanon model, TCs advocate long-term residential stays, frequently lasting up to two years (although

funding shortages have reduced the length of stay offered by many programs to only a year) (NIDA, 2005). Although there are numerous distinct TC programs (e.g., Walden House, Gateway House, Daytop Village, Marathon House), TCs can be distinguished from other approaches to drug treatment in two fundamental ways. As noted by DeLeon (1994), TCs are distinct because "first, the TC offers a systematic approach that is guided by an explicit perspective on the drug use disorder, the person, recovery, and right living. Second, the primary therapist and teacher in the TC is the community itself" (p. 18).

In practice, several elements or principles are emphasized in TC drug treatment programs. These include community sepa-rateness; fostering of a community environment; the participation of members in community activities; peers and staff as community members; a highly structured work day; work as therapy and education; and, most distinguishing, purposive use of the peer community to facilitate social and psychological change in individuals (DeLeon, 1995). As part of this, abstinence from drugs is a central norm espoused in the TC, so these programs are typically "completely drug free" (although the use of caffeine and nicotine are sometimes exceptions to this rule) (DeLeon, 1994). Importantly, the emphasis placed on "complete abstinence" means that recovering opiate addicts who are being treated with methadone cannot simultaneously be treated in a TC.

An additional central trait of TCs is that they typically do not view drug abuse as the main problem in need of treatment, but rather as one symptom of broader problems that afflict the individual (DeLeon, 1994). As DeLeon comments,

> Drug abuse is regarded as a disorder of the whole person. . . . Although individuals differ in their choice of substances, abuse involves some or all of the areas of functioning. Cognitive,

behavioral, and mood disturbances appear, as do medical problems; thinking may be unrealistic or disorganized; and values are confused, non-existent, or antisocial. . . . Finally, whether couched in existential or psychological terms, moral issues are apparent, (p. 18)

Thus, TCs are based on the assumption that the person seeking treatment is in some way deficient; as a result, treatment "may be characterized as an organized effort to resocialize the client" (Tims, Jainchill, &C DeLeon, 1994, p. 2). Resocialization is termed either "habilitation" or "rehabilitation," depending on whether the particular client has "ever" adopted values that are believed to be "associated with socialized living" (NIDA, 2005), and this socialization process emphasizes the importance of "right living" (DeLeon, 1994). According to the TC model, "right living" means adhering to specific values and includes "truth and honesty (in work and deed), the work ethic, learning to learn, personal accountability, economic self-reliance, responsible concern for peers, family responsibility* community involvement, and good citizenry" (DeLeon, 1994, p. 20).

As noted, the process of resocializing individuals towards "right living" involves the use of the peer community; thus, other members of the TC are seen as central in achieving social and psychological change in the particular person (DeLeon, 1994). In practice, this involves the use of confrontation therapy as developed in the Synanon model, and as with Synanon, in the TC as a whole, but particularly in group sessions, "authentic" and brutally honest observations and reactions are considered to be the responsibility of all members of the group (DeLeon, 1994). The objective of this process of confrontation is believed to be important as it serves to "heighten individual awareness of specific attitudes or behavioral patterns that should be modified"

(DeLeon, 1994, p. 26). Thus, it is thought that if the person is continually forced to confront the issues he has not wanted to confront, he will eventually correct the "deficiencies in his character" that have caused him problems throughout his life, including his substance dependency (Tims et al., 1994).

As the individual increasingly adopts the values and norms of the community— honesty, responsibility, personal accountability, and the like—he assumes more independence and begins the "re-entry" process to the broader society (DeLeon, 1994). Re-entry into society typically requires the person to be enrolled in school or to be employed, and once leaving the TC the individual generally remains involved in "post-residence aftercare services" (such as counseling) through his TC (NIDA, 2005).

TC members are also often encouraged to attend self-help support groups, such as Alcoholics or Narcotics Anonymous, upon returning to the broader society.

As might be expected, due to the long-term, round-the-clock care associated with treatment in a TC, the cost of this approach is substantially higher than the cost of other forms of drug treatment (Hubbard et al., 1989; Roebuck et al, 2003). However, TCs have been found to be effective in treating many substance abusers. Although the efficacy of TCs in terms of their self-prescribed goals to "resocialize the client" into total abstinence, good citizenry, and similar outcomes are difficult to empirically assess, we can assess the effectiveness of TCs in terms of more traditional measures. As noted earlier, these measures of treatment efficacy include reduced drug use, reduced criminal activity, and increased steady employment, Condelli and Hubbard (1994) examined these issues by comparing and summarizing the results of four large-scale studies of TC effectiveness. In general, these studies concluded that TCs were effective at producing moderate reductions in drug use, criminal activity, and unemployment in the months following treatment, but that length of stay was important for positive outcomes, particularly among the most disadvantaged clients.

More recently, research by Hubbard et al. (2003) examined the effectiveness of several forms of drug treatment and found that long-term residential drug treatment was associated with positive outcomes at both one year and five years following the completion of treatment. As can be seen in Table 9.1, Hubbard et al. (2003) found long-term residential treatment to be effective in reducing a wide variety of drug use, predatory criminal behavior, risky sexual behavior, and unemployment. Although rates of cocaine and especially heroin use increased substantially between the one-and five-year follow-ups, five-year levels of use still remained far below rates of use prior to the individual's admission to treatment.

While these and other studies provide support for the efficacy of residential programs and especially TCs in treating substance abuse, it is important to note that many of the studies do not include outcome measures for patients who drop out of treatment in the early stages of the program. As such, treatment "success" figures apply only to a subset of the drug treatment population and likely exclude some of the "hardest to treat" (Hubbard et al., 2003).

Compulsory Treatment Programs

The term "compulsory treatment" is used here to describe a wide variety of legally coerced drug treatment strategies. As Faupel et al. (2004) note, compulsory treatment is based on the philosophy that certain populations of drug users will not seek treatment themselves or will not remain in treatment once they have entered it. Such individuals must be forced to enter drug treatment "for

their own benefit but especially for the benefit of the community" (p. 396). Although broad in its application, the term "compulsory treatment" is used to refer to

> required drug treatment and also a variety of legal and quasi-legal incentives for such treatment. It might refer to a probation officer's recommendation to enter treatment; a judge's order to enter treatment as a condition of probation; the option provided by a judge of entering treatment as an alternative to prison; or a mandatory treatment program while in prison, (p. 395)

Among the earliest forms of compulsory treatment were the federal narcotics hospitals or "narcotics farms" that opened in Lexington, Kentucky, in 1935 and Fort Worth, Texas, in 1938. Following the passage of the Harrison Act in 1914 (and similar to the present situation), federal prisons had become increasingly overcrowded with drug offenders, and the facilities in Lexington and Fort Worth offered the government an alternative for dealing with such offenders (Musto,. 1999). Because the narcotics hospitals were intended primarily for convicted drug offenders, they were designed and run like minimum security prisons, but at any given time about half the patients in these facilities were voluntary patients (Musto, 1999). Treatment in these facilities "consisted primarily of gradually weaning patients from heroin with decreasing dosages of morphine" and later, methadone (Faupel et al., 2004, p. 377), and research on their effectiveness found exceptionally high relapse/failure rates, with six-month relapse rates often exceeding 90% (for reviews see Musto, 1999; Task Force on Narcotics and Drug Abuse, 1967). As state and local drug treatment alternatives became more widely available, the facilities in Fort Worth and Lexington were eventually

TABLE 1. Effectiveness of Drug Treatment: Behaviors and Outcomes One and Five Years After Treatment

Behavior or Outcome	Outpatient Methadone (n = 432)			Long-Term Residential (n = 331)			Short-Term Inpatient (n = 266)			Outpatient Drug Free (n = 364)		
	Pre-admission (%)	1-year follow-up (%)	5-year follow-up (%)	Pre-admission (%)	1-year follow-up (%)	5-year follow-up (%)	Pre-admission (%)	1-year follow-up (%)	5-year follow-up (%)	Pre-admission (%)	1-year follow-up (%)	5-year follow-up (%)
Heroin use	91.0	24.1	31.1	.17.3	2.5	9.7**	9.0	3.8	4.2	7.7	3.9	5.5
Cocaine use	45.1	21.7	20.9	65.4	18.2	26.0**	61.7	18.2	16.2	37.4	13.8	17.3
Marijuana use	15.8	13.1	13.9	24.5	11.9	16.3	34.2	12.6	14.0	27.0	11.6	18.7*
Problem alcohol use	16.4	15.9	10.2	36.3	14.4	14.2	51.3	21.1	16.5	32.5	14.9	13.2
Suicidal thought/ attempt	14.6	12.3	14.8	22.7	10.2	10.3	30.8	15.4	16.9	21.7'	11.3	15.4
Predatory illegal acts	31.2	14.3	12.7	40.1	15.3	15.7	16.3	7.7	5.6	24.3	9.8	8.5
Sexual risk behavior	27.3	12.7	17.6	48.5	26.7	26.7	37.0	20.2	20.8	33.3	25.4	17.9*
Full-time work	14.9	19.1	25.1*	10.6	25.5	36.4**	51.4	43.9	54.3**	18.0	33.2	42.3*
Health limitations	37.5	32.6	34.7*	29.3	21.8	13.3*	30.5	22.6	13.2**	31.6	19.0	19.2

SOURCE: From Hubbard, R., S.G. Craddock, and J. Anderson. "Overview of 5-Year Follow-Up Outcomes in the Drug Abuse Treatment Outcome Studies (DATOS)." Journal of Substance Abuse Treatment 25;125-134, © 2003. Reprinted with permission of Elsevier.

* p < .05; ** p < .01—Differences between 1-year and 5-year follow-up percentages tested using paired t-tests.

closed and transformed into formal prisons in 1971 and 1974, respectively (Kosten & Gorelick, 2002).

Compulsory treatment strategies have become increasingly popular in recent years due in part to the tremendous economic strain placed on federal and state governments by the War on Drugs and the resulting need to find more economically feasible options for addressing societal drug problems (NIDA, 1999).

Although it is essential to discuss compulsory drug treatment strategies in any comprehensive discussion of drug treatment, it is also important to recognize that because this form of treatment is legally coerced, it is distinct from the other treatment modalities discussed in this chapter. Compulsory treatment is controversial for a variety of reasons. Among these is the fact that it raises ethical and legal questions regarding whether it is appropriate to "force" someone to accept treatment for drug use (Gomart, 2002). In addition, it is difficult to determine whether compulsory treatment is effective (Faupel et al., 2004; Hubbard et al., 1989). The efficacy of this form of treatment is difficult to assess partly because it involves elements that both hamper and encourage positive treatment outcomes (Hubbard et al., 1989; Lipton, 1995). As noted earlier, one of the most important predictors of positive treatment outcomes is the motivation of the individual to change. Because individuals in compulsory treatment are, in some fashion, under the supervision of the criminal justice system, "they may not be

willing participants in the treatment process" (Hubbard et al., 1989, p. 130). Accordingly, the effect that coercion has on individuals' willingness to engage in treatment is likely to influence treatment outcomes—particularly long-term outcomes—among some patients. However, aside from motivation to change, the length of time spent in treatment is one of the most important factors in terms of treatment outcomes, and in this respect the coercive element can be seen as beneficial because "clients under legal coercion generally stay in treatment longer than those who are not" (Lipton, 1995, p. 46).

Although the efficacy of compulsory treatment is to some degree debated (as discussed in more detail below), the economic benefits of this approach when compared to incarceration (without treatment) has prompted an increasing emphasis on it in recent years (Lipton, 1995; NIDA, 1999). Despite this, there remains a large discrepancy between the number of individuals in the criminal justice system who need treatment and the number of treatment slots available (Gerstein & Harwood, 1990; Harlow, 1991; Hser, Longshore, & Anglin, 1994; Mosher & Phillips, 2006). State corrections officials estimate that between 70% and 85% of inmates need some form of substance abuse treatment (ONDCP, 2001), but resources in this area remain scarce. For example, in approximately 7,600 correctional facilities surveyed in 1997, only 172,851 inmates were participating in drug treatment programs, representing less than 11% of the total inmate population. A recent

---

The recent expansion of pharmacotherapeutic approaches to drug treatment (discussed earlier in this chapter) has led some to question whether these drugs might be forced upon the substantial number of individuals in jail or prison who have substance abuse problems. There is little doubt that these populations are at particular risk of being forced to take these drugs as an "alternative" to incarceration. A similar approach has been selectively used in the treatment of sex offenders with medications designed to regulate hormones (CCLE, 2004).

report estimated that states spend an average of 5% of their annual prison budgets on drug and alcohol treatment (National Center on Addiction and Substance Abuse, 1998), and in 1997, the federal government spent $25 million, or 0.9% of the federal prison budget, on drug treatment programs.

There are many distinct forms of compulsory treatment, but these can be generally categorized into those that are "prison-based" and those that are "community-based." Prison-based programs obviously take place within prisons, but their specific approach to drug treatment might involve drug education classes, self-help programs, treatment based on the therapeutic community model, or some combination of these (NIDA, 1999). One of the more notable prison-based programs is "Stay 'N out," a prison-based therapeutic community that isolates prisoners enrolled in the program from the general prison population (Lipton, 1995; NIDA, 1999). Research has found Stay'N Out and similar prison-based therapeutic communities to be effective in reducing rates of recidivism among released prisoners (Knight, Simpson, & Hiller, 1999; Mosher &c Phillips, 2006; Wexler, Falkin, Lipton, & Rosenbaum, 1992; Wexler, Melnick, Lowe, & Peters, 1999; Wexler & Williams, 1986).

In contrast to prison-based programs that largely involve the application of "traditional" treatment strategies to incarcerated populations, community-based treatment strategies are diversionary programs designed to allow substance-abusing offenders to avoid incarceration. Among the most popular and widespread of these diversionary programs are "drug courts." The first drug court was created in Miami, Florida in 1989, and as of 2005, drug courts existed in all 50 states, with 1,481 fully operational adult drug courts and 453 in the planning stages. In addition, 388 juvenile, 154 family, and 13 combined (juvenile and family drug courts) were in operation (National Criminal Justice Reference Service, 2005). Although there

is considerable variation across programs with respect to who is eligible to participate, drug courts typically deal with "offenders with a long history of drug use and criminal justice system contacts, previous treatment failures, and high rates of health and social problems" (Belenko, 2001, p. 1). In comparison to the traditional legal model, drug courts are based on more of a "restorative justice" or "therapeutic jurisprudence" paradigm, meaning that the legal process in these courts is less about assigning blame and punishment and more about achieving positive change in the life of the offender (Jensen & Mosher, 2006; Turner et al., 2002). Offenders are expected to participate in drug treatment as a condition of avoiding prison, with the understanding that sanctions (including the possibility of incarceration) may result if they do not comply with the requirements of the treatment program as agreed upon in court (Turner et al, 2002). Drug courts use this threat of sanctions to help keep the offender motivated to participate in treatment. Although there are differences in the specifics of particular drug courts, offenders in such programs

> appear more frequently in front of judges; are required to enter into an intensive treatment program; undergo frequent, random urinalysis; undergo sanctions for failure to comply with program requirements; are encouraged to become drug-free; develop vocational and other skills to promote reentry into the community, (p. 1492)

Most studies assessing the effectiveness of drug courts have found, them to be reasonably effective at reducing drug use and recidivism among treated populations, at least in the short term (Belenko, 2001; Brewster, 2001; Creswell & Deschenes, 2001; Goldkamp, White, & Robinson, 2001; Harrell & Roman, 2001; Turner et al., 2002).

Judges in many states are using technology to prevent alcohol use among problem drinkers. Offenders charged with crimes such as DUI or domestic assault, who are prohibited from drinking, may be ordered to wear an anklet that can detect alcohol consumption. The monitoring system tests a person s perspiration every hour for signs of alcohol consumption and sends the data over the Internet, sending an alert if it detects the presence of alcohol or if someone attempts to disable the device by blocking it with a sock or cellophane (Franceschina, 2005).

Perhaps more importantly, however, virtually every study of drug courts has concluded that they result in significant cost savings for the criminal justice system (Washington State Institute for Public Policy, 2002). For example, the California Department of Alcohol and Drug Programs released a report in 2002 showing that the $15 million that the state spent annually on drug courts resulted in at least a $43 million saving for taxpayers. These savings were derived from keeping people out of prisons and jails and helping parents to avoid drug abuse, thereby keeping their children out of foster care. Similarly, since their inception in the state of New York, drug courts have processed 18,000 drug offenders, saving that state an estimated $254 million in prison-related expenses (von Zielbauer, 2003a).

A belief that alternatives to incarceration for substance abusing offenders would be more cost effective was also the motivation behind California's Proposition 36 (the Substance Abuse and Crime Prevention Act [SACPA]), supported by 61% of voters in that state and passed in 2000. This legislation allows individuals convicted of their first or second nonviolent drug possession offense to receive drug treatment in lieu of incarceration. It also allows people on probation or parole for certain offenses to receive treatment instead of reincarceration after violations of drug-related conditions of their probation or parole (Uelmen et al., 2002). Individuals are not eligible for this program if they are convicted of drug trafficking or other felony offenses.

Proposition 36 was estimated to have saved the state of California $275 million in its first year of operation (Drug Policy Alliance, 2006'c); however, there were numerous unintended and negative consequences associated with this law. In the first three months after the legislation was passed, 30% of the offenders who pled guilty and agreed to enter drug treatment had bench warrants issued for their arrests because they failed to show up at treatment centers or did not return to court for a review of their progress (Butterfield, 2001a). In addition, a considerable number of offenders who were eligible to be sentenced under Proposition 36 chose to plead guilty under the old law, where the sentence often consisted of simple probation or a few weeks in jail. If such individuals pled guilty under the provisions of Proposition 36, they would be provided treatment but it could last for several months and they would be on probation for three years. Perhaps more importantly from the offenders' perspective, if they violated the terms of their probation, they could be sent to prison (Butterfield, 2001a).

A recent evaluation of Proposition 36 compared the rearrest outcomes for the initial sample of offenders treated under the legislation in 13 California counties with those of other clients referred to drug treatment through the criminal justice system and clients who entered drug treatment voluntarily. While this study found that Proposition 36 clients were more likely to be rearrested for a drug crime (Farabee, Hser, Anglin, & Huang, 2005), thus questioning the efficacy of the program, as Appel, Backes, and Robbins (2005) note, these higher rates of recidivism should not be taken as indications that the program is a failure. Over 60,000 people who previously would have been subject to incarceration received drug treatment in just the first two years of implementation of Proposition 36 (Longshore et al., 2004), resulting in substantial cost savings for the state of California. In addition, the most commonly misused drug among SACPA clients was methamphetamine, which can present greater problems with respect to treatment; this may partially explain the higher recidivism rates among these clients (Appel et al., 2005). Although programs such as California's SACPA and Arizona's Drug Medicalization, Prevention, and Control Act (Proposition 200, passed by Arizona voters in 1996) remain controversial, a number of states, including Hawaii, Kansas, Texas, and Maryland, have implemented similar legislation.

The wide variety of compulsory drug treatment strategies currently in use are unique because they involve coercive treatment and thus must be considered and evaluated differently than other forms of drug treatment. Although the coercive nature of these programs may discourage positive outcomes among some patients, their compulsory nature also increases the amount of time typically spent in treatment, and this can have a positive effect on later outcomes. These programs are diverse and the efficacy of individual programs varies, but in general, compulsory treatment is more effective than addressing drug problems with criminal justice responses that do not include treatment (ONDCP, 2001). Additionally, compulsory drug treatment is far more cost effective than incarceration for addressing drug problems (NIDA, 1999), and because of their economic feasibility, compulsory drug treatment programs are likely to continue to expand in the future.

Alcoholics Anonymous

Alcoholics Anonymous (A.A.) represents by far the largest drug treatment "program" in the world. Approximately one in 10 adults in the United States have attended an A.A. meeting (for themselves or on behalf of another) (Doweiko, 1999), and although A.A. does not keep formal membership files or attendance records, the organization has estimated its current membership at over two million members, dispersed across more than 150 countries and more than 100,000 separate support groups (A.A., 2005). Although we are aware that A.A. has helped many individuals deal with their problem drinking, it is important to engage in a critical discussion of the central philosophies and tenets of the A.A. model and to examine scientific research on the effectiveness of A.A. in treating those identified as alcoholics.

As discussed in Chapter 2, A.A. was founded in 1935 by Bill Wilson and Robert Smith, alcoholics who had been unable to quit drinking on their own but succeeded with the help and support of each other. Accordingly, A.A. and related groups such as Narcotics Anonymous (N.A.) are peer-based "self-help" groups in which individuals identified as alcoholics/addicts can attend meetings in their community with other individuals identified as alcoholics addicts, enabling them to draw on each other for support and understanding in their

---

Despite the strong abstinence norm of A.A., founder Bill Wilson was an enthusiastic LSD user, believing that the drug could eliminate the "barriers that stood in the way of direct contact with the cosmos and Cod" (Lemanski, 1999, p. 60). When his use of the drug became public, he claimed that since he had stepped down as the leader of A.A. he should be allowed to live as he chose, but under pressure from A.A. members he eventually quit the use of LSD (Cheever, 2004).

---

struggle with addiction. As A.A. members are informed on the utility of this practice in the "Big Book" (the official "manual" of A.A.), "nothing will so much insure immunity from drinking as intensive work with other alcoholics" (A.A., 2005, p. 89).

Based on this philosophy, A.A. meetings are conducted by recovering alcoholics who have been in the program for some time but (typically) have no formal training in counseling or therapy (McCaul & Furst, 1994). New A.A. members are expected to attend 90 meetings in their first 90 days as part of their "early recovery" phase, with the more experienced members expected to act as "sponsors" who advise and mentor members who have recently joined (McCaul & Furst, 1994). A.A. meetings can be conducted in either an "open" or "closed" format. The former are open to non-alcoholics as well as alcoholics and typically involve talks by one or more speakers who share their experiences with alcoholism and their recovery through A.A. (A.A., 2005). Conversely, closed meetings are only for those identified as alcoholics and to emphasize their anonymous nature, these meetings are typically concluded with the motto "Who you see here, what you hear here, when you leave here, let it stay here" (Faupel et al., 2004).

As noted in Chapter 2, A.A. is based on the "disease model" of addiction, which considers addiction to be an incurable, degenerative disease (perhaps genetic in origin) that is often fatal if left untreated (Jellinek, 1960). However, critics of the disease model note that the classification of alcoholism/addiction as a disease is problematic because this classification is not based on any measurable physical effects on the body, as is the case with physical illness, or with measured thoughts, feelings, and behaviors, as is the case with mental illness (Peele, 1998).

Because the A.A. philosophy views the alcoholic as being afflicted with an incurable disease that is characterized by a loss of control over alcohol, total abstinence from the drug is seen as the only effective means of treatment (A.A., 2005). This constitutes one of the most controversial aspects of the A.A. model, and a considerable amount of research has concluded that individuals who have been identified as alcoholics are capable of controlling their drinking and leading normal lives without having to resort to complete abstinence from the drug.

One of the first researchers to challenge the abstinence-only philosophy of A.A. was Davies (1962), who found that 7 of 93 male alcoholics who were followed for a period of from 7 to 11 years following treatment reported being able to control their drinking and function normally in society. According to Davies, these individuals had never been "drunk" over the follow-up period and demonstrated improved human functioning in the domains of employment and family relationships. Subsequent to Davies's study, two studies conducted under the auspices of the Rand Corporation provided further support for controlled drinking. The first Rand study, involving an 18-month follow-up of alcoholics treated at 44 treatment centers in the United States, concluded that "the majority of improved clients are either drinking moderate amounts of alcohol—but at levels far below what could be described as alcoholic drinking—or engaging in alternating periods of drinking and abstention"

"In the United States, we hold out the hope that all alcoholics will stop drinking entirely. So far, this has not occurred. But as with sex education aimed at having all children remain virgins, we are committed to the ideal."

-Peele (2000)

(Armor, Polich, & Stambul, 1976, p. v). A further four-year follow-up of these same individuals also found that a substantial proportion were still engaged in non-problem drinking. The findings of this study were seen as a threat to A.A. and its focus on abstinence, and without even having the opportunity to read the full report, the National Council on Alcoholism denounced the report on the morning it was released, describing it as "dangerous" (Peele, 1983).

Also in the 1970s, Mark and Linda Sobell conducted research on alternative treatments for alcoholism, which generally involved training subjects who had been identified as dependent on alcohol to drink in a controlled fashion. Individuals who were trained to control their drinking had significantly more "days functioning well" during a two-year follow-up period than those who had experienced abstinence-based treatment (Sobell & Sobell, 1973, 1978). These researchers were criticized by another group, headed by the psychologist Mary Pendery, who conducted a 10-year follow-up of subjects in the Sobells's study. In an article published in the prestigious journal Science in 1982, Pendery, Maltzman, and West essentially accused the Sobells of engaging in fraudulent research, and concluded "a review of the evidence, including official records and new interviews, reveals that most subjects trained to do controlled drinking failed from the outset" (p. 169). The popular CBS show 60 Minutes also featured a segment that was extremely critical of the Sobells's research. At one point in the program, the narrator (Harry Reasoner) was shown at the grave of one of the patients who had been placed in the original controlled drinking treatment condition; the implication, of course, being that the controlled drinking option for those identified as alcoholics results in death. However, as Marlatt (1983) notes, "why didn't [Mr. Reasoner] also visit the graves of patients in the control group who received the abstinence-oriented treatment?" (p. 1106). Although the Pendery et al. article noted that four of the original 20 subjects in the controlled drinking condition eventually died from alcohol-related causes, they neglected to note that six out of the 20 control (abstinence) subjects also died within the same period. But as Miller (1986) notes, "American professionals who advocate any alternative to abstinence are likely to be (and have been) attacked as naive fools, unwitting murderers, or perhaps themselves alcoholics denying their own disease" (p. 117).

The issue of whether individuals identified as alcoholics can engage in controlled drinking continues to be a controversial one, and at least part of-the reason for this controversy is that some of the research on controlled drinking has

Balanced placebo design studies conducted by Alan Marlatt and his colleagues involved subjects who were identified as alcoholics being deceived about whether they were drinking an alcoholic beverage. Marlatt asked individuals to "taste-rate" three different brands of the same beverage. Unknown to the subjects, they had been assigned to one of four groups. One group was told that the beverage was tonic water, which was true. Individuals in the second group were told that the beverage was vodka and tonic, although it was actually pure tonic water. Those in the third group were told that the beverage was vodka and tonic, which it was; finally, those in the fourth group were told it was tonic water only, when in fact it was vodka and tonic. Importantly, in the context of the central tenet of disease theory and its notion of loss of control, none of the alcoholic subjects drank all of the beverage, even though, according to disease theory, those who were drinking vodka ought to have proceeded to drink uncontrollably (Fingarette, 1990).

been misinterpreted. As Marlatt (1983) notes, the Rand studies essentially suggested that (a) controlled drinking may be a more appropriate goal than abstinence for individuals who are not severely dependent on alcohol; and (b) for those who are older and show signs of chronic physical dependence, abstinence may be the treatment goal of choice. Similarly, Sobell and Sobell (1995) suggest that research on controlled drinking can be summarized by the following statements: (1) recoveries of individuals who have been severely dependent on alcohol primarily involve abstinence; (2) recoveries of individuals who have not been severely dependent on alcohol predominately involve reduced drinking. Marlatt (1983) effectively sums up the central paradox in the disease model of alcoholism in commenting,

> Patients in treatment are first told that alcoholism is a disease characterized by an inability to exercise voluntary control over drinking. Once they have accepted the diagnosis they are then told that the only way to arrest the development of this progressive disease is to stop drinking—to assert control by abstaining, (p. 1105)

The fact that controlled drinking programs for those with alcohol-related problems have not been widely promoted in the United States is yet another example of American exceptionalism with respect to the approach to drugs. In Canada, 43% of treatment programs allow for moderate drinking for some clients (Shute, 1997). In Norway (and several other European countries), there is less emphasis on "alcoholism" as a problem associated with sick individuals and more emphasis on the drinking culture at large and restrictions on the availability of alcohol (Duckert, 1995). A survey of alcohol treatment centers in Norway found that 90% of them allowed their clients to choose

between abstinence and reduced consumption when the clients were inpatients, and 59% when they were treating outpatients (Duckert, 1995). Those concerned with engaging problem drinkers in treatment also argue that offering goals other than abstinence may attract more individuals to participate in treatment (Hersey, 2001). As Marlatt, Larimer, Baer, and Quigley (1993) comment, "offering controlled drinking alternatives to the general public may act as a motivating push to get people 'in the door,' a low threshold strategy that is consistent with the principles of harm reduction" (p. 483).

The 12 Steps of Alcoholics Anonymous

The 12 steps that supposedly guide recovery from alcoholism under A.A. are as follows:

1. We admitted that we were powerless over alcohol—that our lives had become unmanageable.
2. Came to believe that a Power greater than ourselves could restore us to sanity.
3. Made a decision to turn our will and our lives over to the care of God as we understood Him.
4. Made a searching and fearless moral inventory of ourselves.
5. Admitted to God, to ourselves, and to another human being the exact nature of our wrongs.
6. Were entirely ready to have God remove all these defects of character.
7. Humbly asked Him to remove our shortcomings.
8. Made a list of all persons we had harmed, and became willing to make amends to them all.
9. Made direct amends to such people wherever possible, except when to do so would injure them or others.

10. Continued to take personal inventory and when we were wrong promptly admitted it.
11. Sought through prayer and meditation to improve our conscious contact with God, as we understood Him, praying only for knowledge of His will for us and the power to carry that out.
12. Having had a spiritual awakening as the result of these steps, we tried to carry this message to alcoholics, and to practice these principles in all our affairs. (A.A., 2004, pp. 59-60)

NOTE: The Twelve Steps and a brief excerpt from the pamphlet A Newcomer Asks are reprinted with permission of Alcoholics Anonymous World Services, Inc. (AAWS). Permission to reprint a brief excerpt from the pamphlet A Newcomer Asks and the Twelve Steps does not mean that AAWS has reviewed or approved the contents of this publication or that AAWS necessarily agrees with the views expressed herein. A.A. is a program of recovery from alcoholism only—use of the Twelve Steps in connection with programs and activities which are patterned after A.A. but which address other problems, or in any other non-A.A. context, does not imply otherwise.

As is evident in these 12 steps, treatment in A.A. is deeply spiritual in nature; half of the steps explicitly mention "God," "a power greater than ourselves," or "Him." and Bill Wilson apparently believed he was acting under divine "guidance" when he wrote the 12 steps (Ragge, 1992). Clearly, then, the central tenet of A.A. philosophy is that for an alcoholic to be effectively treated, he or she must give up control of his or her life to "a power greater than one's self." This has been one of the central critiques of A. A., but despite the heavy spiritual influence present in A.A., efforts have been made to make the organization more accessible to individuals who have no belief in God. As the A.A. homepage comments on the role of spirituality in treatment:

The majority of A.A. members believe that we have found the solution to our drinking problem not through individual willpower, but through a power greater than ourselves. However, everyone defines this power as he or she wishes. Many people call it God, others think it is the A.A. group, still others don't believe in it at all. There is room in A.A. for people of all shades of belief and nonbelief. (A.A., 2005)

Despite this, many (e.g., especially those forced to attend A.A. meetings as a result of court sanctions for drinking and driving offenses) have found the spiritual/religious element incompatible with their personal beliefs. As a result, a separate although related groups "Alcoholics Anonymous for Atheists and Agnostics" (called "Quad A") has formed as well. This group adheres to the 12-step program, with the exception that the "Power Greater than Ourselves" element is de-emphasized; instead, the group stresses the key sources of support present in the individual's life. Other alternatives to A.A. include "Secular Organizations for Sobriety," which is a recovery program for individuals dependent on alcohol or other drugs who are similarly not comfortable with the religious aspects of A.A. This organization, founded by James Christopher in 1985, maintains that sobriety is a separate issue from religion or spirituality, and rather than relying on a "higher power," credits the individual for achieving and maintaining his or her sobriety (Secular Organizations for Sobriety, 2003).

It is also instructive to examine some of the logical inconsistencies in certain A.A. steps. The first step requires individuals to concede their powerlessness over their addiction to alcohol, while the second step asserts that belief in a higher power can restore the sanity of the same individual. However, a logical error occurs when these two steps are considered in the context of the third step, which requires the alcoholic to make a decision to turn his or her will over to the "higher power." The question becomes, How can an individual make a decision to turn his will over to a higher power if he is powerless and completely dependent on that same higher power for change? The inconsistent logic here is related to the fact that under A.A. philosophy, people are responsible for some behaviors, but not others. In considering the 12 steps in their entirety, Ragge (1992) argues, "the 12 steps are not a road to recovery, let alone the road to recovery. They are, instead, a road to substitute dependency—a dependency upon A.A. rather than upon alcohol."

Additional critiques of A.A. have characterized the organization as analogous to a "fanatical religious cult" (Trice & Staudenmeier, 1989). As Marc Galanter comments, "from the start, A.A. displayed characteristics of a charismatic sect: strongly felt shared beliefs, intense cohesiveness, experiences of altered consciousness, and a potent influence on members' behavior" (as quoted in Ragels, 2000). Similarly, George E. Vaillant, a prominent researcher and actual supporter of A.A., acknowledged that "A.A. certainly functions as a cult and systematically indoctrinates its members in ways common to cults the world over" (as quoted in Ragels, 2000). To a certain extent, the idea that A.A. constitutes a cult has been recognized by A.A. members themselves in one of their cliches, which states, "if A.A. uses

brainwashing, then our brains must need to be washed" (Ragels, 2000). While many will not agree with the characterization of A.A. as a cult, it is notable that in every court case initiated by individuals challenging their mandatory A.A. attendance—in Wisconsin, Colorado, Alaska, and Maryland—the courts have ruled that A.A. is equivalent to a religion for First Amendment purposes (Brodsky & Peele, 1991).

Although these critiques of A.A. may seem trivial, the problem is that an increasing number of individuals in the United States are being coerced into A.A. treatment, primarily as a result of being convicted of drunk driving offenses and through employee assistance programs. As Brodsky and Peele (1991) suggest, "A.A. and the alcoholism as disease movement it inspired translated American evangelism into a medical world view. . . . We have given government support to group indoctrination, coerced confessions, and massive invasions of privacy" (p. 36).

Many treatment practitioners strongly support the use of A.A.; however, the scientific evidence on the efficacy of A.A. as a treatment for alcoholism is mixed. Although the preface to the "Big Book" states that "inquiry by scientific, medical, and religious societies will be welcomed" (A.A., 2005, p. xiv), rigorous empirical research on the efficacy of A.A. is relatively limited considering the number of individuals who participate in A.A. programs. This is at least partially due to. the emphasis placed on anonymity and the A.A. norm that members should "utilize, not analyze." A limited number of studies have found participation

The 12-step model of Alcoholics Anonymous has spawned several other 12-step programs, including Narcotics Anonymous, Cocaine Anonymous, Marijuana Anonymous, Nicotine Anonymous, Over-Eaters Anonymous, Gamblers Anonymous, Sex Addicts Anonymous, and Workaholics Anonymous. Narcotics Anonymous (NA), founded in 1953, has a 290-page manual, similar in focus to AA's "Big Book." In 1979, there were fewer than 200 NA chapters in three countries, while in 2003, there were approximately 20,000 registered groups in 106 countries (Garfield, 2003).

in A.A. to be effective at reducing alcohol-related problems (Bond, Kaskutas, & Weisner, 2003; Cross, Morgan, Mooney, Martin, & Rafter, 1990), particularly for A.A. sponsors (Pagano, Friend, Tonigan, & Stout, 2004; Zemore, Kaskutas, &C Ammon, 2004). However, it is important to note that the "failure" rate of first-time A.A. members is extremely high. Research has found that at least half of new A.A. members quit attending meetings within three months of joining, and this figure increases to 95% by the end of the first year (Dorsman, 1996). In addition, most research on the effectiveness of A.A. programs has compared outcomes for individuals who did or did not become involved in A.A. While such research generally reports an association between voluntary A.A. participation and abstinence (Fuller & Hiller-Sturmhofel, 1999), it is important to note that because subjects are not randomly assigned to A.A., some factor other than participation (as discussed earlier, motivation could be a potential factor) in A.A. could be responsible for the outcome.

As we noted in the introduction to this section, we are aware of the fact that A.A. has assisted many people in dealing with their dependence on alcohol. But given the critiques of A.A. discussed above, it is interring to consider why this form of treatment for alcoholism retains its popularity and, in fact, continues to grow in the United States. Perhaps, as Gusfield (2003) asserts, A.A.'s continued popularity is related to the growth in the larger "drug treatment industry," an industry that includes hundreds of thousands of individuals whose livelihood is dependent on the continuance of this model of treatment.

Outpatient Drug Treatment

"Outpatient drug treatment" refers to a broad and diverse category of substance abuse treatment strategies that enable the patient to receive treatment while remaining in the larger community (Hubbard et al., 1989). The outpatient model developed in the 1960s in the form of "crisis clinics" and community mental health centers that, as noted by Ray and Ksir (2004), provided

> alternatives to the emergency room for a person who was frightened and needed someone to talk to until the drug wore off. These facilities ranged from telephone hotlines, to emergency room-assisted clinics with medical support available, to "crash pads[59] where people could sleep off a drug's effects and receive some nonjudgmental advice and counseling, (p. 62)

From these foundations, the outpatient model developed into a diverse and flexible form of drug treatment that might involve the use of one or more distinct therapeutic approaches. The programs usually entail some form of mental health counseling or psychotherapy, but they can range from "drop-in rap" centers to highly structured programs (Hubbard et al., 1989). Partly as a function of this, the intensity of the outpatient model also varies substantially from program to program, with some facilities "offering little more than drug education and admonition," while others, such as intensive day treatment, are "comparable to residential programs in service and effectiveness" (NIDA, 1999, p. 27).

The diverse range of treatment options and the convenience of the outpatient model continues to make it one of the most popular and widely used methods of drug treatment (Ray & Ksir, 2004). This model is particularly popular with and well-suited to those individuals who are in need of drug treatment but also have stable employment, which might be disrupted by having to participate in inpatient treatment (NIDA, 1999).

However, despite their popularity, there is not much research on the effectiveness of outpatient programs (Fiorentine, 1997; Hubbard et al., 1989). In large part, this lack of research is due to the substantial diversity that exists among outpatient programs; because the programs involve so many distinct approaches and treatment modalities, it is difficult to assess them collectively (Fiorentine, 1997).

Hubbard et al. (2003; see Table 9.1) do provide some information on the effectiveness of outpatient treatment in their comparison of the major (non-compulsory) treatment modalities currently employed. Their comparison found outpatient to be among the least effective of the major treatment modalities in terms of later drug use (comparing pre-admission figures to one-and five-year outcomes) but also found these programs to have a small positive effect. In contrast, outpatient programs were among the most effective at outcomes not specifically related to drug use, such as rates of employment and levels of criminal behavior. However, as with other findings regarding effectiveness discussed in this chapter, it is important to place such findings in their proper context. Each treatment modality is likely to serve a particular population of substance abusers, and the outpatient program is one of the more informal modes of treatment, particularly in comparison to methadone maintenance and long-term residential programs (Hubbard et al., 1989). As such, in comparison to those programs, outpatient treatment clients are likely to have fewer and less severe problems with substance abuse and fewer problems in general (e.g., employment, mental illness, social adjustment), and these characteristics are likely to have an impact on later substance use and levels of social functioning.

Conclusion

As we have discussed in this chapter, the need for drug treatment, from both a humanitarian and economic standpoint, is clear, and we have therefore assessed drug treatment programs in terms of their approach to treatment and the level of empirical research support each program has received. We provided a discussion of the five primary models of treatment, including pharmacological treatment, a strategy that employs the use of drugs or medications to treat substance abuse; residential drug treatment programs in which patients receive continual care by living in a treatment facility for a long period of time; compulsory drug treatment, which involves forcing individuals with drug problems to accept treatment in lieu of incarceration or another penalty; Alcoholics Anonymous and other peer-based self-help programs; and outpatient drug treatment, which involves a diverse array of treatment options individuals receive while they reside in the community. Although the issues discussed earlier limit all studies of treatment efficacy, most of the treatment models addressed here were found to be useful at reducing drug use, reducing criminal activity, and increasing levels of employment.

In his 2003.State of the Union address, President George W. Bush signaled that his administration would devote more funds to drug treatment. While this message could be construed as encouraging, consistent with the Bush administration's approach to other social issues, the Office of National Drug Control Policy has begun to promote, and devote additional funding to, treatment programs that are "faith based." Drug czar John Walters claimed "youth often turn to their faith communities to seek spiritual guidance about issues such as peer pressure and drugs. Faith communities can help parents instill anti-drug values and shape teens' decisions not to use marijuana and other drugs" (as quoted in

ONDCP, 2003b). One example of a faith-based drug treatment program is the in-prison program known as "Inner Change." In this program, addiction is presented as a sin that can be permanently cured through a connection with Jesus. As Shapiro (2003) notes, this program is typical of faith-based substance abuse programs supported by the Bush administration. When he was governor of Texas, Bush defended another faith-based program, Teen Challenge, against charges that it violated state and health department codes, saying, "I believe that conversion to religion, in this case Christianity, by its very nature promotes sobriety" (as quoted in Shapiro, 2003). While we should thus applaud President Bush and the ONDCP for their apparent commitment to drug treatment programs, we must question whether it is sensible to devote funding to these programs at the expense of other treatment programs that have been proven to have a positive impact on the lives of individuals who experience drug problems.